Metals in Bone

This symposium was organised by the Internal Emitters Committee of the European Late Effects Project Group (EULEP). It was co-sponsored by the Commission of the European Communities, Directorate-General for Research, Science and Education, Biology, Radiological Protection and Medical Research, Brussels, Belgium and by the Commissariat à l' Énergie Atomique, Institut de Protection et de Sureté Nucléaire, Bruyeres-le-Chatel, France.

COMMISSION OF THE EUROPEAN COMMUNITIES
Radiation Protection

METALS IN BONE

Proceedings of a EULEP symposium on the deposition, retention and effects of radioactive and stable metals in bone and bone marrow tissues, October 11th – 13th 1984, Angers, France.

Editor
Nicholas D. Priest

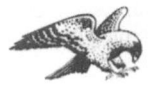 **MTP PRESS LIMITED**
a member of the KLUWER ACADEMIC PUBLISHERS GROUP
LANCASTER / BOSTON / THE HAGUE / DORDRECHT

for the Commission of the European Communities

Published in the UK and Europe by
MTP Press Limited
Falcon House
Lancaster, England

British Library Cataloguing in Publication Data

Metals in bone : radiation protection : proceedings of a EULEP symposium on the deposition, retention
and effects of radioactive and stable metals in bone and marrow tissues : EULEP Symposium
October 11th – 13th 1984, Angers, France.
1. Bones   2. Metals
  I. Priest, Nicholas D.   II. EULEP
  III. Commission of the European Communities
  612'.75   QP88.2

Published in the USA by
MTP Press
A division of Kluwer Boston Inc
190 Old Derby Street
Hingham, MA 02043, USA

Library of Congress Cataloging in Publication Data

EULEP Symposium (1984 : Angers, France)
  Metals in bone.
  At head of title: Commission of the European Communities.
  At head of title: Radiation protection.
  Includes bibliographies and index.
1. Bones – Congresses. 2. Metals in the body – Congresses. 3. Metals – Metabolism – Congresses. 4.
Radioisotopes in the body – Congresses. I. Priest, Nicholas D. II. Commission of the European
Communities. [DNLM: 1. Bone and Bones – metabolism – congresses. 2. Bone Marrow – metabolism
– congresses. 3. Metals – adverse effects – congresses. 4. Metals – metabolism – congresses. 5.
Radioisotopes – adverse effects – congresses. 6. Radioisotopes – metabolism – congresses. WE 200
E88m 1984]
QP88.2.E75 1984   599'.01852   85-5244

ISBN-13: 978-94-010-8680-6   e-ISBN-13: 978-94-009-4920-1
DOI: 10.1007/978-94-009-4920-1

© ECSC, EEC, EAEC, Brussels and Luxembourg, 1985
EUR 9250 EN

Softcover reprint of the hardcover 1st edition 1985

Legal Notice
Neither the Commission of the European Communities nor any person acting on behalf of the
Commission is responsible for the use which might be made of the following information.

Publication arranged by
Commission of the European Communities
Directorate-General Information Market and Innovation-
Scientific and Technical Communication
Brussels and Luxembourg.

Contents

v

PART 5 MICRODOSIMETRY OF RADIONUCLIDES IN BONE

Introduction

In 1980 the Internal Emitters Committee of EULEP organised a symposium in Rotterdam on Bone and Bone Seeking Radionuclides: Their Physiology, Dosimetry and Effects. The speakers for this meeting, mostly from EULEP associated laboratories, were chosen to review this field of scientific research mostly for the benefit of interested scientists who were not actively researching with bone-seeking radionuclides. This meeting was a success and its proceedings were subsequently published in the form of a book by the Commission of the European Communities, reflecting the great importance that both EULEP and the Radiological Protection Programme of the Commission of the European Communities attaches to the study of radionuclides that deposit in bone.

The Metals in Bone symposium in Angers was intended to serve a different function from that of the meeting held in Rotterdam in that, while these proceedings will certainly be of interest to non-involved scientists, the meeting was intended to be of most benefit to those actively researching the metabolism and effects of bone-seeking metals. Moreover, in an attempt to increase the value of its discussions and the number of interested and participating scientists, the remit of the meeting was broader and set to include papers on stable as well as radioactive metals. It is hoped that in this form the meeting provided a forum for discussion and the exchange of ideas between groups of scientists and clinicians who normally never meet, but all of whom share a common interest in the distribution and effects of metals in skeletal tissues. It was intended that the symposium would, in line with the aims of EULEP, foster inter-laboratory cooperation and communication as well as the occasional exchange of personnel, all of which are now necessary for the continuation of effective research in the face of dwindling resources.

The organisers are grateful for the help and encouragement given by many individuals and organisations during the preparations for the symposium. In particular we are grateful for that given by Dr. Henri Mehvier and Mrs. Gill Wilkinson, the Commissariat a l'Énergie Atomique (France) and by the National Radiological Protection Board (UK) and the European Calcified Tissue Society.

N. D. Priest (Editor)
V. Volf (Chairman Internal Emitters Committee, EULEP)

List of Contributors

U. ANDREOZZI
ENEA, CRE Casaccia, PAS-FIBI
Laboratorio Tossicologia
Casella Postale 2400, 00100 Roma
Italy

S. BANG
Institut de Morphologie
Centre Médical Universitaire
1211 Genève 4
Switzerland

C. A. BAUD
Institut de Morphologie
Centre Médical Universitaire
1211 Genève 4
Switzerland

M. BLANUŠA
Institute for Medical Research
and Occupational Health
158 M. Pijade, 41001 Zagreb
Yugoslavia

N. C. BLUMENTHAL
The Hospital for Special Surgery
Cornell University Medical College
New York,. N.Y. 10021
USA

G. E. DAGLE
Biology & Chemistry Department
Battelle Pacific N. W. Laboratory
PO. Box 999
Richland, WA 99352
USA

R. DEHOS
Institute for Radiation Hygiene of the Federal
Health Office
Ingolstädter Landstrasse 1
D-8042 Neuherberg
F.R. Germany

J. DONIEC
Institute of Occupational Medicine
PO. Box 199
90-950 Łódź
Poland

B. ENGFELDT
Department of Pathology II
Karolinska Institute
Huddinge University Hospital
S-141 86 Huddinge
Sweden

P. GERASIMO
CRSSA
1 Bis Rue du Lieutenant Raoul Batany
F-92141 Clamart
France

M. GIBSON
Department of Renal Medicine
King's College Hospital
London
UK

W. GÖSSNER
Abteilung für Pathologie
Gesellschaft für
Strahlen- und Umweltforschung
D-8042 Neuherberg
F.R. Germany

D. GREEN
MRC Radiobiology Unit
Harwell, Didcot
Oxfordshire OX11 0RD
UK

J. W. HAINES
National Radiological Protection Board
Chilton, Didcot
Oxfordshire OX11 0RQ
UK

E. R. HUMPHREYS
MRC Radiobiology Unit
Harwell, Didcot
Oxfordshire OX11 0RD
UK

G. INGRAO
ENEA, CRE Casaccia PAS-SCAMB
P.O. Box 2400
00100 Roma
Italy

A. JACOBS
Department of Haematology
University of Wales College of
Medicine, Heath Park,
Cardiff
UK

Z. JAWOROWSKI
Centre d'Etudes Nucléaires
Fontenay-aux-Roses
F-92260
France

W. S. S. JEE
Division of Radiobiology
Department of Pharmacology
University of Utah School of
Medicine, Salt Lake City
Utah 84112
USA

V. JOVANOVIĆ
Institute for Medical Research and
Occupational Health
158 M. Pijade
41000 Zagreb
Yugoslavia

P. J. MARIE
Unité 18 INSERM
Hôpital Lariboisière
6 Rue Guy Patin
F-75010 Paris
France

J. F. McINROY
Los Alamos National Laboratory
Mail Stop K484, Los Alamos
New Mexico 87545
USA

P. MOCETTI
Department of Human Biopathology
Division of Pathological Anatomy
"La Sapienza" University
00161 Rome
Italy

N. J. PARKS
Laboratory for Energy Related Health
Research, University of California,
Davis, CA. 95616
USA

E. POLIG
IGT/Kernforschungszentrum
Karlsruhe, Postfach 3640
D-7500 Karlsruhe 1
F.R. Germany

N. D. PRIEST
National Radiological Protection
Board, Chilton, Didcot
Oxfordshire OX11 0RQ
UK

J. RUNDO
Argonne National Laboratory
9700 South Cass Avenue
Argonne IL 60439
USA

P. N. SAMBROOK
MRC Clinical Research Centre and
Northwick Park Hospital
Watford Road, Harrow
Middlesex HA1 3UJ
UK

T. J. F. SAVELKOUL
Department of Internal Medicine
University Hospital, PO. 16250
3500 CG Utrecht
The Netherlands

R. A. SCHLENKER
Biological and Medical Research Division
Argonne National Laboratory
9700 South Cass Avenue
Argonne, IL 60439
USA

G. SCHOETERS
Radiobiology Department
SCK/Belgium Nuclear Centre
B-2400 Mol
Belgium

J. L. SEBERT
Service de Néphrologie
Laboratoire d'Anatomie Pathologique
Laboratoire de Biochemie
Hôpital Nord
F-80030 Amiens
France

G. SILVESTRINI
Department of Human Biopathology
Division of Pathological Anatomy
"La Sapienza" University
00161 Rome
Italy

N. P. SINGH
Radiobiology Division
Department of Pharmacology
University of Utah School of
Medicine, Salt Lake City
Utah 84112
USA

W. SONTAG
IGT/Kernforschungszentrum
Karlsruhe, Postfach 3640
D-7500 Karlsruhe 1
F.R. Germany

M. V. STACK
MRC Dental Unit
University of Bristol Dental School
Bristol BS1 2LY
UK

D. M. TAYLOR
IGT/Kernforschungszentrum
Karlsruhe, Postfach 3640
D-7500 Karlsruhe 1
F.R. Germany

M. C. THORNE
Associated Nuclear Services
123 High Street, Epsom
Surrey KT19 8EB
UK

P. TOTHILL
Department of Medical Physics
University of Edinburgh
Royal Infirmary
Edinburgh EH3 9YW
UK

J. T. TRIFFITT
MRC, Bone Research Laboratory
Nuffield Orthopaedic Centre
Oxford OX12 0JH
UK

R. VAN DEN HEUVEL
Radiobiology Department
SCK/Belgium Nuclear Centre
B-2400 Mol
Belgium

M. C. de VERNEJOUL
Unité INSERM 18
Hôpital Lariboisière
6 Rue Guy Patin
F-75010 Paris
France

V. VERNOIS
Laboratoire d'Histologie
Faculté de Chirurgie Dentaire
Paris VI
F-92120 Montrouge
France

W. J. VISSER
Clinical Research Group for Bone
Metabolism, University Hospital
PO. Box 16250
3500 CG Utrecht
The Netherlands

V. VOLF
IGT/Kernforschungszentrum
Karlsruhe, Postfach 3640
D-7500 Karlsruhe 1
F.R. Germany

S. WALLACH
Medical Service
VA Medical Center
Bay Pines
FL 33504
USA

E. WERNER
Gesellschaft für Strahlen-
und Umweltforschung
Paul-Erlichstrasse 20
D-6000 Frankfurt am Main 70
F.R. Germany

Part 1
Bone Mineralization and Turnover

1

Receptor Molecules, Coprecipitation and Ion Exchange Processes in the Deposition of Metal Ions in Bone

J. T. TRIFFITT

The functions of bone include mechanical and protective roles and the involvement in mineral metabolism and marrow development. As a connective tissue bone is a special case in that it contains calcium phosphate mineral, is remodelled continuously and it is capable of regeneration without production of scar tissue, [1]. The peculiar constituents of bone tissue, particularly the mineral phase of calcium phosphate, inevitably results in accumulation of many materials introduced into the blood circulation by either natural processes or artificial means. This fact, together with the reasonably long life of newly-synthesized bone in all but the youngest individuals, allows this tissue to act as a sink for a wide variety of substances.

In tissue fluids many ions are present that can substitute for calcium or phosphate especially at the surfaces of bone crystals. As a result bone mineral is an impure calcium phosphate with the major ionic contaminants being carbonate (6%, ^{w}/w), citrate (1%, ^{w}/w), sodium (0.7%, ^{w}/w), magnesium (0.7%, ^{w}/w) with a trace of fluoride. If calcium phosphate precipitates are produced in solutions of ions of similar composition to serum the precipitates resemble bone mineral in composition [2]. The ionic contaminants in bone mineral, therefore, appear to be a result of a passive, physico-chemical consequence of the presence of these ions in the fluids in which the crystals form [3]. In any event, bone is a storage site in the body for calcium,

3

phosphate, magnesium, sodium, carbonate and possibly other ions.
This function as an ion reservoir aids the maintenance of tissue
fluid concentrations of these ions, which are of physiological
importance in cell metabolic reactions.

Bone is a very heterogeneous and complex tissue made up of various
proportions of mineral, matrix and cells. Depending on the species
and age of the animal and the type and location of bone, the cellular
content, extracellular matrix composition and mineral content varies.
The least heterogeneous sample of bone tissue that can be obtained
for gross analysis is the compact bone of the shafts of long bones.
From analyses of this material the inorganic fraction makes up to 70%
of the tissue weight of the mature bone with about 20% of the weight
being organic material and water accounting for the remaining 10%.

Studies on the exact nature of the structure and chemistry of bone
mineral have been pursued for many years. The calcium phosphate
mineral is present in the matrix as minute crystals of approximate
dimensions 15-35 Å x 50-100 Å x 400-500 Å of poorly crystalline
hydroxyapatite [4]. The surface area of these crystals is up to
200 m^2/g and the possibilities for adsorption and surface exchange
and interaction are tremendous. This adsorption capacity has been
used for decades in the chromatographic separation of proteins,
nucleic acids and lipids [5,6]. In addition many ions are able to
interact at the crystal surfaces, with Mg , Sr , Ra , Pb and Na
exchanging at calcium sites, and carbonate, citrate, phosphate esters,
diphosphonates, pyrophosphates and amino-acids exchanging at
phosphate sites.

After its initial deposition the mineral undergoes extensive
structural and chemical changes and the nature of the first phase
produced has long been a controversial subject. The amorphous
calcium phosphate theory [7] proposed bone mineral was composed of a
poorly crystalline hydroxyapatite together with an additional
amorphous phase possessing no long range three dimensional order of
the constituent ions as determined by x-ray defraction techniques.
It was postulated that the amorphous phase predominated in early bone
and was superceded by, and transformed into, crystalline apatite as

the bone matured [8]. Recently Glimcher [9] has concluded from x-ray
analysis and plots of atomic density against atomic separation
(radial distribution function analyses) that the amorphous calcium
phosphate theory is incorrect, and that bone mineral is best defined
as a poorly crystalline non-stoichiometric hydroxyapatite, which
becomes more crystalline with increased stoichiometry with time.
Nevertheless, whatever the structure, the physicochemical reactivity
of the hydroxyapatite mineral is of primary importance to bone uptake
of many substances, not only metal ions.

The organic matrix of bone is composed of many diverse materials
but a single protein, collagen, makes up to 90% of the matrix of the
tissue. The remaining 10% (^{W}/w),   the non-collagenous material,is
made up of proteins, glycoproteins, proteoglycans, lipids and other
substances with the bulk being non-collagenous proteins. With regard
to the organic matrix of bone, its general contribution to the
structure of the tissue is the most obvious. In addition, the
relationship between the mineral and matrix may play a role in mineral
homeostasis by affecting the availability of the constituent calcium
and phosphate ions to the circulatory fluids. Furthermore, components of the organic matrix have been suggested to initiate the
deposition of mineral in bone by a process of heterogeneous nucleation.
In bone,initial crystals of mineral are formed within the collagen
fibrils at specific hole zone regions within each fibril [9]. However, the presence of native type I collagen fibrils, which are
present in many tissues, does not adequately explain why mineralisation occurs in vivo in skeletal sites and consideration of the interactions of collagen with other proteins has been necessitated. Also
a variety of collagens from rat tail tendon and skin, which do not
normally mineralise can be demonstrated to exhibit hydroxyapatite
nucleation properties, and in vivo specificity may require activation
of particular sites by the presence of specific molecules or the
phosphorylation of collagen fibrillar sites [10]. Most of the non-
collagenous proteins isolated from bone tissue to date, at least
initially upon their discovery, have been suggested to fulfill the
nucleation role. Recently there has been a remarkable increase in
attention paid to these non-collagenous bone constituents. Before

describing the nature of these interesting materials, other factors
influencing deposition of any moiety in any tissue site must be
considered. The delivery to the site of deposition, the relative
affinities for tissue constituents and the use or substitution in
anabolic processes are major factors controlling this accumulation.
So blood flow, vascular permeability, tissue-fluid flow and the
presence of specific inorganic and organic materials are of great
importance with respect to the skeletal uptake of metal ions and
other substances. Cellular metabolism also modifies the localisation
of these materials by receptor molecule and active transport processes
and the patterns of accumulation in the tissue changes with time.

The vascular anatomy of bone has been studied extensively [11,12],
particularly with respect to the tubular bones and the vascular
pattern is dependent on the particular bone and the nature of the
constituent type of bone tissue. However, as most types of tissue,
all bone tissue is fed by afferent arteries that supply a vascular
lattice which is drained by efferent veins. Bone tissue is normally
formed and broken down in relation to blood vessels, and these latter
have an important influence on bone shape and structure [11]. The
measurement of blood flow to bone tissue has been determined by
several methods. These have included measurement of venous outflow
[13,14,15] uptake or clearance of radioisotopes [16,17,18] fractionation of diffusible indicators [19,20] erythrocyte labelling [21,11]
and microsphere techniques using microspheres labelled with gamma
emitting-isotopes (^{46}Sc, ^{95}Nb, ^{85}Sr, ^{141}Ce, ^{125}I and ^{113}Sn) [22]. The
latter method is the only one that allows repeated measurements of
regional blood flow to bone in experimental animals. Many stimuli
such as exercise, physiological stress, humoral effects and sympathe-
tic tone can alter the vascular resistance in bones and marrow, so it
is probable that skeletal circulation actively participates when
physiological conditions require circulatory adjustment [22]. In dogs
estimates of about 5 to 11% of the cardiac output [12,23,24] goes to
bone tissue. In the long bones a flow rate of about 2-7 ml/100 g/min
occurs in the cortex (the higher figure in less mature bone) in a
centrifugal direction from marrow towards the periosteum, while the
flow in hemopoietic marrow and hemopoietic cancellous bone can be up

to 38 ml/100 g/min [12]. Consequently blood flow within the skeleton
is not very homogeneous [25]. Venous drainage of bone cortex is by
the periosteal veins and by large emissary veins that penetrate the
cortex, with the nutrient vein of the dog transmitting only about 10%
of the blood from the tibial diaphysis [26]. As has been stated
previously,the blood flow, the plasma concentration of a particular
ion and the number of potential binding sites for bone accumulation
are important items for the ionic exchange of metal ions [27].
Particularly for those metals present in low concentrations in the
plasma, blood flow is a limiting factor in this uptake and an appreciable amount of time is required to supply the exchangeable bed in
bone in this case.

Once presented to the site, diffusion across the blood capillary
wall is related to the permeability and surface area of this potential
barrier. Studies by Kelly and Bassingthwaighte [28] suggest that the
walls of bone blood capillaries function similarly to those in the
muscle. In marrow the capillaries have large gaps between the endothelial cells [29], whereas the capillaries of bone haversian canals
have closed, continuous endothelia. In bone and muscle tissues the
electrolytes and lipid insoluble substances are believed to diffuse
through the capillary walls through pores made up of chains of
vesicles or through clefts between the endothelial cells. Also free
diffusion is the principle mechanism whereby ions and solutes move
into bone [30]. This diffusion depends on the size of the moieties
diffusing and on the volume of the extravascular space. The extravascular space in bone is composed of a number of compartments. If
they can penetrate the blood vessel walls and the continuous cellular
membrane of bone cells, molecules originating from the blood plasma
can penetrate into the regions outside the blood vessels and outside
cells in bone tissue. These regions are essentially divided into two
further areas; the calcified matrix itself and the remaining extracellular space between the cells and the calcified matrix. This
latter has been termed the 'bone fluid' space [31] and is probably
similar in composition and characteristics to the gel-like extracellular matrices of soft tissues. The high surface charge and low
water content of the calcified matrix, restricts diffusion of

molecular species particularly those of high charge density such as the multivalent metal ions.

Studies with larger molecules than metal ions has resulted in increased knowledge with respect to the lacunar-canalicular network. It is likely that this syncytium of cells and the surrounding fluid space are important pathways for ionic passage also. Horseradish peroxidase (molecular weight 40,000) appears in canaliculi 15 mins after intravenous injection and in lacunae within 30 mins [32]. In other connective tissues plasma proteins circulate through the interstitial fluids and an analogous situation is seen in bone [33]. These results from the time-sequence localisation of these macromolecules in bone suggest that there is a net movement of macromolecules in tissue fluid from endosteum to the periosteum via the canalicular-lacunar network and the surfaces of Volksman and haversian canals. Furthermore, there is a high vascular pressure within marrow [34,35], so that a net drainage of some tissue fluid from marrow through the bone wall is conceivable. Clearly further studies are required before the characteristics of bone tissue fluid flow are fully understood. This net direction of flow is supported by the work of Seliger [36] on the passage of thorotrast after its release in the tibial marrow cavity of the cat. Here general tissue fluid drainage was shown to be from the endosteum to the periosteal surface and its removal was suggested to be by lymphatic vessels. Several authors state that no lymph vessels can be seen in bone marrow or bone cortex [37,38,39] and any definite periosteal lymphatics have not been described in detail. Nevertheless the circulation of materials through bone interstitial fluid matrix is of obvious importance for the carriage of essential factors to and from the bone cells. As one of their important roles, plasma proteins are generally considered to act as transporters of hormones, metals, ions and other metabolites. The presence of these and other proteins in the interstitial fluid space could significantly influence movement of ions and other molecules and their deposition in and removal from bone tissue. Some of the proteins present in the interstitial space are known to be synthesised by bone cells as well as being derived from the plasma. As stated earlier, these materials are under active investigation at the present time and numerous new components have been discovered   [31,40,41,42,43].

Interest in the non-collagenous substances of bone began over 20 years ago when the large group of bone seeking elements, including yttrium, cerium, americium and plutonium that concentrate on bone surfaces, were beginning to be investigated. Herring, Vaughan and Williamson [44] observed that under certain conditions the resorbing and quiescent surfaces where yttrium, plutonium and americium concentrate, stain strongly with periodic acid-Schiff reagent. After isolating from bone a protein containing 16% (^{w}/w) sialic acid it was suggested that the acidic nature of this protein may be important in binding of these metals. Subsequently, other bone fractions were found to bind plutonium and americium with equal avidity [45,46]. It is not surprising to find that a metal ion may be chelated by more than one tissue constituent, albeit with variable affinity. Constituent anions of the extracellular matrix of bone may require very specific structures for complex formation with metal ions. But in the case of calcium and certain other ions it appears that any phosphate-containing compound has a strong attraction.

In the original work of Herring [45], buffered solutions of the calcium chelating agent ethylenediamine tetraacetic acid (EDTA) were used to decalcify the bone powders and extract the associated organic constituents. Recently dissociative methods of extraction, firstly in guanidinium chloride solutions containing protease inhibitors and then in similar solutions containing EDTA, have been employed and suggested to diminish degredation of the constituent organic molecules [40]. What effect this denaturation has on the properties of the recovered molecular species has not been considered in any detail. The materials obtained in higher yield by the second extraction, which contains EDTA in the solution, are those that are released by the demineralization and are likely to have been associated with the mineral phase. They are probably not exclusively localised in this compartment, however.

Collagen type I fibres constitute the majority of the bone matrix and are arranged generally as parallel fibrils of even diameter. The orientation changes through the thickness of the tissue, presumably

related to the secretory cell. The strong bonds that crosslink and
stabilize the molecules result in the relative insolubility of bone
collagen. Differences in crosslinking patterns and hydroxylysine
content of bone collagen have been found compared with non-minerali-
sing tissues.

The non-collagenous constituents of the organic matrix of bone
are mainly proteinaceous in nature, although lipids and carbohydrates
are also present. The following discussion relates only to the major
proteins that have been characterised in some detail as being present
in bone matrix. After bone mineral and collagen these constituents
are likely to be the next most important potential receptor molecules
for ionic interaction in bone.

Sialoprotein as originally described [45] is a 23,000 molecular
weight, bone-specific glycoprotein containing up to 20% (^{w}/w) sialic
acid with over 40% of the polypeptide chain, that makes up about one
third the weight of the molecule, being acidic amino acids. Phosphate
groups also make up 1% of the weight of the protein. Investigation
of the sialoproteins of developing bovine bone [47] has suggested a
foetal form of this protein, which has a higher molecular weight
(70-80,000) but has very similar composition to the adult form.
Proteolysis of the larger molecule leads to smaller components
(20-3,000 M.W.) that are enriched in the adult bone and may well be
the sialoprotein Herring originally described [45]. Antibodies have
been produced against the larger molecule and immunofluorescent
techniques have shown localisation of the sialoprotein in the entire
osteoid seam and trabeculae of growing bone. Its function is unknown
and the metal binding characteristics of the parent molecule have not
been determined.

The second bone protein to be isolated and studied in great detail
has been named osteocalcin or BGP, (bone γ-carboxyglutamic acid containing protein) [42,43]. This is a quantitatively major constituent
of the non-collagenous protein fraction. It contains 2-3 molecules
of the unusual amino acid γ-carboxyglutamic acid (Gla) per molecule
of protein. This amino acid is derived from glutamate by a post-
translational enzymatic synthesis requiring vitamin K. It was

discovered first in the blood clotting proteins and is important in haemostasis as specific interaction of Ca^{++} ions with this moiety allows the clotting factors to interact with phospholipid vesicles released by blood platelets at the site of blood vessel damage [48]. It is therefore described as a calcium binding amino acid and, although osteocalcin shows only weak binding to this ion, the binding results in a compact α-helical conformational change. In the resultant structure the Gla residues become aligned at distances approximating the Ca^{++}-hydroxyapatite lattice spacings. Its affinity for hydroxyapatite is far greater than its affinity for Ca^{++} ions and this fact explains its accumulation in calcified bone matrix, as has been noted for other proteins. Competition studies show Ba^{++} and Sr^{++} do not compete significantly for the Ca^{++} sites in the protein, while Mg^{++} shows weak affinity. Other ions show variable inhibition of Ca^{++} binding and trivalent lanthanide ions (La^{+++}, Tb^{+++}) completely inhibit the Ca^{++} binding [49]. Depending on the species, this protein contains about 50 amino-acid residues and has a molecular weight of about 5-6,000. It is probably synthesized by the osteoblast and appears with onset of mineralisation. Osteocalcin is detected at ng levels in the serum and urine and is a result of leakage from the site of bone synthesis. Measurement of the blood and urine levels may have some relevance clinically in determining particular bone disease states. Vitamin D has been shown to affect the synthesis and distribution of osteocalcin and this protein could play some role in mediating the action of this vitamin on bone tissue. Osteocalcin is now the most extensively characterised non-collagenous protein and it is found also in dentine and possibly other mineralised tissues, but its physiological function has not been determined. Other, high molecular weight components containing Gla are found in bone matrix [50] and some higher molecular weight precursors are involved in osteocalcin biosynthesis [51,52].

Phosphoproteins have been isolated from bone where they make up to 1% (^{W}/w) of the organic matrix and have been extensively characterised [53]. They were first isolated by Spector and Glimcher [54] from bovine and chicken bone and are now known to contain phosphoserine and phosphotyrosine as the sole organic phosphorus content.

In addition,in the major component of molecular weight 28-30,000, the carboxylic acid side chain groups and the organic phosphorus groups make up almost one half the total amino acid residues. These sites have the potential capacity for interaction with calcium ions and possibly function as a crystal nucleator. The phosphoproteins are synthesized by the bone tissue and are located at mineralising sites. Once mineralization has started, however, it appears to proceed as a secondary nucleation phenomenon by the mineral crystals themselves without the need for more phosphoprotein nucleation.

Recently one of the most abundant bone glycoproteins, which makes up to 25% (^{W}/w) of the non-collagenous matrix in foetal calf bone, was isolated, characterised chemically and named osteonectin [55]. This name was suggested because of its possible function of linking the organic and mineral phases together. It shows binding to collagen and to hydroxyapatite and promotes the mineralisation of type I collagen in vitro. The protein contains 3% sialic acid, 1.6% hexosamine and 0.5% organic phosphate and has a molecular weight of 32,000. The bone forming cells, osteoblasts, seem to synthesize this protein, but other fibroblastic cells in vitro have been found to produce this constituent [56]. It is also found in plasma but this level changes with age. Its localisation in bone tissue is similar to that seen for bovine sialoprotein, being found in the osteoid seam and trabeculae of the growing bone. Apart from its strong association with calcium the metal binding characteristics of osteonectin have not been determined.

The proteoglycans of bone are carbohydrate-protein conjugates which make up about 2% of the non-collagenous matrix of bone. In early studies Herring [57] proposed structures for the major bone proteoglycan where one or two chondroitin sulphate chains are linked to a protein core. He considered the possibility that the sialoprotein was this protein core because of the similar amino acid compositions of the two isolated species. However, many amino acid analyses show similarities between widely different proteins. This fraction has been studied in much greater detail recently [58] and the protein core shows no identity with sialoprotein. Fisher et al [58] purified and characterised the bone proteoglycans from foetal calves, growing rats and human foetuses. The major proteoglycan in the foetal bone, and the sole proteoglycan in compact bone was found to be of small molecular weight (80-120,000) with 20-30% protein and either one or two chondroitin sulphate chains of 40,000 molecular weight attached to the small molecular weight (38,000) protein core, similar to the tentative structures proposed by Herring [45]. Antibodies against the protein core do not show reaction with cartilage, skin, cornea or basement membrane proteoglycans, and indirect immunofluorescence localizes the molecule to bone trabeculae and dentine but not to other tissues. Similar in location to osteonectin and sialoprotein, the bone proteoglycan also appears to mark preosteoblastic as well as osteoblastic activity. Proteoglycans are important structural components in many tissues but in bone they appear to be inhibitory to calcification processes.

It has been mentioned earlier that plasma proteins penetrate into the bone tissue fluid compartment. They are also found in calcified matrix with albumin and α_2HS-glycoprotein in greatest abundance [31] and are accumulated in bone as mineralisation proceeds. The role of the plasma proteins in transporting ions to the bone depository is probably of some importance, for example, in the case of the transport of plutonium in the blood by its adsorption to transferrin [59]. More than twenty plasma-derived proteins have been detected in bovine bone extracts [41], but quantitatively the majority will have been derived from the blood vessels in the tissue. Using two dimensional electrophoresis in polyacrylamide gels it was also found that twelve previously unidentified non-serum proteins were present in these bone extracts [41]. With the application of the monoclonal antibody technique to the field of non-collagenous bone proteins the possibility of developing a complete library of reagents for the study of each bone-specific protein is apparent [60].

Even without this technique, however, progress has been made in defining some of these new constituents. As a further example we have recently investigated one of the major small molecular weight components of rat bone of molecular weight 19,000. This has been named BP2 and its distribution investigated by the production of antibodies to purified material produced by polyacrylamide gel

electrophoresis [61]. This material has been localised by immunofluorescence and immunoperoxidase-labelling techniques to bone matrix,
osteoid and calcifying cartilage in calcified and decalcified sections
of rat neonatal calvaria, and in rat neonatal and adult femora. It is
not found in soft tissues such as spleen, kidney, thymus, bone marrow,
gut, eye, or skin. From this work BP2 has a tissue distribution
specific to calcified matrix and osteogenic tissue. Its function is
unknown, as is the case with all the non-collagenous proteins
described. It is a further example of one of the interesting bone
constituents that will be useful in future work in defining when a
developing tissue becomes osteogenic, when a cell becomes a bone cell
and how disease processes alter bone metabolism. The question, "Do
any of these minor organic constituents significantly influence
accumulation of particular metal ions in bone?", should be answerable
as the physicochemical and physiological properties of the components
of this group of substances are more clearly defined.

SUMMARY

In addition to its protective, structural and homeostatic functions,
bone acts as a sink for many materials introduced into the circulation
either naturally or artificially. Accumulation of certain of these
materials is of continuing concern to toxicologists and radiobiologists. Bone is a very heterogeneous tissue and depending on age and
bone type, it has various proportions of mineral, matrix and cells.
The mineral phase is considered to be analogous to a highly substi-
tuted, poorly crystalline hydroxyapatite, with the crystallinity
increasing with age. Type I collagen makes up the majority of the
organic matrix and recent studies of the non-collagenous proteins have
shown a number of proteins are specific to bone tissue. As with all
moieties deposited in any tissue site, the delivery to the site, the
relative affinities for tissue constituents and the use or substitution in anabolic processes are major factors controlling this accumulation. The influence of blood flow, tissue fluid flow, vascular
permeability and the presence of specific inorganic and organic
materials are thus of paramount importance with respect to the
skeletal uptake of metal ions. Cellular metabolism also modifies the

localisation of these materials by receptor molecule and active transport processes and the patterns of accumulation in the tissue changes with time. This review has concentrated on the recent advances that have been made in determining the nature of the materials present in the organic matrix of bone. What effect particular constituents have on metal ion uptake is relatively unknown, but unique components of the organic matrix of bone may initiate mineralization of the tissue.

REFERENCES

1. Urist, M. R., DeLange, R. J. and Finerman, G. A. M. (1983). Bone cell differentiation and growth factors. Science, 220, 680-686.

2. Engstrom, A. (1956). Structure of bone from the anatomical to the molecular level. In: Wolstenholme, G. E. W. and O'Connor, C. M. (eds). Bone Structure and Metabolism. pp. 3-13. (Boston: Little, Brown and Co.)

3. Neuman, W. F. and Neuman, M. W. (1953). The nature of the mineral phase of bone. Chem. Rev., 53, 1-45.

4. DeJong, W. F. (1926). La substance minerale dans les os. Recl. Trav. Chim. Pays-Bas Belg., 45, 445-448.

5. Moreno, E. C., Kresak, M. and Hay, D. I. (1984). Adsorption of molecules of biological interest onto hydroxyapatite. Calcif. Tissue Int., 36, 48-59.

6. Bio-Rad Catalogue J. (1984). Hydroxylapatite applications. pp. 41-44. (Watford, U. K.: Bio-Rad Laboratories Ltd.)

7. Posner, A. S. (1969). Crystal chemistry of bone mineral. Physiol. Rev., 49, 760-792.

8. Termine, J. D. and Posner, A. S. (1967). Amorphous/crystalline interrelationships in bone mineral. Calcif. Tissue Int., 1, 8-23.

9. Glimcher, M. J. (1981). On the form and function of bone: From molecules to organs. Wolff's law revisited. In: Veis, A. (ed.). The Chemistry and Biology of Mineralised Connective Tissues. pp. 618-673. (New York: Elsevier)

10. Neuman, W. F. (1980). Bone material and calcification mechanisms. In: Urist, M. R. (ed.). Fundamental and Clinical Bone Physiology. pp. 83-107. (Philadelphia: Lippincott)

11. Brookes, M. (1971). The Blood Supply of Bone. (London: Butterworths)

12. Kelly, P. J. (1983). Pathways of transport in bone. In: Handbook of Physiology - The Cardiovascular System III, Chapter 12. pp. 371-396.

13. Cumming, J. D. (1962). A study of blood flow through bone marrow by a method of venous effluent collection. J. Physiol., 162, 13-20.

14. Post, M. and Shoemaker, W.C. (1964). Method for measuring bone metabolism in vivo. J. Bone Jt Surg., 46A, 111-120.

15. Shim, S. S. and Patterson, F. P. (1967). A direct method of qualitative study of bone blood circulation. Surg. Gynec. & Obstet., 125, 261-268.

16. Copp, D. H. and Shim, S. S. (1965). Extraction ratio and bone clearance of ^{85}Sr as a measure of effective bone blood flow. Circ. Res., 16, 461-467.

17. Kelly, P. J., Xipintsoi, T. and Bassingthwaighte, J. B. (1971). Blood flow in canine tibial diaphysis estimated by iodoantipyrine ^{125}I-washout. J. Appl. Physiol., 31, 38-47.

18. Paradis, G. R. and Kelly, P. J. (1975). Blood flow and mineral deposition in canine tibial fractures. J. Bone Jt Surg., 57A, 200-226.

19. Kane, W. J. (1968). Fundamental concepts in bone blood flow studies. J. Bone Jt Surg., 50A, 801-811.

20. McElfresh, E. C. and Kelly, P. J. (1974). Simultaneous determination of blood flow in cortical bone, marrow and muscle in canine-hind-leg by femoral artery catheterization. Calcif. Tissue Res., 14, 301-307.

21. Brookes, M. (1967). Blood flow rates in compact and cancellous bone and bone marrow. J. Anat., 101, 533-541.

22. Gross, P. M., Marcus, M. L. and Heistad, D. D. (1981). Measurement of blood flow to bone and marrow in experimental animals by means of the microsphere technique. J. Bone Jt Surg., 63A, 1028-1033.

23. Shim, S. S., Copp, D. H. and Patterson, F.P. (1967). An indirect method of blood flow measurement based on the bone clearance of circulating bone seeking radioisotope. J. Bone Jt Surg., 49A, 693-702.

24. Gross, P. M., Heistad, D. D. and Marcus, M. L. (1979). Neurohumoral regulation of blood flow to bones and marrow. Am. J. Physiol., 237, H440-H448.

25. Falkow, B. and Neil, E. (1971). Circulation. pp. 518-523. (London: Oxford Univ. Press)

26. Cofield, R. H., Bassingthwaighte, J. B. and Kelly, P. J. (1975). Strontium-85 extraction during transcapillary passage in tibial bone. J. Appl. Physiol., 39, 596-602.

27. Neuman, W. F., Terepka, A. R., Canas, F. and Triffitt, J. T. (1968). The cycling concept of exchange in bone. Calcif. Tissue Res. 2, 262-270.

28. Kelly, P. J. and Bassingthwaighte, J. B. (1977). Studies on bone ion exchange using multiple tracer indicator dilution techniques. Fed. Proc., 36, 2634-2639.

29. Zamboni, L. and Pease, D.C. (1961). The vascular bed of red bone marrow. J. Ultrast. Res., 5, 65-85.

30. Davies, D. R., Bassingthwaighte, J. B. and Kelly, P. J. (1976). Transcapillary exchange of strontium and sucrose in canine tibia. J. Appl. Physiol., 40, 17-22.

31. Triffitt, J. T. (1980). The organic matrix of bone tissue. In: Urist, M. R. (ed.). Fundamental and Clinical Bone Physiology. pp. 45-82. (Philadelphia: Lippincott)

32. Doty, S. B. and Schofield, B. H. (1972). Metabolic and structural changes within osteocytes of rat bone. In: Calcium, Parathyroid Hormone and the Calcitonins, Proc. Parathyroid Conf., 4th, Chapel Hill N. Carolina. pp. 353-364. (Amsterdam: Excerpta Med. Fd.)

33. Owen, M., Howlett, C.R. and Triffitt, J.T. (1977). Movement of ^{125}I albumin and ^{125}I polyvinylpyrrolidone through bone tissue fluid. Calcif. Tissue Res., 23, 103-112.

34. Michelsen, K. (1967). Pressure relationships in the bone marrow vascular bed. Acta physiol. Scand., 71, 12-29.

35. Shim, S. S., Hawk, H. E. and Yu, W. Y. (1972). The relationship between blood flow and marrow cavity pressure of bone. Surg. Gynec. and Obstet., 135, 353-360.

36. Seliger, W. G. (1970). Tissue fluid movement in compact bone. Anat. Rec. 166, 247-255.

37. Anderson, D. W. (1960). Studies of the lymphatic pathways of bone and bone marrow. J. Bone Jt Surg., 42A, 716-717.

38. Cooper, R. R., Milgram, J. W. and Robinson, R. A. (1966). Morphology of the osteon. J. Bone Jt Surg., 48, 1239-1271.

39. Yoffey, J. M. and Courtice, F. C. (1956). Lymphatics, Lymph and Lymphoid Tissue. (London: Edward Arnold)

40. Termine, J. D. (1983). Osteonectin and other newly described proteins of developing bone. In: Peck, W. A. (ed.). Bone and Mineral Research, Annual 1. pp. 144-156. (Amsterdam: Excerpta Medica)

41. Delmas, P. D., Tracy, R. P., Riggs, B. L., and Mann, K. G. (1984) Identification of the noncollagenous proteins of bovine bone by two-dimensional gel electrophoresis. Calcif. Tissue Int., 36, 308-316.

42. Gundberg, C. M., Hauschka, P. V., Lian, J. B., and Gallop, P. M. (1984). Osteocalcin: isolation and characterization. Methods Enzymol. In press.

43. Price, P. (1983). Osteocalcin. In: Peck, W. A. (ed.). Bone and Mineral Research, Annual 1. pp. 157-190. Amsterdam: Excerpta Medica.

44. Herring, G. M., Vaughan, J., and Williamson, M. (1962). Preliminary report on the site of localization and possible binding agent for yttrium, americium and plutonium in cortical bone. Health Phys., 8, 717-724.

45. Herring, G. M. (1972). The organic matrix of bone. In: Bourne, G. H. (ed.). The Biochemistry and Physiology of Bone, 2nd edit., 1. pp. 128-189. London: Academic Press.

46. Chipperfield, A. R. and Taylor, D. M. (1972). The binding of thorium (IV), plutonium (IV), americium (III) and curium (III) to the constituents of bovine cortical bone in vitro. Rad. Res. 51, 15-30.

47. Fisher, L. W., Whitson, S. W., Avioli, L. V. and Termine, J. D. (1983). Matrix sialoprotein of developing bone. J. biol. Chem., 258, 12723-12727.

48. Stenflo, J. and Suttie, J. W. (1977). Vitamin K-dependent formation of γ-carboxyglutamic acid. Ann. Rev. Biochem., 46, 157-172.

49. Hauschka, P. V. and Gallop, P. M. (1977). Purification and calcium-binding properties of osteocalcin, the γ-carboxyglutamate-containing protein of bone. In: Wasserman, R. H., Corradino, R. A., Carafoli, E., Kretsinger, R. H., MacLennan, D. H. and Siegel, F. L. (eds). Calcium binding proteins and calcium function. pp. 338-347. (Amsterdam: Elsevier North-Holland Inc.)

50. Price, P. A., Urist, M. R., and Otawara, Y. (1983). Matrix Gla protein, a new γ-carboxyglutamic acid-containing protein which is associated with the organic matrix of bone. Biochem. Biophys. Res. Comm., 117, 765-771.

51. Hauschka, P. V. (1979). Osteocalcin in developing bone systems. In: Suttie, J. W. (ed.). Vitamin K metabolism and vitamin K-dependent proteins. pp. 227-236. Baltimore: University Park Press.

52. Nishimoto, S. K., Cotter, T. M., and Nimni, M. E. (1984). Presence of bone Gla protein and higher molecular weight immuno-reactive molecules in extracts of rat bone. Trans. Orthop. Res. Soc., Abst. 194.

53. Glimcher, M. J. (1984). Recent studies of the mineral phase in bone and its possible linkage to the organic matrix by protein-bound phosphate bonds. Phil. Trans. R. Soc. Lond. B304, 409-588.

54. Spector, A. R. and Glimcher, M. J. (1972). The extraction and characterization of soluble anionic proteins from bone. Biochim. biophys. Acta, 263, 593-603.

55. Termine, J. D., Kleinman, H. K., Whitson, S. W., Conn, K. M., McGarvey, M. L., and Martin, G. R. (1981). Osteonectin a bone-specific protein linking mineral to collagen. Cell, 26, 99-105.

56. Wasi, S., Tung, P., Otsuka, K., Yao, K. L., Sodek, J., and Termine, J. D. (1983). Synthesis of an osteonectin-like protein by various connective tissue cells in culture. Calcif. Tissue Int., 35, 652.

57. Herring, G. M. (1968). Studies on the protein bound chondroitin sulphate of bovine cortical bone. Biochem. J., 107, 41-49.

58. Fisher, L. W., Termine, J. D., Dejter, S. W., Whitson, S. W., Yanagishita, M., Kimura, J. H., Hascall, V. C., Kleinman, H. K., Hassell, J. R., and Nilsson, B. (1983). Proteoglycans of developing bone. J. biol. Chem., 258, 6588-6594.

59. Priest, N. D. (1980). Plutonium in bone: the effects of bone remodelling. In: Bone and Bone Seeking Radionuclides: Physiology, Dosimetry and Effects, EULEP Symposium, Rotterdam. pp. 39-55. London: Harwood Academic Publishers.

60. Stenner, D. D., Romberg, R. W., Tracy, R. P., Katzman, J. A., Riggs, B. L., and Mann, K. G. (1984). Monoclonal antibodies to native noncollagenous bone-specific proteins. Proc. Natl. Acad. Sci. U.S.A., 81, 2868-2872.

61. Mardon, H. J., and Triffitt, J. T. (1984). The expression of a new bone-specific, bone matrix-derived protein by osteogenic cells. Proceedings British Connective Tissue Society, St. Catharine's College Oxford.

2

Localization of ^{99m} Technetium in Bone

T. J. F. SAVELKOUL, W. J. VISSER, S. J. OLDENBURG and S. A. Duursma

INTRODUCTION

Skeletal scintigraphy is a routine procedure in the evaluation of bone disease. One of the agents of choice is methylene diphosphonate labeled with ^{99m}Technetium (^{99m}Tc-MDP) (1). The uptake of ^{99m}Technetium at sites of active bone formation is higher in comparison with normal bone (2-7). The mechanism of uptake is still controversial (8-15). Micro-autoradiography is a possibility to evaluate the localization in bone and some macro and micro-autoradiographic studies have been performed (12,15,17-23). Due to the long processing time for embedding in plastic, these studies were mostly performed with frozen bone sections. In other studies wax have been used as embedding material, but in these studies ^{96}Tc and ^{95m}Tc with relatively long physical half-lives were used as the tracer (20-26). The preservation of the bone structure in frozen bone sections or using wax is inferior to the embedding in methylmethacrylate.

Tilden et al (23) used epoxy resin for embedding and reduced the processing time before exposure to 14 hours (2.3 ^{99m}Technetium half-lives). In a previously described study we used a rapid method for preparing undecalcified sections of bone, embedded in methylmethacrylate (24). The processing time before exposure has been reduced to 6 hours. The results of micro-autoradiography of ^{99m}Tc-MDP, prepared after electrolytical reduction of ^{99m}TcO$_4^-$ in the presence of MDP (25),

21

are reported. Bone sections of fetal rat calvaria after administration
of ^{99m}Tc-MDP _in vitro_ and of rat femora after administration _in vivo_
are studied.

MATERIALS AND METHODS

Radiopharmaceutical

^{99m}Tc-MDP was prepared after electrolytical reduction of ^{99m}TcO$_4^-$ in
the presence of MDP, as previously described (25). Before administration ^{99m}Tc-MDP was separated from remaining ^{99m}TcO$_4^-$ by means of
gel chromatography at Biogel P$_4$(Biorad), 100-200 mesh with normal
saline as the eluant in a 0.9 x 28 cm columm. The purity of ^{99m}Tc-MDP
is controlled by means of ascending paper chromatography on Whatman
3MM with 0.5 M acetate buffer (pH 5.0) as the eluant.

Incubation of fetal rat calvaria

Calvaria of fetal Wistar rats on the 19th day of gestation were incubated with 111 MBq (3mCi) of ^{99m}Tc-MDP in Hank's Balanced Salt Solution (PH 7.4, temperature 37°C) for two hours. The calvaria were
clamped in modified Ussing Chambers with their concave site directed
to the compartment B in which the radiopharmaceutical was administered
(Fig. 1).

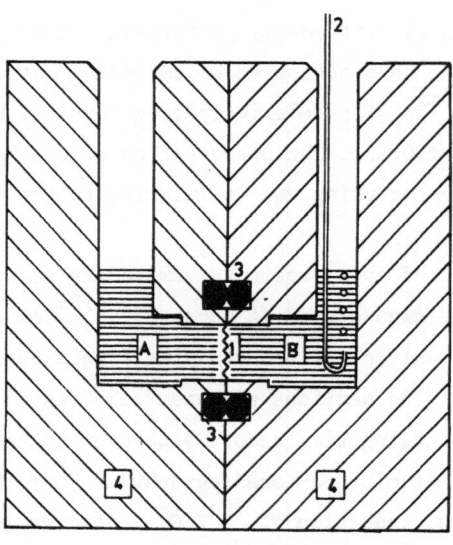

FIGURE 1

During the incubation the radiopharmaceutical was regularly checked
for purity by means of paper chromatography.

Rat femora

Male Wistar rats (6 weeks old) received 185 MBq (5mCi) ^{99m}Tc-MDP,
administered into the tail vein. Two hours after this administration
a scintigram was performed. The rats were killed and the femora were
immediately removed and divided longitudinally with a thin rapidly
rotating saw, cooled with normal saline.

Tissue preparations and micro-autoradiography

All bone specimen were fixated in a mixture of formaline and methanol
according to Burkhardt (26) and further processed as previously described (24). The 4 μm sections were dipped in a nuclear track emulsion
(NTB-2, Kodak) diluted 1:1 with doubly distilled water. The slides
were exposed for 18 hours at 4°C, developed (D-170, Kodak) and fixed
in 24% sodium thiosulfate. For histological staining toluidine blue
and hematoxylin/eosin was used.
In all experiments unlabeled bone sections were subjected to the same
procedures as a control.

RESULTS

During the incubation experiment ^{99m}Tc-MDP remained stable as was shown
by the paper chromatograms. No radioactivity was detected in compartment A. The uptake of radioactivity by the calvarium was 40% of the
administered dose (corrected for the decay). In the calvaria the uptake
of radioactivity is localized in areas of bone formation with a slight
preference for the convex site of the calvarium (Fig. 2).
The scintigrams of the rats showed a normal bone uptake with little
activity in the soft tissues. In the rat femora ^{99m}Technetium is
diffusely localized in the mineralized bone (Fig. 3).
Most radioactivity is localized in the region below the epiphyseal
plate (Fig. 4). In the unlabeled sections the amount of developed
silver grains is equal to the background of the labeled sections.

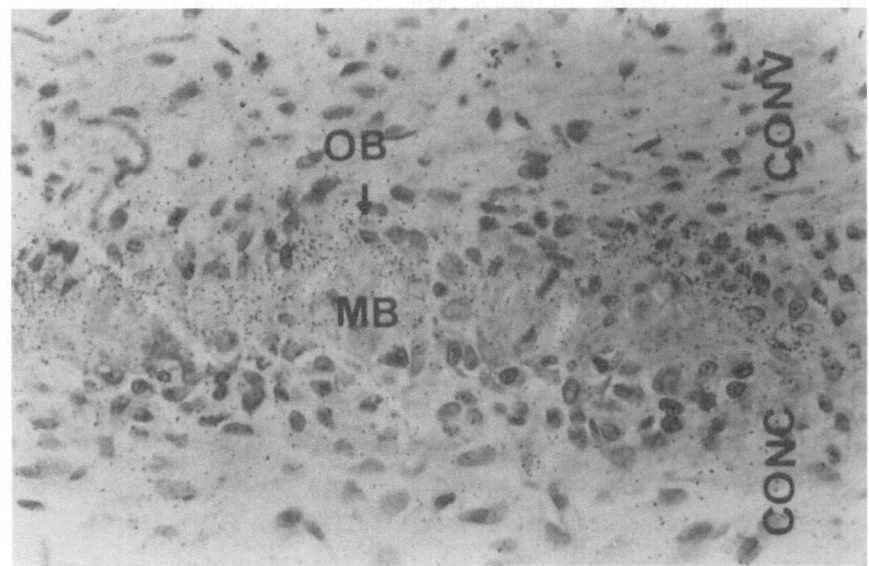

FIGURE 2 Section of fetal rat calvarium incubated with ^{99m}Tc-MDP
(Toluidine blue, 40x). There is a slight preference in the
localization of ^{99m}Technetium for the convex site (CONV)
of the calvarium.
OB= osteoblast, MB= mineralized bone, CONC= concave site

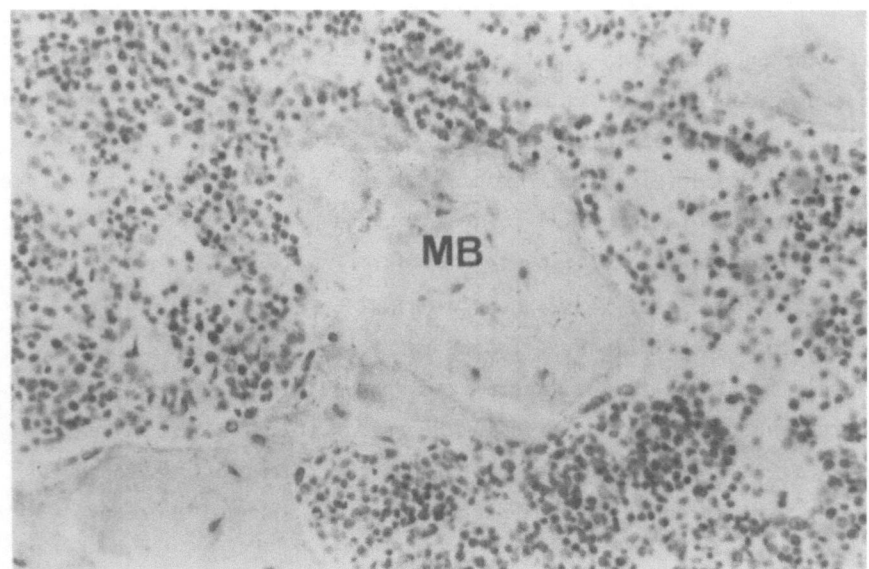

FIGURE 3 Section of the metaphysis of a distal femur of a wistar rat
(Toluidine blue, 40x). Radioactivity is diffusely distributed
in the mineralized bone (MB).

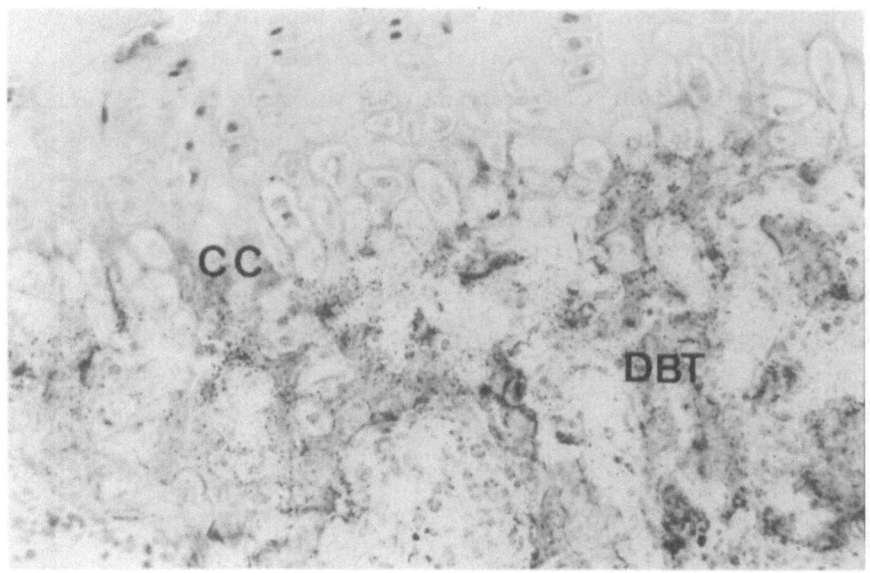

FIGURE 4 Section of a distal femur of a wistar rat containing the
lower part of the epiphyseal plate. There is a high uptake
of ^{99m}Technetium in the calcifying cartilage (CC) and in
the developing bone trabeculae (DBT).

DISCUSSION

With the rapid embedding in methylmethacrylate, histological sections
with a good structural preservation were obtained in combination with
a short processing time. The extranuclear electrons emitted by ^{99m}Tech-
netium are of sufficient low energy for good resolution micro-autoradio-
grams (27). In the fetal rat calvaria a high uptake is detected in the
bone germs especially at the active bone forming sites. At sites of
bone resorbing (concave site of calvarium) fewer developed grains are
seen. The calvaria were placed in the incubation chambers with their
concave sites to the compartment in which the radioactivity was administered. So the radioactivity has passed this site at first. In an
incubation experiment with rat femora, Khan et al (18) concluded to
localization of the tracer adjacent to the epiphyseal plate and also
on the surface of the bone. They found no tracer in established bone,

however, it is not known if there was enough passage from the radio-pharmaceutical through the 5mm bone sections.

In the rat femora a high uptake can be seen beneath the epiphyseal plate and to a lesser extent in bone trabeculae. No distinct cell labeling can be concluded from this study as is described by Guillemart et al (20). The preferent localization for developing trabeculae of the metaphysis and at sites of bone formation is described earlier and is in agreement with our results (15,18,20).

However, we did not find a preference for localization in resorbing areas as is found by Christensen et al (15).

The finding of a high uptake in a skeletal scintigram corresponds with uptake of [99m]Technetium in mineralizing bone in the micro-auto-radiogram.

REFERENCES

1. Fogelman, I. (1982). Diphosphonate bone scanning agents-Current concepts. Eur.J.Nucl.Med., 7, 506-509

2. Matin, P. (1979). Appearance of bone scans following fractures, including immediate and long-term studies. J.Nucl.Med., 20, 1227-1231

3. Batikles, J., Vasilas, A., Pizzi, W.F. et al. (1981). Bone scanning in the detection of occult fractures. J.Trauma, 21, 564-569

4. Miller, S.W., Castronovo, F.P., Pendergrass, H.P. et al. (1974). Technetium-99m labeled diphosphonate bone scanning in Paget's desease. Am.J.Roentgenol., 121, 177-183

5. Lisbona, R., Rosenthall, L. (1977). Radionuclide imaging of septic joints and their differentiations form periarticular osteomyelitis and cullulitis in pediatrics. Clin.Nucl.Med., 2, 337-343

6. McNeil, B.J., (1978). Rationale for use of bone scans in selected metastasis and primary bone tumors. Semin.Nucl.Med., 8, 336-345

7. Rosenthall, L., Kaye, M. (1975). Technetium-99m pyrophosphate kinetics and imaging in metabolic bone disease. J.Nucl.Med., 16, 33-39

8. Yano,Y., McRae, J., van Dyke, D.C. et al. (1973). Technetium-99m-labeled stannous ethane-1-hydroxy-1,1-diphosphonate: a new bone scanning agent. J.Nucl.Med., 14, 73-78

9. Cox, P.H. (1974). ^{99m}Tc-complexes for skeletal scintigraphy. Physi-cochemical factors affecting bone and bone marrow uptake. Br.J.Rad,.

<u>47</u>, 845-850

10. Garnett, E.S., Bowen, B.M., Coates, G. et al. (1975). An Analysis
of factors which influence the local accumulation of bone-seeking
radiopharmaceuticals. Invest.Rad., <u>10</u>, 564-568

11. Kaye, M., Silverton, S., Rosenthall, G. (1975). Technetium-99m-
pyrophosphate: Studies in vivo and in vitro. J.Nucl.Med., <u>16</u>, 40-45

12. Van Langevelde, A., Driessen, O.M.J., Pauwels, E.K.J. et al. (1977)
Aspects of Technetium binding from Ethane-1-hydroxy-1,1-diphosphonate-
^{99m}Tc-complex to Bone. Eur.J.Nucl.Med., <u>2</u>, 47-51

13. Francis, M.D., Ferguson, D.L., Tofe, A.J. et al. (1980).
Comparative evaluation of three diphosphonates: In vitro adsorption
(C-14 labeled) and in vivo osteogenic uptake (Tc-99m labeled).
J.Nucl.Med., <u>21</u>, 1185-1189

14. Billinghurst, M.W., Jette, D., Somers, E. (1981). Investigation of
the interaction of hydroxy-apatite with Technetium in associaton with
stannous pyrophosphate. Int.J.Appl.Radiat.Isot., <u>32</u>, 559-566

15. Christensen, S.B., Krogsgaard, O.W. (1981). Localization of ^{99m}Tc-
Methylene Diphosphonate in epiphyseal Growth plates of rats.
J.Nucl.Med., <u>22</u>, 237-245

16. Schümichen, C., Korfgen, T., Hoffman, G. (1980). Relationship
between complex stability and biokinetics of ^{99m}Tc-phosphate compounds.
Nucl.Med., <u>19</u>, 7-10

17. Rohlin, M., Hammerstrom, L. (1976). Whole-body Autoradiography of
^{99m}Tc-labeled pyrophosphate and related compounds in young rats.
Acta Rad.Ther.Phys.Biol., <u>15</u>, 71-80

18. Kahn, R.A., Hughes, S., Lavender, P. et al. (1979). Autoradiography of Technetium labeled diphosphonate in rat bone.
J.Bone Joint Surg., <u>61-B</u>, 221-224

19. Christensen, S.B., Arnoldi, C.C. (1980). Distribution of ^{99m}Tc-
phosphate compounds in ostearthrytic femoral heads. J.Bone Joint Surg.,
62-A, 90-96

20. Guillemart, A., Besnard, J-C., le Pape, A. et al. (1978). Skeletal
uptake of pyrophosphate labeled with Technetium-95m and Technetium-96,
as evaluated by autoradiography. J.Nucl.Med., <u>19</u>, 895-899

21. Guillemart, A., le Pape, A., Besnard, J-L. (1980). Bone kinetics
of Calcium-45 and pyrophosphate labeled with Technetium-96: An auto-

radiographic evaluation. J.Nucl.Med., 21, 466-470

22. Le Pape, A., Guillemart, A. (1982). Autoradiographic Comparison of ^{96}Tc-pyrophosphate and ^{45}Ca bone uptake. Eur.J.Nucl.Med.J., 7, 127-129

23. Tilden, R.L., Jackson, J., Enneking, W.F. et al. (1973). ^{99m}Tc-polyphosphate: Histological localization in human femurs by autoradiography. J.Nucl.Med., 14, 576-578

24. Savelkoul, T.J.F., Visser, W.J., Roelofs, J.M.M. et al. (1983). A rapid method for preparing undecalcified sections of bone for autoradiographic Investigation with short-lived radionuclides. Stain Techn., 58, 1-5

25. Savelkoul, T.J.F., Oldenburg, S.J., van Oort, W.J.et al. (1984). Electrolytically Labeled (^{99m}Tc)MDP: Chromatographic Pattern, Stability and Biodistribution in Rats. Int.J.Appl.Radiat.Isot., 8, 709-713

26. Burkhardt, R. (1966). Präparative Voraussetzungen zum klinische Histologie des menschliches Knochenmarkes. Blut, 14, 30-46

27. Barth, R.F., Clancy, J., Pugh, J.M. (1976). Autoradiographic studies on the cellular uptake of Technetium-99m and Chromium-51. J.Microsc., 109, 211-222

The Pattern of Calcium Deposition in Rat Bone as demonstrated by Calcein Labeling

W. SONTAG

Introduction

Many heavy metals reaching the skeleton are initially deposited non-uniformly on internal and external bone edges. Some metals are bound so strongly (Am,Pu), that only bone remodeling changes this initial pattern (Po81, Pr83), whereas others are bound more weakly (Ra), so that bone remodeling together with diffusion or ion exchange can vary this pattern (Pr83). There is also evidence to suggest that after contamination with bone seeking radionuclides the risk of osteosarcoma induction may be more likely in bones with a high turnover rate (Je78).

Thus a detailed knowledge of bone turnover rates in selected bones is not only of great interest in the understanding of bone development under normal and pathological conditions, but also for the understanding of changing radionuclide deposition patterns and osteosaracoma induction. Newly forming bone tissue can be measured after vital staining with fluorochromes, such as calcein or tetracycline (Su66), which form fluorescent complexes with calcium and can be measured with a high accurancy by use of a fluorescence microscope. Whereas in a previously publication the bone turnover rate has been studied in the diaphysis as an example of cortical bone (So81), the aim of the present investigation was to obtain detailed information on the femoral epiphysis and metaphysis of growing rats, as an example of predominantly spongy bone; plus information on both the anatomical regions sites and extent of bone remodeling.

Material and Methods

The experiments were performed with 60-day-old and 100-day-old female and male rats of the Heiligenberg strain. The rats received subcutaneous injections of calcein twice weekly until death. The dose injected was 20 mg/kg body mass in 0.24 M $NaHCO_3$. The rats were killed between 2 and 75 days after injection; the femur was removed, halved, embedded in methyl-methacrylate and cut, on a Leitz sawing microtome, into about 60 μm thick sections. The sections were mounted on glass slides and the fluorescence was measured in incident light with a Leitz microphotometer (MPV II). After measurement of the fluorescence intensity, the surface of the bone was stained with alizarin red S and in a second measurement the structure of the bone was determined in digitized form by processing the photometer signal in transmitted green light. The measuring field was 20 μm square. After the measurements, the two data sets, representing the information on the fluorescence intensity and the bone structure, respectively, were combined and the combined data file was the basis for calculation of morphological and bone turnover parameters by using different FORTRAN programmes, which were described in detail in a previous publication (So80). For every time point two animals were used and from each animal two sections were analysed, to eliminate most of the variation resulting from the different cut positions.

To calculate the remodeling rate from the experimental data it has been assumed that within the time interval between the start of the experiment and sacrificing the animals the remodeling rate decreased exponentially with increasing age, then the differential equation of the new forming bone V_F can be written as:

$$dV_F/dt = B_F e^{-\alpha t} V_B \qquad (1a)$$

where $B_F e^{-\alpha t}$ and V_B are the bone formation rate at the age t and the total hard tissue, respectively. The integrated differential equation 1b describes the new forming bone volume V_F as a function of the labeling time t and the age t_0 at the start of the experiment

$$V_F(t,t_0) = B_F e^{-\alpha t_0} V_B(1 - e^{-\alpha t})/\alpha \qquad (1b)$$

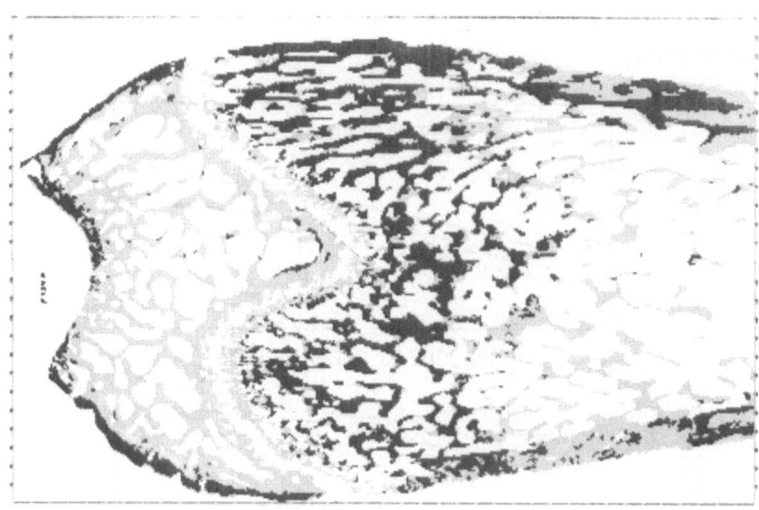

Fig.1. Computer printout of the distal femur of a female rat labeled between age 60 and 92 days with calcein. The grey area is unlabeled bone and the darker area is calcein-labeled bone. The measurement field was 20 μm square.

The scan area was over the whole width of the distal femora and 8 mm in length from the articular cartilage in the direction of the diaphysis. This area contains the whole epiphysis and most of the metaphysis (Fig.1). Whereas epiphysis and metaphysis were digitized as a whole, for calculation there were separated, with the border taken as the middle of the epiphyseal plate.

Additionally to the automatic analysis, some selected bone samples were analysed using a digitizer (Digiplan, Kontron) to measure the thickness of the trabeculae. To obtain the real thickness the experimental values are multiplied by the isotrop factor $\pi/4=0.785$.

Results and Discussion

In the age region examined between 60 and 130 days both bodyweight as well as the mass and volume of all organs including the skeleton are growing rapidly. Most of the bones of the skeleton can be divided into epiphysis, metaphysis and diaphysis (Ba83); the distal femora has been picked as an example of this morphological part of bone, because many investigations have studied the distribution of incorporated radionuclides in this bone region, so that a comparison between bone turnover and nuclide distribution gives us a deeper understanding of the mechanisms of initial nuclide deposition, distribution change and tumour induction.

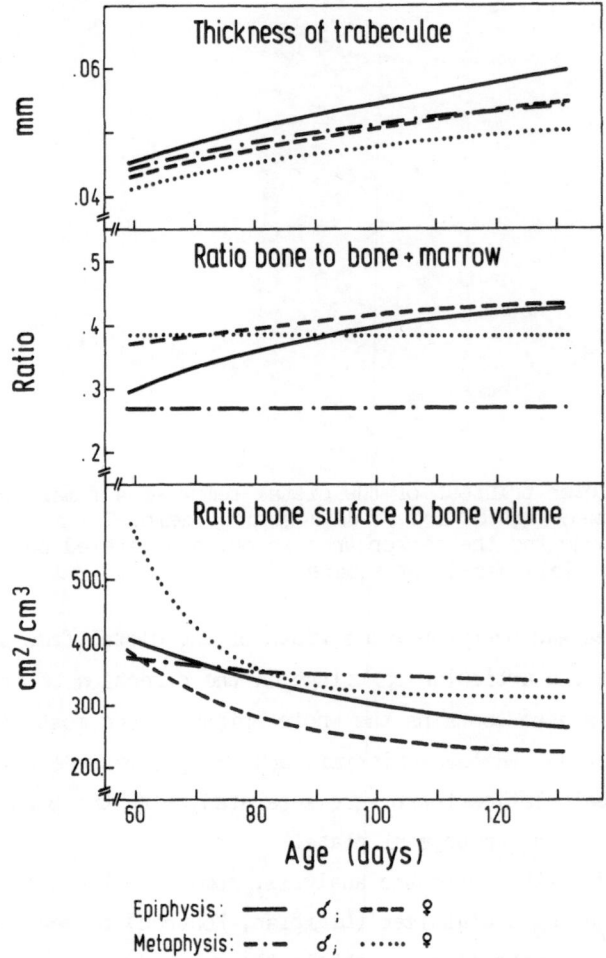

Fig.2. Morphological parameters in the distal femora of male and female rats as a function of age. The upper picture shows the trabecular thickness, the middle picture the ratio bone to total volume and the lower picture the surface to volume ratio.

Epiphysis

In this age range the epiphysis increases in outside diameter and length by the progressive addition of new bone to its periosteal surface with simultaneous resorption from its cortical-endosteal surface (Fig.1); therefore the growth in length occurs more on the articular cartilage than on the epiphyseal plate. With increasing age the mean trabeculae thickness increases in both sexes from about 45 μm (60 days) up to 57 μm at 130 days (Fig.2); in male rats the thickness is greater than the corresponding values in female rats. For sawing, the bone samples were orientated in such a manner that the cut area is longitudinal through the middle of the diaphysis; nevertheless, the variation of the the absolute values of bone and marrow volume in different animals of equal ages is greater than the variation with age. Figure 2 presents the proportion of mineralized tissue from the total tissue; as can be seen for both sexes the fraction of mineralized tissue increases with increasing age simultaneously with the thickness of trabeculae and at age 130 days, at 0.43, is comparable for both sexes. The Surface/Volume(S/V)-ratio shows the opposite effect; with increasing age it decreases from 400 cm^{-1} to 250 cm^{-1}.

From Fig.3 it can be seen that the calcein labeled bone area increases continuously with increasing time after labeling for both sexes and both age groups. The bone formation rate (Fig.4) - i.e. the area of newly growing bone, expressed as per cent of total bone in one year - calculated by use of equation 1b, decreases with increasing age, the diminution being greatest in female rats.

Metaphysis

The growth in length of the femora takes place in the metaphysis by forming new trabeculae in the primary metaphysis near the epiphyseal plate (Fig.1) and simultaneous resorption of trabeculae in the seqondary metaphysis near the diaphysis. Comparison between the growth in length of the whole femora and the growth of the distal epiphyseal plate show, that the rate of growth in length in the distal metaphysis is about two-fold higher than in the proximal metaphysis. Additionally to growth in length, the old metaphyseal cortical bone decreases in outside diameter by the progressive resorption of periosteal bone surfaces with simultaneous addition of new bone to its opposite endosteal surfaces (Fig.1).

With increasing age the mean trabeculae thickness increases for both sexes from about 43 μm (60 days) to 53 μm at age 130 days (Fig.2), whereas the ratio of bone to total volume is constant over the whole age region examined. The S/V-ratio is greatest in female rats, but decreases for both sexes with increasing age. The fractional bone

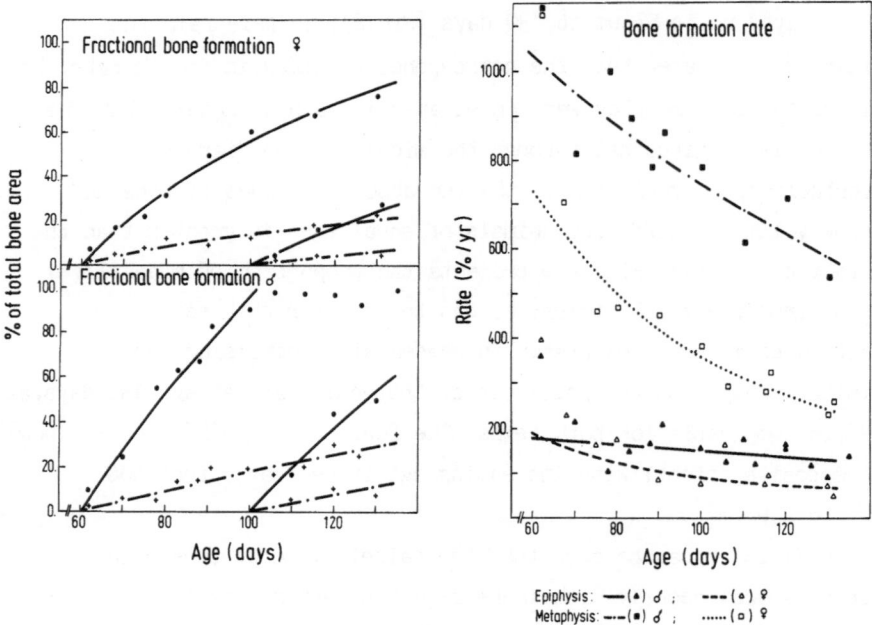

Fig.3.(Left figure) The fractional bone formation rate in the distal femora of 60 and 100-day-old male and female rats as a function of the time of labeling, the symbols (*) and (+) indicate the values of the metaphysis and epiphysis, respectively. Each symbol is the mean value of four measurements, whereas the lines represents the regression analysis using equation 1b.

Fig.4.(Right figure) Bone formation rate as a function of age in the epiphysis and metaphysis of male and female rats calculated from the data presented in Fig.3.

formation area increases continuously with increasing time after start of labeling for both sexes and both age groups; except in the 60-day-old male rats, where from age 100 days the whole bone is labeled and no measurement is possible. The bone formation rate, 1000%/yr, in the 60-day-old male rats is 40% higher than in the corresponding female rats and decreases between 60 days and 130 days by a factor of two.

Comparison of the morphological parameters in the epiphyses and metaphyses show a similar behaviour of the trabeculae thickness and the S/V-ratio (Fig.2); whereas the bone to total volume ratio increases in the epiphysis, but is constant in the metaphysis. This can be explained by the fact that in the epiphysis the augmentation of spongy bone is greater than the augmentation of the total volume; this means that the marrow cavities have been drawn together with increasing age; in the metaphysis the absolute bone volume increases with increasing age, therefore with a constant ratio both hard tissue and marrow have been expanded by the same amount.

The fractional bone formation (Fig.3) and the bone formation rate (Fig.4) are considerably higher in the metaphysis than in the epiphysis. Estimation of the bone formation rate in the metaphysis resulting from the increasing thickness of spongy bone and the re-modeling of the cortical bone gave values comparable to those in the epiphysis, i.e. between 75% and 80% of bone turnover comes from the longitudinal growth of the metaphysis. The bone formation rate, which is higher in male than in female rats and is higher in the metaphysis than in the epiphysis, can be approximated in the age region examined by a decreasing exponential function.

In contrast to the diaphysis where regions of forming and resorbing surfaces are separated over a long period of observation (Ba70), this cannot be presupposed in the epiphysis and metaphysis. Comparison of the bone turnover rate in the overlapping interval between 100 and 130 days show a good agreement, within statistical error, between the two age groups, except in the metaphysis of the 60-day-old male rats; additionally, observations of the fluorescence bands after single injection of calcein (unpublished observation) show at different times after injection, and therefore at different distances from the epiphyseal plate in the metaphysis, little change in their lengths relative to the lengths of the surface; from this finding it can be concluded that the resorption of labeled bone -if it occurs- is probably of minor importance. On the other hand, in the primary metaphysis there is some evidence that the processes of bone formation and resorbtion are occurring in the same regions (Ba83, Ki80). If there is resorption of labeled bone proportional to new forming bone over the whole observation time, equation 1b cannot distinguishes between formation and resorption, so that bone turnover calculated from calcein labelled hard tissue, can result in an underestimation, thus the bone formation rates presented in Fig.4 are the minimum bone formation rates.

Conclusions

Morphological and bone turnover parameters have been measured in the epiphysis and metaphysis of male and female rats between age 60 and 130 days.

In this age region the trabecular thickness increases on everage by 25%, whereas the S/V-ratio decreases. The fraction of mineralized tissue increases, as a function of age, only in the epiphysis, whereas in the metaphysis it remains constant.

The bone formation rate decreases exponentially with increasing age and decreases in the different parts of the femora in the order metaphysis (male) > metaphysis (female) > epiphysis (male) > epiphysis (female). The four-fold higher bone formation rate in the metaphysis is a result of the longitudinal growth starting from the epiphyseal plate.

References

Ba70 Baylink D., Staufer M., Wergedal J. and Rich C.,1970, Formation, mineralization, and resorption of bone in vitamin D-deficient rats , J.Clin.Invest. 49, 1122-1134.

Ba83 Balmein N., Moscofian A. and Cuisinier-Gleizes P., 1983, Metaphyseal pattern: Uniqueness of this structure in growing bones originating from cartilaginous anlage. A microradiographic study , Calcif.Tiss.Int. 35, 225-231.

Je78 Jee W. S. S.,1978, The relationship of trabecular bone surface areas, bone turnover rates, and initial uptake of Pu and Ra to sites of occurrence of osteosarcoma in beagles , Annual report of the Radiobiology Devision of Utah, College of Medicine, Salt Lake City, COO-119- 253, pp.220-223.

Ki80 Kimmel D. B. and Jee W. S. S.,1980, A quantitative histological analysis of the growing long bone metaphysis , Calcif.Tiss.Int. 32, 113-122.

Po81 Polig E. and Sontag W.,1981, Alpha-dosimetry and fluorescence label analysis in bone , Bone and bone seeking radionuclides: Physiology, dosimetry and effects, pp.73-90 (Brussels: Harwood Academic).

Pr83 Priest N. D., Howells G., Green D. and Haines J. W., 1983,
    Pattern of uptake of americium-241 by the rat skeleton and its
    subsequent redistribution and retention: Implications for human
    dosimetry and toxicology , Human Toxicol. 2, 101-120.
Pr83 Priest N. D., Howells G., Green D. and Haines J. W., 1983,
    Autoradiographic studies of the distribution of radium-226 in rat
    bone: Their implications for human radiation dosimetry and
    toxicity , Human Toxicol. 3, 479-496.
So80 Sontag W.,1980, An automatic microspectrometric scanning method
    for the measuring of bone formation rates in vivo , Calc.Tiss.Int.
    32, 63-68.
So81 Sontag W.,1981, Bone turnover rate in the midshaft of the femur
    - A comparative study of male and female rats , Biennial Report
    1979/80, pp.38-45, KFK-Report 3200.
Su66 Suzuki H. K. and Mathews A.,1966, Two colour fluorescent
    labeling of mineralizing tissues with tetracycline and
    2,4-bis(N,N-dicarboxymethyl)aminomethyl- fluorescein , Stain Technol.
    41, 57-60.

Part 2
Metals and the Bone Marrow

4

Iron Metabolism in the Bone Marrow

A. JACOBS

Iron is an important element in human metabolism. It has a central role in erythropoiesis and is associated with intracellular processes in all the tissues of the body. Its study has been stimulated by the common occurrence of iron deficiency and its consequent clinical manifestations. More recently there has been an increasing awareness of the problems of iron overload. Our understanding of the pathology of these conditions has been greatly aided by an increasing knowledge of the biochemistry and physiology of iron metabolism (Bo 1, Ci 2, Ja 3, Ja 4, Ja 5. Ur 6).

BIOCHEMISTRY

Iron is one of the group of transition metals which share two important properties, the ability to exist in several oxidation states and to form stable complexes. These properties have made iron an important component of electron and oxygen carrying proteins. In acid solution Fe^{2+} and Fe^{3+} ions can exist in the free form surrounded by six molecules of water. On neutralisation such solutions gradually hydrolyse with precipitation of ferric hydroxide. If, however, water molecules are replaced by appropriate ligands a stable complex can be formed which is soluble at neutral pH. The biochemistry of iron is the chemistry of these complexes and although they may be formed with many sugars, amino acids and nucleotides, almost all the iron in the body is found in relation to specific proteins.

Many of the known iron compounds in the body are haemoproteins, some of which are directly involved in oxygen transport. The haemoglobin molecule itself has a molecular weight of 64,500 and consists of 4 haem groups linked to 4 polypeptide chains. It combines with 4 molecules of oxygen. Most of the iron in the body is present as haemoglobin and this is synthesised entirely in the immature erythroid cells of the bone marrow before they are released into the peripheral circulation. Myoglobin in muscle has a molecular weight of 17,000 and consists of a single peptide chain with 1 haem group. It has a higher affinity for oxygen than haemoglobin and behaves as an oxygen store in muscle cells. This comprises up to 8% of the total body iron. If oxygen supply is limited it is released to cytochrome-oxidase, which has a higher affinity for oxygen than myoglobin. Mitochondria contain a system for the transport of electrons from intracellular substrates to molecular oxygen with a simultaneous generation of ATP. This pathway contains a number of iron compounds, including the cytochromes, which transmit electrons by means of reversible valency changes of their iron atoms. Failure in this system due to lack of oxygen supplied to the tissues, enzyme depletion or blocking with metabolic inhibitors such as cyanide, leads to a failure of energy production and an accumulation of inter-mediate metabolites with eventual cell death. One of the most closely studied cytochromes, cytochrome C, has a molecular weight of 12,500 and contains a single haem group together with an associated poly-peptide chain. The free binding sites of its haem iron are linked to histidine and methionine and the haem complex is placed deeply within the molecule. These characteristics prevent cytochrome C from binding free oxygen while allowing the iron atom to alternate between the ferric and ferrous states. Cytochrome P450 occurs in endoplasmic reticulum and in adrenal mitochondria. It takes part in hydroxylation reactions associated with drug detoxication and also with steroid synthesis. Other iron compounds or iron dependent enzymes are associated with DNA synthesis (ribonucleotide reductase), catecholamine metabolism (monoamine oxidase), and collagen formation (proline hydroxylase).

Storage iron   When any cell takes up more iron than is needed for its specific metabolic requirements the excess stimulates ferritin synthesis and a small intracellular store is formed. The storage iron compounds, ferritin and haemosiderin, are found mainly in the reticuloendothelial (RE) cells of the liver, spleen and bone marrow, where iron is released following haemoglobin degradation, but they are also found in many parenchymal cells. Liver parenchymal cells contain visible amounts of iron and muscle contains storage iron both in the muscle cells themselves and in the RE cells between fibres. Storage compounds represent a reserve that can be mobilised when requirements elsewhere in the body are increasing. Storage iron in the bone marrow is clearly visible as ferritin or haemosiderin accummulations on staining, when the RE cells are seen to be almost the only site of deposit. Minimal amounts of ferritin may be visualised in some erythroid precursors where it forms an intermediate on the pathway to haemoglobin synthesis.

Ferritin   Ferritin is a well defined molecule consisting of a protein shell containing an iron core of variable size. Haemosiderin appears to be a degraded form of ferritin in which polymerisation and intra-lysosomal digestion of the protein shell has allowed the iron cores to aggregate, forming an intracellular mass. Haemosiderin deposits are readily seen with the aid of the light microscope as areas of Prussian blue staining when tissue sections or smears are stained with potassium ferrocyanide in the presence of iron. Normally much of the body store of iron is present as ferritin but with increasing iron deposition in the tissues the proportion present as haemosiderin increases. Ferritin is a soluble protein with a unique configuration. Its outer protein shell, consisting of 24 subunits of molecular weight 18,500 encloses an inner core consisting of a variable amount of iron in the form of a ferric hydroxyphosphate complex. Apoferritin has a molecular weight of about 480,000 and the iron filled molecule, containing over 4000 atoms of iron, has a molecular weight of about 900,000 and an iron content of over 20%. Synthesis of the protein is stimulated by the presence of iron and degradation occurs when no iron is incorporated.

Transferrin   Circulating iron in the plasma is bound entirely to transferrin, a   globulin of molecular weight about 80,000 containing

6% carbohydrate.   Transferrin has two binding sites each able to bind one atom of Fe^{3+}.   The iron-transferrin complex has a characteristic salmon-pink colour with an absorption maximum at 470 nm.   At pH 7.0 the affinity of transferrin for iron is very high but there is 50% dissociation at pH 4.8 and this is complete at pH 4.5.   The plasma concentration of transferrin is normally about 2.4 g/l and each milligram of transferrin binds 1.45 µg iron.   The iron binding sites are usually about 30% saturated and a total of about 3 mg of iron is found circulating in the plasma of adults.   Over 80% of circulating transferrin iron is delivered to bone marrow erythroid precursors for haemoglobin synthesis.

Serum transferrin consists of a single polypeptide chain, the amino acid sequence of which has been determined.   There are 679 residues and comparison of the C and N terminal portions reveals strong internal homology with approximately 40% of the amino acids in corresponding positions being identical.   It has been suggested that transferrin may have evolved from a precursor with a single binding site.   The carbohydrate is present in the form of two identical and nearly symmetrical branched heterosaccharide chains each ending with N-acetyl-neuraminic acid, and both of which are present in the C terminal portion of the protein.   One iron binding site is on the C terminal portion of the molecule and one on the N terminal portion. There has been much speculation about possible functional differences between the iron binding sites of transferrin.   Recent evidence from the use of urea electrophoresis reveals four species of transferrin in vivo; apotransferrin, diferric transferrin and two different monoferric transferrins with iron on the C terminal and N terminal sites, respectively.   The distribution of iron between the two sites is dependent on the form of iron presented to the protein and in vivo there appears to be preferential binding to the N terminal site. Formation constants for the various iron-transferrin species are of the order of 10^{20} mols^{-1} under physiological conditions of pH and pCO_2.

IRON BALANCE

The iron content of the body is normally kept constant by a delicate balance between the amount absorbed and the amount lost.   Iron losses from the body are limited and there is no physiological mechanism for regulating the excretion of excess amounts. This is a reflection of the ease with which iron forms intracellular complexes and the absence of loosely bound iron in the body. The factors determining balance are complex and relate to the subject, the diet and the environment. The mean iron loss in men is about 0.9 - 1.0 mg daily. In menstruating women there is a variable blood loss which may be equivalent to over 1.4 mg iron daily giving a mean daily total iron loss in excess of 2.3 mg.

Iron Absorption   Physiological control over iron balance is normally maintained by the regulation of iron absorption which occurs primarily in the duodenum and upper jejunum. Three separate processes appear to be involved, all of which may be subject to separate regulatory mechanisms. These are: iron uptake by the brush border membrane of small intestinal epithelial cells, binding of iron to intra-cellular carrier proteins or other complexing agents, and transfer across the serosal border of the cell to transferrin.

Although the increase in iron absorption found in iron deficient subjects, and the decrease found in subjects with iron overload, is well documented, the control mechanisms responsible for this sensitive response of the intestinal mucosa have not been defined. They could relate to the rate of ferritin synthesis, the degree of saturation of a carrier, or the iron requirement of the cell for haem synthesis.

IRON TRANSPORT

Iron is transported around the body by the plasma and extravascular fluids. Plasma iron has been studied rather more thoroughly than that of extravascular fluids. Although only about 4 mg of iron is present in the plasma at one time, the daily turnover is about 30 mg. Approximately equal amounts of transferrin are present in the intravascular and extravascular compartments. About 85% of ^{59}Fe bound to transferrin is taken up by developing red cell precursors in the bone marrow. In normal subjects about 34% of the iron leaving the plasma pool refluxes from a non-fixed extravascular compartment and is only incorporated in mature red cells after recycling.

INTRACELLULAR IRON TRANSPORT

The lack of clear agrement on many aspects of intracellular iron metabolism is impressive. All mammalian cells probably have surface receptors for transferrin and their density may be related to the needs of that cell for iron. For any one cell type the number of transferrin receptors increases with the rate of proliferation, and it has been suggested that receptor numbers are a useful indicator of dividing cells in malignant tissue. The transferrin receptor appears to be the target for the natural killer cells and may be involved in their in vivo function. Cellular iron in bone marrow erythroblasts, and probably in most other cells, is derived from receptor bound transferrin though there is some disagreement as to the exact mechanism. While most workers suggest that transferrin enters the cell through a process of endocytosis there is conflicting evidence regarding the possible fusion of these endocytotic vesicles with lysosomes prior to the release of iron and the recycling of transferrin and its receptor to the surface of the cell. The contrary view is that iron may be released from transferrin and reduced to a ferrous form on the surface of the cell without any internalisation. RE cells including those in the bone marrow, derive most of their iron from the ingestion and breakdown of effete red cells at the end of their limited life span. Iron released as a result of haem oxygenase activity may be incorporated into ferritin or recycled to transferrin for return to the haem synthetic pathway. The RE cells play a focal role in iron metabolism as the major site of haem breakdown and the major source of plasma iron as well as containing the major compound of storage iron.

The nature of intracellular iron after its release from transferrin or haem breakdown is not known. It has been postulated that there is a 'labile' or 'chelatable' pool of iron which behaves as an intermediate in intracellular exchange and this may be in the form of complexes with sugars, nucleotides, amino acids, or may be loosely associated with protein. The concentrations of such iron compounds are likely to be extremely low and inferred from knowledge of the chemistry of iron rather than from direct observation. It is likely that iron in this pool is available for uptake by mitochondria, ferritin and for the synthesis of specific iron compounds as well as being potentially chelatable.

MEASUREMENT OF IRON STATUS

Variations in iron balance may sometimes lead to considerable changes in the total amount of iron in the body with a consequent iron deficiency or overload. Ferritin and haemosiderin are usually thought to be reserve compounds which are synthesised when the amount of iron present in the body is in excess of active metabolic requirements. Iron does not stimulate haemoglobin formation. During iron depletion all the iron containing compounds in the body may be reduced in amount though not simultaneously and the parameter of iron status chosen for study in any given situation will depend on the precise objective and whether iron overload or iron deficiency is suspected.

STORAGE IRON

The most direct method for measuring this is to determine the amount available for haemoglobin formation following vigorous phlebotomy. This method is rarely practicable and it has been suggested that storage iron in muscle is not readily available for mobilisation in this way. The mean level of mobilisable iron found for men using this technique varies from 600 to 900 mg and for females is usually about 230 mg. In blood donors very much lower levels of iron stores are found. The liver and bone marrow are the most important storage sites for iron and the amount present in these organs can be estimated chemically, visually, using the Prussian Blue reaction on tissue sections, or indirectly by using chelating agents. The chemical estimation of non-haem iron in human bone marrow aspirates and the use of needle biopsy samples of liver have both been found useful in the diagnosis of iron overload. In a study of adult Bantu and white subjects dying in hospital, the concentration of non-haem iron in the bone marrow showed a close correlation with the concentration in the liver over a wide range. Histological assessment of haemosiderin in bone marrow particles was found to show a good agreement with chemical estimations over a wide range, though greater variation has been found by other workers.

A number of workers have attempted to assess iron stores indirectly by measuring urinary iron excretion following an injection of desferrioxamine or other iron chelating agents. The intramuscular injection of 500 mg of desferrioxamine is followed by an increase in urinary iron excretion during the subsequent 6 hours. The amount is significantly increased in patients with iron overload. In order to improve the relationship between excreted iron in the urine and the amount chelated in vivo the differential ferrioxamine test, involving the simultaneous injection of desferrioxamine and ^{59}Fe ferrioxamine has been devised. Other workers have not found this modification necessary and a close linear correlation has been observed between desferrioxamine induced iron excretion and iron stores measured by phlebotomy. Measurement of desferrioxamine chelated iron excretion in the urine as a measure of iron stores takes no account of the variable amount of ferrioxamine excreted in the bile. The amount of chelatable iron may be increased in patients with active haemolysis and ineffective erythropoiesis. DTPA (diethylenetriaminepentaacetic acid) has also been used as an iron chelating agent for diagnostic purposes.

Serum Ferritin   Measurement of serum ferritin concentration provides useful information about storage iron levels. Normal adult serum ferritin concentratins are usually within the range of 15 to 300 μg/l but concentrations are both age and sex dependent. At   birth, serum ferritin concentrations are relatively high in parallel with non-haem iron concentrations in the liver. During the first week of life the haemoglobin concentration in the blood falls to 10-11 g/dl due to the removal of foetal cells from the circulation at a time when the rate of erythropoiesis is relatively low. Iron released by the destruction of these red cells is stored in the tissues and causes increased concentrations of serum ferritin reaching a maximum at about 1 month of age. In the next two months, synthesis of adult haemoglobin causes a rapid fall in the concentration of tissue non-haem iron and in serum ferritin. Serum ferritin concentrations remain low throughout childhood and adolescence. In adults there is a good correlation between mobilisable storage iron measured by phlebotomy and serum ferritin concentration in normal subjects. Patients with simple iron deficiency anaemia have serum ferritin concentrations which are invariably less than 15 μg/l. In iron overload, serum ferritin concentrations are high and eventually levels in excess of 10,000 to 20,000 μg/l may be observed. There is some evidence that in iron overload serum ferritin concentrations above

4,000 µg/l may result partly from liver damage and the leakage of proteins from damaged parenchymal cells. Serum ferritin concentrations have been shown to correlate with the amount of stainable iron in the bone marrow and the assay is of value in monitoring iron therapy in patients with iron deficiency.

Serum ferritin may be grossly increased due to causes other than iron overload. In patients with liver disease very high concentrations (up to 30,000µg/l) have been reported but, although some authors have found parallel changes in serum ferritin concentration and aspartate transaminase activity in patients with liver damage there is no universal agreement on this. Acute infection or inflammation causes a rapid drop in serum iron concentration and an increase in serum and bone marrow ferritin. Correlation between stainable iron in the bone marrow and serum ferritin concentration has been demonstrated in patients with inflammation and rheumatoid arthritis, though the serum ferritin concentration may be higher than expected for the grade of stainable iron in the marrow, possibly due to an input from ferritin synthesis at other sites than the bone marrow.

SUMMARY

The bone marrow contains iron in two main forms. Firstly it is the major site of erythropoiesis and red cell precursors take up most of the iron flowing through the plasma pool for haemoglobin synthesis. Secondly, it contains many reticuloendothelial cells which, together with those at other sites in the body, are the site of mature red cell breakdown and haemoglobin catabolism. They contain much of the body's iron stores in the form of ferritin and haemosiderin and are the source of much of the iron circulating in the plasma transferrin pool. The amount of iron in both these forms is affected by iron balance and the iron status of the body. Depression of erythropoiesis is associated with a balancing increase in storage iron.

REFERENCES

Bo1 Bothwell T.H., Charlton R.W., Cook J.D. and Finch C.A., 1979, Iron metabolism in man, Blackwell Scientific Publications, Oxford.

Ci2 Ciba Foundation, Iron Metabolism, Symposium 51, 1977, Elsevier, Amsterdam.

Ja3 Jacobs A. (Ed) Clinics in Haematology, Vol.II, No.2., 1982, Disorders of Iron Metabolism.

Ja4 Jacobs A. and Worwood M. (Eds) Iron in Biochemistry and Medicine, 1974, Academic Press, London.

Ja5 Jacobs A. and Worwood M. (Eds) Iron in Biochemistry and Medicine II, 1980, Academic Press, London.

Ur6 Urushizaki I., Aisen P., Listowskey I. and Drysdale J.W. 1983, Structure and Function of Iron Storage and Transport Proteins, Elsevier, Amsterdam.

5

The Study of Damage to Bone Marrow Cells as a Biological Dosimeter after Contamination with Osteotropic α Emitters

G. SCHOETERS, R. VAN DEN HEUVEL and O. VANDERBORGHT

INTRODUCTION

The occurrence of bone tumors is the most frequently studied long-term radiation effect after contamination of experimental animals with bone-seeking radionuclides. Bone tumors are considered as sensitive parameters for radiation damage at low doses and valuable information is already obtained for extrapolation of the effect to other species and other radiation dose levels (ICRP67). However, recently it became obvious that more information is needed to fill gaps in the existing knowledge in order to explain and predict bone tumor location (Sp 83), latency period and differences in sensitivity for bone tumor induction between species and between ages. One of the reasons for this lack of knowledge is the scarce attention which has been paid to events at the cellular and molecular level which occur after contamination and which may lead to carcinogenesis; even the target cell population for bone tumor induction is not yet identified. In this paper some experiments will be summarized in which bone marrow cell populations are selectively studied and their radiosensitivity at early times after contamination with α emitters is compared with the dose levels at which bone tumors are induced. The goals are to define target cell populations and investigate how valuable they are as early biological indicators of radiation damage at low dose levels. Moreover, studies of haemopoietic stem cells gained importance recently after indications

51

that myeloid leukaemia may be enhanced in ^{224}Ra patients (Wi 83) and ^{224}Ra injected mice (Hu 82).

MATERIALS AND METHODS

The experimental animals were SCK inbred Balb/c and C_{57} Bl mice which were three months old at intraperitoneal radionuclide injection. The short range α-emitting radionuclides ^{226}Ra and ^{241}Am were injected respectively as chloride and citrate solutions and represent respectively bone-volume seekers and bone-surface seekers.

Six parameters were observed for radiation damage.

Peripheral red and white blood cell counts

On each sampling date, blood was taken from the tail vein at 4:00 PM, and cells were counted using an electronic counter (Coulter counter ZF, Coulter Electronics).

Haemopoietic stem cell damage : CFU-s and CFU-c numbers (Sc 81)

Radiation damage was assessed at various times after radionuclide injection from 4 hrs up to 300 days. Marrow cells were collected from various bone sites – sternum, lumbar vertebrae and various parts of the femur.

To obtain marrow cells the dissected bones were ground in a mortar. However, in the femur shaft the central marrow cell population was flushed out and was separately studied from the peripheral marrow cell population which was obtained by grinding the remaining femur shaft. Corresponding bone sites of five animals were pooled in each experiment.

The proliferation capacity of pluripotent stem cells was assessed by the spleen colony technique (Ti 61). The pluripotent stem cells among injected marrow cells which form colonies after 8 days in the spleen of irradiated recipient mice (8 Gy of X-rays, 0.8 Gy/min, 250 kV, focus-skin distance 54 cm, 1 mm Cu filter) were counted and called CFU-s.

The proliferation capacity of granulocyte-macrophage committed stem cells was determined via in vitro cultures of bone marrow cells in a single-layer soft agar system (Br 68).

Stromal bone marrow cells

Bone marrow cells which form adherent layers in liquid cultures were tested after ^{241}Am injection for their colony forming capacity in vitro (Va 84a), and functionally for their capacity to maintain in vitro haemopoietic stem cell proliferation (CFU-c) and to inhibit differentiation of these stem cells (Va 84b).

Bone tumor induction after ^{226}Ra injection

A large scale experiment with 389 male C_{57} Bl mice was performed which were injected with 170, 350 or 920 kBq ^{226}Ra/kg.

At death, after autopsy the carcasses were radiographed. Diagnosis of osteosarcoma was confirmed by histological evaluation of suspicious bone fragments (Sc 83b).

Analyses of the skeletal ^{241}Am and ^{226}Ra content

Ra and Am retention were measured in ashed bones at times corresponding to the observation of radiation damage.

To measure ^{241}Am the ash was dissolved in 1 M HNO_3 and 10 µg $La(NO_3)_3$. $6H_2O$ was added per ml as an Am carrier.

To measure ^{226}Ra the ashed samples were surrounded by active charcoal and suitable equilibration with the daughter products was reached after 21 days. Measurements were performed in a NaI (Tl) well-type crystal (3 x 3 in). For Am measurements pulses were integrated between 30 and 100 keV; ^{226}Ra concentrations were calculated by extrapolation from the ^{214}Bi measurements.

Morphometric measurements

Quantitative measurements were performed of bone and bone marrow structure from selected mouse bones of Balb/c mice, with an electronic image analyser-Quantimet 720 (Imanco, UK) - and with a semi-automatic MOP system (Kontron, B.R.D.).

The percent endosteal bone surface per unit bone volume, and the per cent of bone marrow volume were obtained from these measurements (Sc 82).

RESULTS AND DISCUSSION

<u>Damage to haemopoietic stem cells has been observed in the same dose range as induction of bone tumors</u>

Table 1 presents our data on bone tumors in male C_{57} Bl mice : 170 kBq ^{226}Ra/kg induced an increased amount of bone tumors, 350 kBq ^{226}Ra/kg did not yield a maximum number of bone tumors. Comparison with the other ^{226}Ra experiments indicates an increase in bone tumor incidence till an average skeletal dose of 60 Gy (Sc 83b).

With respect to ^{241}Am induced bone tumors in male CBA mice an increase in bone tumor incidence was observed from 1.5 kBq ^{241}Am/kg till 296 kBq ^{241}Am/kg (Ni 76). Table 1 and 3 demonstrate that peripheral red blood cells are least affected by radiation from the osteotropic α-emitters ^{226}Ra and ^{241}Am; peripheral white blood cell counts (WBC) are more radiosensitive but changes in CFU-s concentration occurred at lower doses. Changes in CFU-s numbers (table 2 and 4) were observed very early after injection even after 230 kBq ^{226}Ra/kg and 138 kBq ^{241}Am/kg mouse. The radiation response of the more differentiated granulocyte, macrophage progenitor cells was slower and less pronounced than that of CFU-s.

The higher the injected radioactivities of ^{241}Am and ^{226}Ra, the more important the changes in number and concentration of blood-forming stem cells (table 1,2,3,4).

The observed changes at high doses were decreases but at lower doses increases in stem cell numbers are often observed. Changes in stem cell numbers are thus not only due to direct radiation killing, but to indirect radiation effects on regulatory mechanisms for cell proliferation and cell functioning. This is demonstrated in an ^{241}Am experiment where 55 kBq ^{241}Am/kg affected the capacity of adherent stromal bone marrow cells to sustain CFU-c proliferation (table 3). Other functional changes may perhaps be detected at lower dose levels than quantitative changes, we only need the proper way to examine them.

<u>A relation exists between bone structure and radiation damage</u>

Comparison of the radiation response of haemopoietic stem cells in various marrow cavities reveals differences, indicating that these

TABLE 1 : CHANGES IN PERIPHERAL RED BLOOD CELL COUNTS (RBC), WHITE BLOOD CELL COUNTS (WBC) AND IN CFU-S CONCENTRATION AFTER ^{226}RA INJECTION.
● CHANGES ARE STATISTICALLY SIGNIFICANT (P < 0.05).
○ THE OBSERVATION IS NOT SIGNIFICANTLY DIFFERENT FROM CONTROLS.

^{226}RA kBq/kg	RBC			WBC			CFU-s/10^5 cells FEMUR			LUMBAR VERTEBRAE	% BONE TUMORS
	8 W.	12 W.	30 W.	8 W.	12 W.	30 W.	8 W.	12 W.	30 W.	8 W.	
148							○			○	
166	○	○	○	○	○	○	○	●	○		
170											7.0
255	○	○	○	●	○	○	○	●	○		
296							○			○	
333	○	○	○	●	○	○	●	●	○		
350											8.7
500	○	○	○	●	○	○	●	●	○		
592							●			●	
888							●			●	
920											20.6

W. = WEEKS

TABLE 2 : DAYS AFTER ^{226}RA INJECTION IN BALB/C MICE AFTER WHICH SIGNIFICANT CHANGES (P < 0.05) IN CFU-S NUMBERS (●) OR CFU-C (▲) NUMBERS ARE OBSERVED.

^{226}RA kBq/kg	DAYS AFTER INJECTION	BONE MARROW SITES				
		FEMUR			LUMBAR VERTEBRAE	STERNUM
		CENTRAL MARROW	PERIPHERAL MARROW	DISTAL END		
230	0.2					
	1		●			
	3		●			
	10					
	24			●		
	100	●	●			
	300		● ▲			
660	0.2		● ▲			
	1		● ▲			
	3				● ▲	●
	10	● ▲	● ▲	● ▲	● ▲	●
	24	● ▲		● ▲		
	100		● ▲	● ▲	● ▲	
	300	● ▲	● ▲	● ▲	● ▲	●

TABLE 3 : SIGNIFICANT CHANGES (P < 0.05) IN HAEMATOLOGICAL PARAMETERS AFTER ^{241}AM CONTAMINATION(●).

^{241}AM kBq/kg	RBC 8 w.	WBC 8 w.	CFU-s/10^5 CELLS		CFU-c/10^5 CELLS		FUNCTIONAL CHANGES IN STROMAL CELL CULTURES				
			LUMBAR VERTEBRAE 8 w.	FEMUR 8 w.	LUMBAR VERTEBRAE 8 w.	FEMUR 8 w.	LUMBAR VERTEBRAE 4 w.	LUMBAR VERTEBRAE 8 w.	STERNUM 4 w.	STERNUM 8 w.	FEMUR 8 w.
55							●		●		
72			0	0	0	0					
94	0	0	0	0							
164			●	●	●	0					
200								●		●	●
205	0	●	●								
223							0		●		
295			●	●	●	0					
425	●	●	●	●							
538			●	●	●	●					
738								●		●	●
887							0		●		
945	●	●	●	●							
960			●	●	●	●					
2047	●	●	●	●							

W. = WEEKS

TABLE 4 : SIGNIFICANT CHANGES (P < 0.05) IN CFU-s ● AND CFU-c ▲ NUMBERS IN VARIOUS MARROW SITES.

^{241}AM kBq/kg	DAYS AFTER INJECTION	FEMUR			LUMBAR VERTEBRAE	STERNUM
		CENTRAL MARROW	PERIPHERAL MARROW	DISTAL END		
138	0.2					
	1		● ▲		●	
	3		●		●	●
	10		● ▲	▲		
	24		● ▲	▲		
	100		● ▲			
552	0.2	▲	● ▲	●		
	1		● ▲			
	3	●	●	●	●	
	10		● ▲		●	
	24	● ▲	● ▲	● ▲	● ▲	●
	100	● ▲	● ▲	● ▲	● ▲	●
768	0.2		● ▲		● ▲	
	1					
	3	● ▲	● ▲	● ▲	● ▲	
	10	● ▲	● ▲	● ▲	● ▲	● ▲
	24	● ▲	● ▲	● ▲	● ▲	▲
	100	●	● ▲	● ▲	● ▲	●

stem cell killing studies can be used to provide information of local radiation conditions (table 2,4). In various bone sites the data on haemopoietic stem cell numbers or concentrations reflect the situation averaged over all marrow spaces in the given bone site,e.g. the marrow cell population of lumbar vertebrae is collected from all the marrow spaces between the trabeculae of the vertebrae. Peripherally located marrow cells close to the endosteum are not separated from marrow cells in the center of a marrow space. In the femur shaft however distinction is made between central marrow cells and peripheral marrow situated within α-range from the endosteal bone surface. Since α particles penetrate from bone surfaces into the bone marrow cavities the ratio of endosteal bone surface to marrow volume may be expected to interfere with the degree of radiation damage.

The ratio of endosteal bone surface to bone marrow volume (table 5) corresponds indeed with the observed stem cell damage. Both are highest in peripheral marrow of femur shaft, intermediate in lumbar vertebrae and distal end of femur, and lowest in sternum and central marrow of the femur shaft (Table 2,4,5).

TABLE 5 : ENDOSTEAL SURFACE AREA/MARROW VOLUME (MM^{-1}).

FEMUR DIAPHYSIS	PERIPHERAL MARROW OF FEMUR DIAPHYSIS	DISTAL END OF FEMUR	LUMBAR VERTEBRAE	STERNUM
6.0	31.6	20.1	19.1	9.8

For bone tumor induction the target cells are assumed to be located close to the endosteum, thus the amount of bone surfaces in a given bone fragment should be important in determining the risk for bone tumor induction in a given bone site. The number of observed bone tumors is too small to draw conclusions but lumbar vertebrae are definitely the highest risk sites and contain the highest amount of endosteal bone surfaces (Table 6).

TABLE 6 : ANATOMIC LOCATION OF BONE TUMORS RELATED TO THE AMOUNT OF ENDOSTEAL BONE SURFACE IN $C_{57}BL$ MICE.

	DIAPHYSIS OF FEMUR	DISTAL END OF FEMUR	LUMBAR VERTEBRAE	STERNUM
NUMBER OF BONE TUMORS	1	1	14	
TOTAL ENDOSTEAL BONE SURFACE (MM^2)	86	313	1044	237

Radiation dose in bone marrow does not always correspond with observed radiation damage at haemopoietic cells

Radionuclide retention is initially highest in bone sites with the largest bone surfaces and remains that way for ^{241}Am but declines and becomes proportional to the amount of bone volume in ^{226}Ra injected mice. Retention measurements and morphometric measurements of endosteal surface, bone and marrow volume allow calculation (Sc 83a) of ^{226}Ra as a bone-volume seeker and ^{241}Am as a bone surface seeker, the cumulative marrow dose averaged over the marrow volume (table 7), and the cumulative marrow dose rate averaged over the α particle range close to the bone surface (table 8).

TABLE 7 : CUMULATIVE MARROW DOSE AVERAGED OVER THE MARROW VOLUME (10^{-2}Gy), 100 DAYS AFTER INJECTION, NORMALIZED TO UNIT ACTIVITY INJECTED (KBQ/KG MOUSE).

	FEMUR DIAPHYSIS	PERIPHERAL MARROW OF FEMUR DIAPHYSIS	DISTAL END OF FEMUR	LUMBAR VERTEBRAE	STERNUM
^{226}Ra	0.12	0.60	0.69	0.63	0.35
^{241}Am	0.47	2.45	2.19	1.68	0.98
MEAN MARROW DOSE ^{241}Am/^{226}Ra	4	4	3	3	3

TABLE 8 : MARROW DOSE RATE (10^{-2} GY/DAY), 100 DAYS AFTER INJECTION AVERAGED OVER THE α-PARTICLE RANGE AND NORMALISED TO UNIT ACTIVITY (KBQ) INJECTED PER KG BODY-WEIGHT.

	FEMUR DIAPHYSIS	DISTAL END OF FEMUR	LUMBAR VERTEBRAE	STERNUM
^{226}Ra	0.005	0.008	0.006	0.006
^{241}Am	0.022	0.029	0.024	0.026
MARROW DOSE RATE FROM AM / MARROW DOSE RATE FROM RA	4	4	4	4

The highest radiation dose as averaged over the bone marrow cavity was calculated for bone sites with small marrow cavities and large inner bone surfaces (Table 5). These bone sites show the highest radiation damage to blood forming stem cells. However, exceptions were observed. After ^{241}Am injection changes to haemopoietic stem cells were more pronounced in marrow from lumbar vertebrae than in that of the distal end of the femur, not only the frequency at which changes were observed (table 4) but also stem cell numbers fell very deep below control values in lumbar vertebrae. Nevertheless, the radiation dose calculated for bone marrow of both bone sites was very similar.

Table 8 indicates that per unit endosteal bone surface the cumulative marrow dose rate averaged over the α particle range is similar in all bone sites. This holds for ^{226}Ra and for ^{241}Am in mice. This emphasizes also that the risk for bone tumor induction in a given bone site is determined by the amount of bone surfaces in the observed bone (table 6).

The relative radiotoxicity of ^{241}Am and ^{226}Ra for haemopoietic stem cells is less than expected

Radiation damage to blood-forming stem cells observed after ^{226}Ra and ^{241}Am injections can be used as a biological indicator for the relative radiotoxicity of ^{241}Am versus ^{226}Ra for radiosensitive cells in the bone marrow. Experimental information on the relative radiotoxicity of ^{241}Am versus ^{226}Ra is scarce. Table 7 predict that ^{241}Am would be 3 to 4 times as toxic as ^{226}Ra for bone marrow cells.

We observed CFU-s changes after ^{226}Ra injection at 166 kBq ^{226}Ra/kg (table 1); the lowest ^{241}Am dose at which CFU-s changes are observed is 138 kBq ^{241}Am/kg (table 5). Within the limits of the utilized radioactivities used in these experiments, it is suggested that the difference in radiotoxicity between ^{241}Am and ^{226}Ra for bone marrow cells is less than expected.

With respect to bone tumor induction table 8 predicts that ^{241}Am would be 4 times as toxic as ^{226}Ra in inducing radiation damage close to bone surfaces.

Our own data in male C_{57}Bl mice for ^{226}Ra induced bone tumors are mentioned in table 1, data on ^{241}Am induced bone tumors in the same mouse strain are under investigation.

These studies demonstrated that beside radionuclide retention anatomical and physiological factors affect the induction of radiation damage from incorporated α-emitting bone seekers to bone marrow.

Detailed studies at cellular and molecular level on functional changes are needed and may help to explain and understand the complicated biological reactions which are observed after irradiation and which are obviously not entirely predictable by radiation dose.

Br 68, Bradley T.R. and Sumner M.A., 1968, Stimulation of mouse bone marrow colony growth in vitro by conditioned medium , Aust. J. Exp. Bio. Med. Sci. 46, 607-618.

ICRP67, International Commission on Radiological Protection, 1968, A review of the radiosensitivity of the tissues in bone , ICRP Publication II.

Hu 82, Humphreys E.R., Loutit J.F., Major I.R. and Stones V.A., 1982, The induction by ^{224}Ra of myeloid leukemia and osteosarcoma in male CBA mice , Eulep Newsletter 31, 12.

Ni 76, Nilsson A. and Broomé-Karlsson A., 1976, The pathology of americium 241 , Acta Radial Ther. Phys. Biol. 15, 49-70.

Sc 81, Schoeters G.E.R. and Vanderborght O.L.J., 1981, Temporal and spatial response of marrow colony-forming cells (CFU-s and CFU-c) after ^{226}Ra incorporation in BALB/c mice , Radiat. Res., 88, 251-265.

Sc 82, Schoeters G.E.R., 1982, Dose delivered to various bone and marrow sites of ^{226}Ra Injected Mice Related to the Observed Heterogeneity in Damage to Haemopoietic Marrow Cells , Brit. J. Radiology 55, 520-529.

Sc 83a, Schoeters G.E.R., 1983a, Haemopoiesis in the bone marrow after contamination with 226-radium and with 241-americium in the mouse , Ph. D. thesis.

Sc 83b, Schoeters G.E.R., Luz A. and Vanderborght O.L.J., 1983, ^{226}Ra induced bone-cancers; the effect of a delayed Na-alginate treatment , Int. J. Radiat. Biol. 43, 231-247.

SP 83 Spiers F.W. and Beddoe A.H., 1983, Sites of incidence of osteosarcoma in the long bone of man and the beagle , Health Phys. 44, suppl. 1, 49-64.

Ti 61, Till J.E. and Mc Culloch E.A., 1961, A direct measurement of the radiosensitivity of normal mouse bone marrow cells , Radiat. Res 14, 213-222.

Va 84a, Van Den Heuvel R.L., Schoeters G.E.R. and Vanderborght O.L.J., 1984, Effect of 241-Am on bone fibroblasts , Radiat. Environ. Biophys. 23, 137-140.

Va 84b, Van Den Heuvel R.L., Schoeters G.E.R. and Vanderborght O.L.J., 1984, Functional damage to bone marrow fibroblasts after contamination with ^{241}americium.

Wi 83, Wick R.R. and Gossner W., 1983, Follow-up study of late effects in ^{224}Ra treated ankylosing spondylitis patients , Health Phys. 44, suppl., 187-196.

6

Functional Damage to Bone Marrow Fibroblasts after Contamination with [241] AMERICIUM

R. VAN DEN HEUVEL, G. SCHOETERS and O. VANDERBORGHT

INTRODUCTION

Fibroblast of the bone marrow are a constituent of the stromal hemopoietic microenvironment. These cells are involved in the regulation of hemopoiesis (De 77). They may have an osteogenic potential and are important for the production of components of the extracellular matrix. Bone marrow fibroblasts are known to be candidate target cells for bone cancer induction (Ha 76).

The goals of our experiments are to study the radiosensitivity of bone marrow fibroblasts with regard to their function in hemopoiesis after contamination of mice with the osteotropic radionuclide [241]Am. The qualitative response of stromal fibroblasts on continuous <u>in vivo</u> α-irradiation will be checked by investigating two aspects :

1. The effect of the stromal cells on the <u>in vitro</u> proliferation of granulocyt-macrophage progenitor cells (CFU-c).

2. The effect of the stromal cells on CFU-c differentiation.

MATERIALS AND METHODS

Treatment of animals

65 male Balb/c (aged 3 months) were injected intraperitoneally with 0.25 ml of an [241]Amcitrate solution (Sc 83). Four dose groups are considered : 0.036 µCi/mouse (55 kBq/kg); 0.148 µCi/mouse (223 kBq/kg);

kBq/kg); 0,59 μCi/mouse (887 kBq/kg) and a control group (mice received an equal volume of isotonic salt solution = 0 μCi ^{241}Am/mouse). All the mice were kept on a normal standard pellet diet and were given water ad libitum.

Collection of bone marrow cells

Mice of each dose group were killed by cervical dislocation at four and ten weeks post contamination. Femur, sternum and 4 lumbar vertebrae were removed. Bones were ground in α-MeM (Flow Laboratories, U.K.). Three cell suspensions per dose group were prepared by pooling the corresponding bone fragments from 5 animals.

Qualitative tests

1. The influence of stromal cells on CFU-c progenitor cell proliferation is examined by means of long-term cultures (De 77). Bone marrow cells (2 x 10^6 nucleated cells/ml medium) of ^{241}Am contaminated mice were inoculated into culture flasks. Cultures were incubated at 37°C in a humidified atmosphere of 5 % CO_2 in air. The cultures were fed at weekly intervals by changing the growth medium. A confluent adherent cell layer was formed in the third week. The growth medium on top of the monolayer was completely removed and flasks were reinoculated with freshly obtained femoral cells (femur of Balb/c, male, 3 month old, non-contaminated) at a concentration of 1 x 10^6 cells/ml α-MeM supplemented with 20 % horse serum (total volume of 8 ml). Cultures were maintained in the same conditions as before. Weekly, half of the medium, which contains non-adherent cells, was removed and replaced with fresh medium (4 ml α-MeM + 20 % HS). The non-adherent cells were counted and assayed for CFU-c concentration.

2. The effect of stromal cells on CFU-c differentiation is tested by mixing bone marrow fibroblasts in CFU-c cultures. Bone marrow adherent cells derived from contaminated mice are detached from the bottom with trypsine treatment. Stromal cells are centrifuged, resuspended in α-MeM, counted and mixed with freshly obtained bone marrow cells (femur of Balb/c mice, male, 3 month old non-contaminated) in CFU-c cultures. By this a direct cell-cell interaction is possible between stromal cells and

haemopoietic unipotent stem cells. A decrease or increase in the number of CFU-c colonies is checked.

CFU-c cultures

Bone marrow cells are inoculated at a concentration of 1×10^5 cells per ml α-MeM medium (Flow Laboratories, U.K.) in a single-layer soft agar system. To stimulate the colony formation we added conditioned serum (100 µl of a 20 % serum solution) derived from mice injected with an endotoxin (lipopolysaccharide B from <u>Salmonella abortus</u> Equi, Difco Lab. USA) and β-mercaptoethanol (50 µl of a 2×10^{-3} M β-mercaptoethanol solution). Quadruplicate cultures were made into 35 mm plastic petri dishes (Lux Sc Coop, Ca USA). Cultures were grown in a humidified atmosphere at 37°C and 5 % CO_2. After 7 days the colonies were stained with INT (2-p-iodophenyl-)-3-(p-nitrophenyl)-5-phenyl tetrazolium chloride, Aldrich-Europe, Beerse, België) and counted using a binocular (magnification 20x).

RESULTS

Effect of α-irradiation on the maintenance of hemopoiesis in long-term bone marrow cultures

Long-term Dexter-type marrow cultures can maintain the CFU-c proliferation <u>in vitro</u>. Tables 1.1, 1.2, 1.3 indicate the CFU-c concentration in the supernatans above the adherent stromal monolayer derived from contaminated mice. Results are obtained 1 week after reinoculation of the adherent monolayer with fresh bone marrow cells. "t" tests were performed to verify if there is a significant difference between the CFU-c numbers in long-term cultures from contaminated or non-contaminated mice.

Table 1.1 : CFU-c proliferation in long-term bone marrow cultures,
stromal layer is derived from bone marrow cells of mice 4
weeks after contamination of the mice with ^{241}Am.
CFU-c/2 x 10^5 cells ($\bar{x}$ ± 95 % confidence limits).
| significantly different (p ≤ 0.05)

^{241}Am(kBq/kg)	Femur	Sternum	Lumbar vertebrae
0		32 ± 15				13 ± 8	
55	32 ± 5		7 ± 2		44 ± 12	||
223	12 ± 21		10 ± 14		17 ± 10	
887		14 ± 3			12 ± 8	

Table 1.2 : CFU-c proliferation in long-term bone marrow cultures,
stromal layer is derived from bone marrow cells of mice 8
weeks after contamination of the mice with ^{241}Am.
CFU-c/2 x 10^5 cells ($\bar{x}$ ± 95 % confidence limits).
| significantly different (p ≤ 0.05)

^{241}Am(kBq/kg)	Femur	Sternum	Lumbar vertebrae
0	348 ± 80	110 ± 40	260 ± 90
200	290 ± 64	44 ± 20	150 ± 56
738	80 ± 18	20 ± 6	40 ± 26

Table 1.3 : CFU-c proliferation in long-term bone marrow cultures,
stromal layer is derived from bone marrow cells of mice 10
weeks after contamination of the mice with ^{241}Am.
CFU-c/2 x 10^5 cells ($\bar{x}$ ± 95 % confidence limits).
| significantly different (p ≤ 0.05)

^{241}Am(kBq/kg)	Femur	Sternum	Lumbar vertebrae
0	110 ± 28	47 ± 6	59 ± 102
55	57 ± 12		40 ± 15
223	22 ± 4		31 ± 9
887	24 ± 11		17 ± 2

Bone marrow of femur, sternum and lumbar vertebrae yielded cultures of adherent stromal bone marrow fibroblasts. These cultures are able to maintain the proliferation of granulocyt-monocyt precursor cells.

A radiation effect was seen on the functional role of the bone marrow fibroblasts in CFU-c proliferation, in long-term cultures obtained from mice with a 4 weeks old ^{241}Am contamination. In the sternum the number of CFU-c in the medium on top of the adherent layer is lower in long-term marrow cultures derived from contaminated mice. In the long-term cultures from stromal cells of the lumbar vertebrae of mice which got a dose of 55 kBq/kg ^{241}Am, the CFU-c number is increased significantly compared with the other doses.

Fibroblast monolayers obtained from marrow of mice with 8 and 10 week old radiocontamination, maintain a number of CFU-c that decreases with increasing dose of ^{241}Am. The lowest dose (55 kBq/kg) has already an effect in the three bone marrow compartments (femur, sternum and lumbar vertebrae).

Influence of α-irradiation on the effect of stromal cells on CFU-c differentiation after mixing bone marrow fibroblasts with fresh bone marrow cells

Table 2 gives the number (%) of CFU-c/2 x 10^5 cells in function of the dose of ^{241}Am and in function of the concentration of added fibroblasts. Two points of time are considered : A = results with fibroblasts from mice with a 4 weeks old contamination, B = results with fibroblasts from mice with a 10 weeks old ^{241}Am contamination.

Results in non-contaminated animals indicate that there is a functional difference between bone marrow fibroblasts from femur compared to bone marrow fibroblasts from sternum and lumbar vertebrae. Increasing concentration of cultured fibroblasts mixed with fresh bone marrow cells causes a decrease in CFU-c number in the femur. This does not occur when cultured fibroblasts derived from sternum and lumbar vertebrae are mixed with freshly obtained femoral bone marrow cells.

There are some indications of possible α-irradiation effects on the function of bone marrow fibroblasts on CFU-c differentiation. There is a partial cancellation of the inhibition in the femur at the highest ^{241}Am dose (887 kBq/kg). In the lumbar vertebrae, an

Table 2 : Influence of ^{241}Am contamination on the effect of stromal fibroblasts on CFU-c differentiation. Number of CFU-c colonies (%) after adding cultured fibroblasts derived from mice with a 4 weeks old contamination (A) and from mice with a 10 weeks old contamination (B).

concentration of bone marrow fibro-blasts (cells/ml)	^{241}Am (kBq/kg)							
	0		55		220		880	
	A	B	A	B	A	B	A	B
Femur 0 x 10^5	100 %	100 %	100 %	100 %	100 %	100 %	100 %	100 %
0,5 x 10^5	74 *	29 *	107		74 *		70	
1 x 10^5	47 *		49 *	42 *	48 *	53 *	65 *	
2 x 10^5	26 *	20 *	23 *		20 *		75 *	60 *
3 x 10^5	22 *					14 *		
4 x 10^5		13 *		3 *				
5 x 10^5						2 *		
6 x 10^5		0 *						
Sternum 0 x 10^5	100 %		100 %		100 %		100 %	
0,1 x 10^5	110				62 *		81	
0,5 x 10^5	106		110		91		99	
1 x 10^5	103		90		87		62 *	
2 x 10^5			70					
Lumbar Vertebrae 0 x 10^5	100 %	100 %	100 %	100 %	100 %	100 %	100 %	
0,5 x 10^5	89				116		68 *	
1 x 10^5	110	124	53	51 *	126 *		50 *	
2 x 10^5	80	54			29 *	73	30 *	
3 x 10^5					14 *			
4 x 10^5					4 *			
5 x 10^5					0 *			

(* significantly different from control (0 x 10^5 bone marrow fibro-blasts/ml), p $\leqslant$ 0.05).

inhibitory effect appears at the highest doses (223, 887 kBq/kg ^{241}Am) when fibroblasts are derived from mice 4 weeks after contamination and at the lowest dose ^{241}Am (55 kBq/kg) when fibroblasts are obtained from mice 10 weeks after contamination. No radiation effect on the regulation of CFU-c differentiation is seen in the sternum.

DISCUSSION

We examined the functional response in vitro of stromal bone marrow fibroblasts after contamination of mice with different doses of the osteotropic α- emitter ^{241}americium. Radiosensitivity of the regulatory function for CFU-c (granulocyt-monocyt progenitor cell) proliferation and differentiation was tested.

CFU-c proliferation

Long-term bone marrow cultures of femur, sternum and lumbar vertebrae obtained from radiocontaminated mice, indicate that the adherent stromal cells are changed functionally after contamination of mice with ^{241}Am. Monolayers of stromal cells obtained from radiocontaminated mice, yield cultures that partly loose their capacity to support CFU-c proliferation. Already at the lowest dose of 55 kBq/kg, the CFU-c proliferation was changed.

CFU-c differentiation

Mixing of fibroblasts, derived from femur and lumbar vertebrae of ^{241}Am contaminated mice, with fresh bone marrow cells induces changes in the CFU-c differentiation. Further experiments are needed to allow a definite conclusion about the radiation effect on stromal cells in CFU-c differentiation.

Results in non-contaminated animals indicate a remarkable difference between the hemopoietic microenvironment of femur and sternum or lumbar vertebrae. Mixing of bone marrow fibroblasts with freshly isolated marrow cells induces an inhibition of CFU-c colony-formation if the fibroblasts are derived from the femur but not from sternum or lumbar vertebrae.

This inhibitory effect of femoral marrow fibroblasts on CFU-c differentiation is also found by Zipori (Zi 81), Greenberg (Gr 81) and Werts (We 80).

CONCLUSION

^{241}Am contamination induces functional changes in the population of stromal cells at low doses (55 kBq/kg ^{241}Am) and after short-time (4 weeks). Stromal cells are radiosensitive for their function on the CFU-c proliferation. It is not yet clear if the influence of stromal fibroblasts on CFU-c differentiation is also changed by a continous α-irradiation.

In non-contaminated mice, the stromal cells of the femur are qualitatively different from the stromal cells of the sternum and lumbar vertebrae with respect to their function in the differentiation of CFU-c.

REFERENCES

De 77   Dexter T.M., Testa N.G., 1977, "Differentiation and proliferation of hemopoietic cells in culture", Methods in cell biology, 14, pp. 387-405.

Ge 81   Greenberg B.R., Wilson F.D., Woo L., 1981, "Granulopoietic Effects of Human Bone Marrow Fibroblastic Cells and Abnormalities in the Granulopoietic Microenvironment", Blood, 58, 3, pp. 557-564.

Ha 76   Hashimoto E.G., Jee W.S.S., 1976, " Cells at risk from bone-seeking radionuclides. A review", in : The health effects of plutonium and radium (Edited by Webster S.S. Jee) pp. 643-656 (Salt Lake City, Univ. of Utah).

Sc 83   Schoeters G.E.R., Vanderborght O.L.J., 1983, "Relative effectiveness of ^{241}Am vs ^{226}Ra approached by haemopoietic stem cells studies in various bone marrow sites of contaminated mice", Health Physics, 44, 1, pp. 555-570.

We 80   Werts E.D., DeGowin R.L., Knapp S.K., Gibson D.P., 1980, "Characterization of Marrow Stromal (Fibroblastoid) Cells and Their Association with Erythropoiesis", Exp. Hemat., 8, 4, pp. 423-433.

Zi 81   Zipori D., 1981, "Cell Interactions in the Bone Marrow microenvironment : role of endogenous colony stimulating activity", Journal of Supramolecular Structure and Cellular Biochemistry, 17, pp. 347-357.

7

The Release of Transportable Plutonium from Macrophages: The Effects of Dietary Iron

J. W. HAINES and N. D. PRIEST

INTRODUCTION: Macrophages in the bone marrow concentrate plutonium released from bone surfaces by resorption during bone remodelling (Pr 81). The dosimetric significance of the bone marrow plutonium deposits, with regard to the risk of damage to radiation sensitive cells, depends upon their retention time. Experiments have shown that the iron status of animals is a potential regulator of the rate of plutonium loss. (Pr 82) (Ha 84). The present experiments were designed to compare the loss of plutonium from macrophages at different sites in the body (experiment 1) and to investigate its dependence on iron status (experiment 2).

METHODS: Experiment 1 Female Wistar rats aged 1½ years were injected intravenously with a Pu-238 labelled ferric hydroxide colloid. This was removed from the blood stream by macrophages and then solubilised, releasing plutonium within the cells in a transportable form. Most of the released plutonium was subsequently either excreted or deposited onto bone surfaces. Animals were killed between 1 day and 3 months after injection, and their liver, spleen and tibiae, removed for the radiochemical determination of plutonium (Ke70). Additionally, concentrations of plutonium in the femoral bone marrow were measured in autoradiographs of longitudinal sections of the rat femora. These were prepared using the solid state plastic detector CR39 (He79). Experiment 2 Male Wistar rats aged 1 year were injected with the

Pu-238 labelled ferric hydroxide colloid. Subsequently, the
injected animals were maintained on one of three diets which
contained either 900, 109 or >1mg kg^{-1} iron. The experimental
animals were killed at 3 months. The plutonium content of their
tissues was determined radiochemically.

RESULTS and CONCLUSIONS: Experiment 1 A similar biphasic loss of
plutonium was found for macrophages at all tissue sites. This
comprised a phase of rapid loss lasting ~ 10 days followed by a
phase of slower loss (Fig.). The overall retention time for

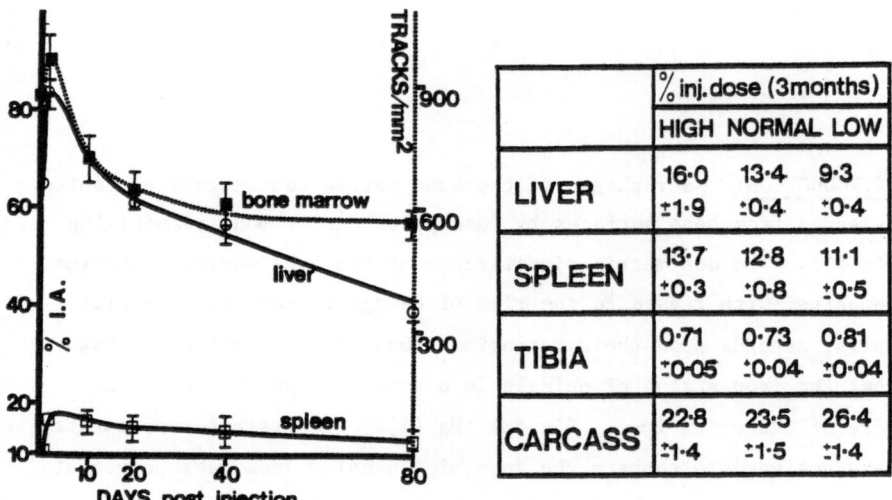

	% inj.dose (3months)		
	HIGH	NORMAL	LOW
LIVER	16·0 ±1·9	13·4 ±0·4	9·3 ±0·4
SPLEEN	13·7 ±0·3	12·8 ±0·8	11·1 ±0·5
TIBIA	0·71 ±0·05	0·73 ±0·04	0·81 ±0·04
CARCASS	22·8 ±1·4	23·5 ±1·5	26·4 ±1·4

Fig. Concentration of plutonium in liver, spleen and bone marrow
of normally fed 1½ year old rats at different times after
injection.
Table. The effect of different levels of dietary iron on the
concentration of plutonium in the liver, spleen, tibia and carcass
at 3 months after injection.

plutonium in the liver was lower than for the bone marrow and
spleen.

Experiment 2 Plutonium loss from hepatic and splenic macrophages
was greatest in those rats fed the low iron diet and least in those
fed the iron rich diet. (Table). This suggests that plutonium
loss in old rats is modified by changes in iron status in the same
way as described previously for young animals (Pr82). However, the
effect was not as large as in the young animals perhaps indicating
their lower demand for, and slower turnover of iron.

REFERENCES

Ha 84.   Haines, J W and Priest, N D, 1984, The loss of
transportable plutonium deposits from the macrophages of the rat
femoral bone marrow . Radiat. Environ. Biophys. 23 133-135.
He 79.   Henshaw, D L, Fens, A P and Webster, D J, 1979, A
Technique for high sensitivity alpha-autoradiography of bronchial
epithelium tissue . Phys. Med. Biol. 24 216.
Ke 70.   Keough, R F and Powers, G J, 1970, Determination of
Plutonium in biological materials by extraction and liquid
scintillation counting , Analyt. Chem. 42, 419.
Pr 81. Priest, N D, 1980, Plutonium in bone: the effects of bone
remodelling . Bone and Bone seeking radionuclides: Physiology,
Dosimetry and effects. EULEP symposium Aug 1980, Rotterdam,
EUR-7168-EN.
Pr 82. Priest, N D and Haines, J W, 1982, The release of
plutonium from macrophages in rats : The effect of changes in
iron status . Health Phys. 42   415-423.

Part 3
Alkaline Earth Metals and Bone

8

Long-Term Retention of Radium in Female Former Dial Workers

J. RUNDO, A. T. KEANE and M. A. Essling

INTRODUCTION

Of all the bone-seeking metals, radium may well be unique in more than one respect. It is the only such element with alpha particle emitting isotopes that has unequivocally produced serious biological effects, in particular bone sarcomas, in persons who acquired burdens of 3.66-day ^{224}Ra (Ma84) or the longer-lived ^{226}Ra (half-life 1600 years) with or without 5.75-year ^{228}Ra (Ro83). Furthermore, it is the only bone-seeking element whose metabolism in man has been studied in both the short and the very long terms. This paper is a contribution to our knowledge of the long-term metabolism. It presents strong presumptive evidence for an effect of radiation on the late retention of radium-226 in man.

SOURCE OF DATA

Studies in the U.S.A. of the late effects of radium in man were consolidated in 1969 in the newly created Center for Human Radiobiology (CHR), whose charter included metabolic and dosimetric studies. The current status of these studies is the subject of a recent paper (Ru84). An expandable computerized database, the CHR Information System (CHRIS), was established at an early stage. All new data were entered into the CHRIS, as were data that had been

---

*Work supported by U.S. Department of Energy

accumulated by previous contributors in the field of radium studies at Argonne National Laboratory/Argonne Cancer Research Hospital, at the Massachusetts Institute of Technology Radioactivity Center, and in the New Jersey Radium Research Project. One of the CHRIS files, VVRA, contains all the data on the measurements of radium in vivo, including those for 1916 former dial workers, the vast majority of whom were women.

THE DATA

The file VVRA was searched for the results of serial measurements of the radium contents of individuals, meeting certain criteria: (1) each individual must have been a female former dial worker; (2) there were to have been at least four observations of each individual's radium content starting in the 1950s with at least one in each completed decade since; and (3) the contents were to be at least 10 nCi to ensure a degree of reliability and to minimize statistical errors. Surprisingly, there were only 13 women who met all these criteria, and they had all worked at studios of the same Illinois dial company. Relevant data for these women are summarized in Table 1.

Table 1. Exposure and measurement data for 13 former dial workers.

Parameter	Median	Range
Age at first exposure	19	15–28
Year of first exposure	1922	1921–1925
Duration of exposure, y	2.0	0.4–4.0
Time from first exposure to first measurement, y	34.7	29–38
Age at first measurement	54	45–61
Year of first measurement	1958	1952–1959
Number of measurements	8	5–11
Most recent estimate of ^{226}Ra body content, nCi	230	12–1200

Six of the women continued working in the radium dial industry after 1925 but we do not include such employment in calculating the duration of exposure because recommendations were made in 1925 against the "pointing" of the radium-laden brush between the lips

(BLS29); radium intakes dropped rapidly for persons whose year of first exposure was subsequent to 1925 (Ru84).

With one exception, the periods of observation were >20 years; the exception was a 19.2-year period for one woman where the first of five measurements was made in January 1959 and the last in April 1978. Thus, the case still met the criteria for selection.

ANALYSIS OF DATA

It was assumed that the retention of radium 30-60 years after intake could be described by an exponential function of time, and such a function was fitted to the data for each woman by a computer method of least squares analysis, to yield values of the biological half-life, $t_{1/2}$ (years), and of the intercept, A_0 (nCi), at zero time. The data and fitted curves for the cases giving the shortest (15 y), the longest (90 y), and an intermediate value (31 y) for $t_{1/2}$ are plotted in Figure 1 to show the general quality of the data.

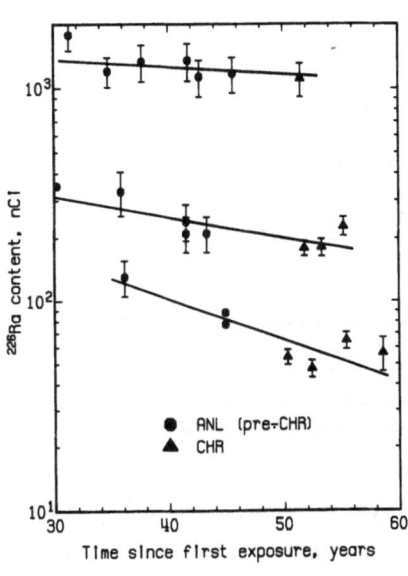

FIGURE 1 Data and fitted curves for subjects with biological half-lives of 90 y, 31 y and 15 y.

It is obvious from Figure 1 that the uncertainties on the half-lives are substantial. In this connection, some comments should be made on the standard errors represented by the vertical bars in Figure 1, and on the weighting used in the least squares analysis. The standard errors stored in the file VVRA and indicated in Figure 1 represent our best estimates of the absolute accuracy of the values for the radium contents, each being considered in isolation. For the intercomparison of estimates of the radium content of an individual, made by one investigator under comparable conditions, relative standard errors should be smaller, perhaps

approaching the statistical error of counting. We have been unable
to establish any kind of intercalibration between the results of the
earlier investigators whose work is included with ours in the
data. It is for this reason that the estimated errors of absolute
accuracy are indicated in Figure 1, whereas weights in the least
squares analyses were taken as the reciprocals of the values of the
body contents.

RESULTS AND DISCUSSION

Values of λ, the elimination rate in percent of body content per
year, were calculated from the relation,

$$\lambda = 69.3/t_{1/2} \quad .$$

In Figure 2, λ is plotted as a function of the body content at 45
years post-exposure, the latter being calculated from the
expression,

$$A_{45} = A_0 e^{-0.45\lambda} \quad . \quad \text{There is a strong}$$

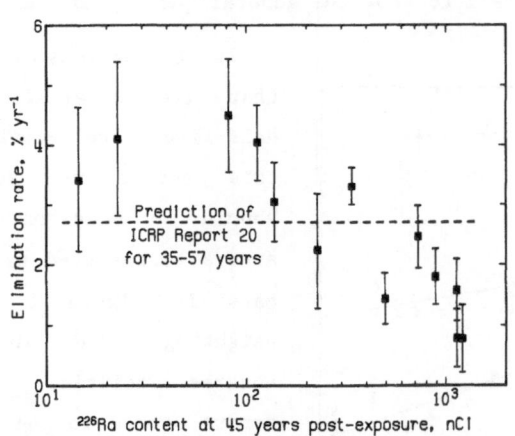

FIGURE 2   Elimination rate of radium at late times
as a function of calculated radium content
at 45 years (see text).

negative correlation between λ and A_{45} ($r = -0.88$, $p < 0.001$ for a
two-tailed test), indicating an effect of radiation in the expected
direction, i.e. an inhibition of bone resorption or remodelling at
the higher radium contents. The horizontal dashed line in Figure 2
represents the average excretion rate ($2.74 \% \ yr^{-1}$) for the interval
35-57 years predicted by the International Commission on
Radiological Protection (ICRP) model of alkaline earth metabolism in
man (IC73). It is in good agreement with the mean of the 13 values

for λ (2.58 % y^{-1}) but no allowances were made in the model for the effects of radiation, although the possibility was recognized.

A consequence of the correlation shown in Figure 2 is that the value of the intercept A_0 was proportionately greater than A_{45} for those subjects with the higher elimination rates, than for those with lower values of λ. Consequently, it can be argued that some of the persons with low values of A_{45} would have higher values of A_0 than some of those with high values of A_{45}, where we claim to have observed an effect of radiation. We would then have a paradox. Certainly the order of the subjects when they are sorted according to the values of A_{45} is different from the order when they are sorted according to A_0. However, there is still a reasonable correlation between λ and A_0 ($r = -0.64$, $p < 0.02$), supporting our hypothesis of an effect of radiation on the elimination rate.

There exists a measure of bone damage that has been shown to be strongly correlated with systemic intake of radium. This measure is the so-called "x-ray score" (Ke83), the sum of numbers assigned according to size, to lesions observed radiographically in 20 skeletal areas. Such scores exist for the 13 women of this study. When the score excludes values for bone sarcoma or pathological fracture, it is termed the "reduced x-ray score," and in Figure 3 this "reduced" score is plotted as the independent variable to show the strong correlation between it and the elimination rate, λ. A

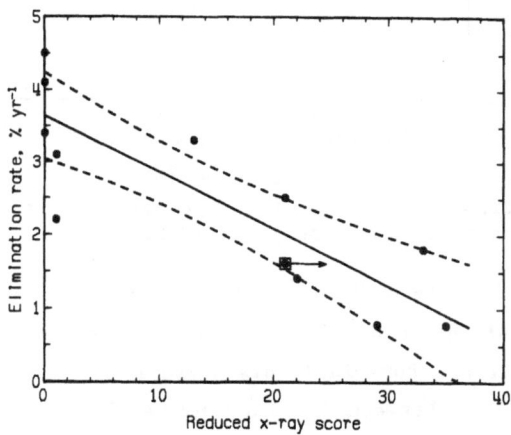

FIGURE 3   Elimination rate as a function of reduced x-ray score for the 13 subjects.

linear relationship was assumed and a least squares analysis yielded the plotted regression line; its upper and lower 95% confidence limits are drawn as dashed lines. The outlined point at a score of 21 was for a case where only 13 skeletal areas were examined. Had 20 areas been scored, a higher value might well have resulted, a possibility indicated by the arrow, but it is clear that the effect on the regression analysis would have been slight.

The results summarized in Figures 2 and 3 represent strong but not conclusive evidence for an effect of the radiation on the late retention of radium in these subjects. We can add one further piece of evidence derived from data on radium concentrations in soft tissues from eight different subjects who died 40–53 years post-exposure (Sc82). If the fractional rate of elimination of radium does vary as the inverse of the total amount present, then the levels in blood and soft tissues should be proportionately lower at the higher body contents. Figure 4 shows that this is the case for soft tissues.

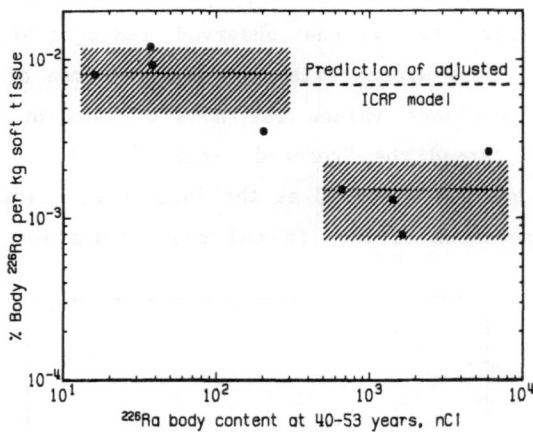

FIGURE 4   Relative concentration of ^{226}Ra in soft tissues as a function of terminal body content, for 8 subjects (Sc82).

It is tempting to draw a straight line through the data but there is no rationale for doing so when both axes have logarithmic scales. Also the results are for widely disparate numbers of samples; seven of the subjects had between one and four samples analyzed, while for one subject the number was 29. The data were divided into two groups by body content (below and above 400 nCi ^{226}Ra) and mean values were calculated. In Figure 4 these values are indicated as dotted lines at 8.2×10^{-3} % kg^{-1} and 1.5×10^{-3} % kg^{-1} for the two groups respectively. The shaded areas represent the spread of two standard errors on either side of the mean values. The prediction of the ICRP model was 3.6×10^{-2} % kg^{-1}, above the range of the ordinate scale in Figure 4, but an adjusted model (Sc82) that improved the fit to experimental data yielded an expected value of 7.0×10^{-3} % kg^{-1} as indicated by the dashed line.

There remain two other possibilities to explain the trend shown in Figure 2, namely, the age at which radium was acquired and the length of the exposure period. The analysis made in the development of the ICRP model of alkaline earth metabolism demonstrated an age-effect on retention depending on whether the subject was younger or older than 24 at the time of radium intake (IC73). In our series, six of the 13 women were aged 18 or less at the time they started work with radium paint so skeletal growth may have been incomplete.

Variability in the duration of exposure may also affect long-term retention by virtue of different dose rates: intake of a given amount in a short period may result in higher local concentrations ("hot spots") and higher dose rates compared to intake of the same amount over a protracted period.

As a test of the possible contributions to the causes of the variability in λ, a multivariate analysis was performed. The prediction equation was: $\lambda = a + bA_{45} + cY_{fxp} + dD_w$, where a, b, c, and d were constants to be determined, A_{45} was as already defined, Y_{fxp} was the age in years at first exposure, and D_w was the duration of exposure in weeks. The results, summarized in Table 2, confirm that the body content at late times is by far the most important factor controlling the variability in λ, the contributions of the others not being significant. We conclude that we have detected an effect of radiation on the long-term retention of radium.

Qualitatively similar findings have been reported for radium in dogs (L176, Pa78). However, the doses were higher and the periods of observation were much smaller fractions of the lifespan, so it is not possible to make a detailed comparison.

Table 2. Results of multivariate analysis for the prediction of λ.

Parameter	Constant	Estimate	± S.E.	Significance level
Intercept	a	4.99	0.95	0.0005
^{226}Ra content at 45 yrs	b	−0.0027	0.0004	0.0001
Age at first exposure	c	−0.07	0.05	0.14
Duration of exposure	d	0.003	0.003	0.26

$$r^2 = 0.83, \ p < 0.0008$$

SUMMARY

The results of measurements of the radium contents of 13 women made over periods of about 20 or more years have been extracted from our files. The women were all employed at different studios of the same Illinois plant as luminous dial workers for periods of up to 4 years, starting at ages 15 to 28 in the early 1920s. The data for each woman were fitted by an exponential function of time, yielding a value for the biological half-life at roughly 30–60 years after first exposure to radium. There was a strong negative correlation between the elimination rate and the body content, suggesting an effect of radiation on bone resorption or remodelling.

We also observed a strong negative correlation between the elimination rate and the "reduced x-ray score," a measure of bone damage observed radiographically in the same subjects. Age at first exposure and duration of exposure were not significantly correlated with the elimination rate. The concentration of radium in soft tissues from eight other subjects, expressed as a percentage of the terminal radium content, decreased with increasing body content, providing further evidence that radiation was affecting the elimination rate. We conclude that an effect of radiation on the late retention of radium has been demonstrated.

ACKNOWLEDGMENTS

Determinations of radium in vivo at ANL in the early 1950s were made by W. P. Norris. Subsequent measurements at ANL prior to the formation of CHR were made by Miller (Mi69).

REFERENCES

BLS29 U.S. Bureau of Labor Statistics, 1929, Radium poisoning , Monthly Labor Rev., **28**, 1200-1275.

IC73 International Commission on Radiological Protection, 1973, Alkaline earth metabolism in adult man , **ICRP Publication 20** (Oxford: Pergamon Press).

Ke83 Keane, A. T., Kirsh, I. E., Lucas, H. F., Schlenker, R. A. and Stehney, A. F., (1983), Non-stochastic effects of ^{226}Ra and ^{228}Ra in the human skeleton , in: **Biological Effects of Low-Level Radiation**, pp. 329-350 (Vienna: International Atomic Energy Agency).

Ll76 Lloyd, R. D., Mays, C.W., Atherton, D. R., Taylor, G. N. and Van Dilla, M. A., 1976, Retention and skeletal dosimetry of injected ^{226}Ra, ^{228}Ra, and ^{90}Sr in beagles , Radiat. Res., **66**, 274-287.

Ma84 Mays, C. W. and Spiess, H., 1984, Bone sarcomas in patients given Ra-224 , in: **Radiation Carcinogenesis: Epidemiology and Biological Significance.** (Edited by J. D. Boice, Jr. and J. F. Fraumeni, Jr.), pp. 241-252 (New York: Raven Press).

Mi69 Miller, C. E., Hasterlik, R. J. and Finkel, A. J., 1969, THE ARGONNE RADIUM STUDIES - Summary of Fundamental Data , Argonne National Laboratory and Argonne Cancer Research Hospital Report ANL-7531 and ACRH-106.

Pa78 Parks, N. J., Pool, R. R., Williams, J. R. and Wolf, H. G., 1978, Age and dosage-level dependence of radium retention in beagles , Radiat. Res., **75**, 617-632.

Ro83 Rowland, R. E., Stehney, A. F. and Lucas, H. F., 1983, Dose-response relationships for radium-induced bone sarcomas , Health Phys., **44**, Suppl. 1, 14-31.

Ru84 Rundo, J., Keane, A. T., Lucas, H. F., Schlenker, R. A., Stebbings, J. H. and Stehney, A.F., 1984, Current (1984) status of the study of ^{226}Ra and ^{228}Ra in humans at the Center for Human Radiobiology , to be presented at the Symposium on **The Radiobiology of Radium and Thorotrast**, Neuherberg, Federal Republic of Germany, 29-31 October 1984.

Sc82 Schlenker, R. A., Keane, A. T. and Holtzman, R. B., 1982, The retention of ^{226}Ra in human soft tissue and bone; implications for the ICRP 20 alkaline earth model , Health Phys., **42**, 671-693.

9

Strontium-90 Content in Human Bone in West German Residents

R. DEHOS and H. SCHMIER

INTRODUCTION

Quantitative assessments of the radionuclide Sr-90 in human diet originating from the fallout of atmospheric nuclear weapon tests are still carried out today all over the world. To gain an insight into the transfer of Sr-90 in the food chain and the discrimination between strontium and calcium, examinations of human bone samples are a necessary addition to assessments of this radionuclide in food.

Extensive studies on the Sr-90 content of human tissues were conducted in the Federal Republic of Germany from 1958 to 1971 by Prof. Dr. Pribilla's work group at the Institute for Forensic and Social Medicine of the University of Kiel. Within the scope of these studies it was possible to demonstrate that there is a correlation between the age-dependent Sr-90 content of defined sections of the compact bone (tibia or femur) and the Sr-90 uptake via the food chain which showed increased amounts of the Sr-90 and other decay products due to the fallout from the nuclear weapon tests in 1961/62. The maximum contamination of food products occured in 1963/64 approximately, and was found in human bone in 1964/65 approximately.

The measurement conducted in the Federal Republic of Germany to assess the Sr-90 content of human bone samples first covered a period of several years up to 1971 only. The results of these measurements served as a basis for calculating the radiation exposure according to the recommendations of the ICRP and were published in the Annual Reports "Environmental Radioactivity and Radiation Exposure" issued by the Federal Minister of the Interior. These results were also included in the Reports of the United Nations' Scientific Committee on the Effects of Atomic Radiation (UNSCEAR) and were of importance with regard to the obligations within the scope of the EURATOM contract.

In 1977 the Institute for Radiation Hygiene of the Federal Health Office started another series of measurements within the scope of a research project supported by the Federal Minister of the Interior, in cooperation with the Institute for Forensic Medicine and the Institute for Pathology, both of the University of Munich, the Institute for Forensic Medicine and the Institute for Pathology both of the University of the Saarland in Homburg.

The objective of this study was to complete the basic data needed for future dose assessments by measurements of bone samples from West German residents to observe the further course of the age dependence of the Sr-90 content in human bone. The research project has been concluded in the meantime, and data from a period of 7 years are available now.

MATERIALS AND METHODS

In 1960 Kulp et al. (Ku60) observed an anisotropic distribution of Sr-90 in the human skeleton. This may be due to the varying turnover of mineral substances in different parts of the skeleton. For example spongious bone sections show a higher turnover rate than the compact bone substance. Consequently, the radionuclide incorporation and decorporation is slower in the compact bone (such as the tibia or femur diaphysis) than in spongious bone (such as ribs or vertebrae).

Since there has been a significant decrease in the Sr-90 content of human diet from the maximum observed in 1963/64 to the present value, only bone sections with a low turnover rate were expected to show increased Sr-90 concentrations today. However, there are varying turnover rates in the different sections of the tibia and femur. The turnover rate of mineral substances in the centre of these bones is lower than in the epiphyses. Therefore only bone sections from the centre of the tibia and femur were analyzed. For this purpose, samples from forensic examinations were preferred to section material from university clinics, since it can not be excluded that the bone turnover has been influenced by previous treatment with pharmaceutical drugs in the case of the latter.

From 1977 to 1983, defined sections of the femur or tibia diaphysis were taken from dead male and female persons of all age groups, and deep-frozen after removal of the surrounding tissues. The samples collected in this manner were wet ashed with hydrogen peroxide and nitric acid during the first study period or later on mineralized by heating to 700 $^{\circ}$C.

The radiochemical separation was performed according to the procedures suggested by the Environmental Measurements Laboratory (Em82) in a slightly modified way. The content of natural strontium as well as the chemical yield of the strontium carrier was estimated by atomic absorption spectrophotometry in the nitrous oxide/acetylene flame. Calcium was titrated with EDTA, and the beta-

activity of the separated yttrium-90 was measured using
a low-level Omniguard-Geiger-Müller counter.

RESULTS AND DISCUSSION

The results from 1977 (Fig. 1) suggest that the uptake
of strontium-90 by human bone was significantly increased
in the age group of about 15 to 25 years compared to the
25 to 55 years' age group. This may be attributed to the
fact that those in the 15-25 years age group were in the
first stage of bone growth at the time of maximum fallout
in 1963/64 and therefore showed an increased incorporation
of the radionuclide. As compared to other bones of the
human body, the femural or tibial sections selected for
examinations (i.e. the diaphyses) show only a low turnover
rate, and the deposited strontium-90 therefore is eliminated from the bone at a very slow rate. Since the fallout
has considerably decreased in the meantime, only small
amounts of Sr-90 are incorporated into human bone today.
If the Sr-90 content shown in Fig. 1 is compared with that
observed in 1980 (Fig. 2) and 1982 (Fig. 3), it becomes
evident that the radionuclide concentration of the bone
slowly decreases and that there is a simultaneous shift of
the concentration maximum to the higher age groups (De84)
(Fig. 4).

In 1982 an increased number of bone samples from persons aged 55 and more could be examined, and a higher
uptake of Sr-90 was observed also in this age group. This
might be attributed to increased osteoporotic or postcli-
macteric processes in the skeleton occurring in this age
group which caused higher bone turnover rates and thus
gave rise to a higher incorporation of Sr-90 during or
after the period of maximum fallout. Natural strontium,
however, is absorbed from food and incorporated into
the skeleton at constant levels of concentration, whereby
there is a discrimination between strontium and calcium.

For this reason, an age-dependent concentration of natural strontium was not observed in the bone sections examined (see Fig. 5).

A complete right femur of a 72-year-old woman was divided into eight sections and examined (De84) (Fig. 6). The measurement results showed that the strontium-90 concentration was lowest in the bone section from slightly below the centre towards the knee joint and increased by about 60 % in the direction of the epiphyses. This may be explained by the fact that bone growth of the femur in this case was already complete at the time of maximum fallout in 1964/65 and strontium-90 was incorporated into (and eliminated from) the medium bone section only at a low bone turnover rate. The increased turnover rate in the direction of the epiphyses caused a higher intake of the fission product. Although the bone matrix showed an increased elimination (of Sr-90 as well), a higher concentration is still observed today in this region compared to the centre of the femoral diaphyis.

According to current studies conducted in other countries, the Sr-90 content of bone samples (such as vertebrae or ribs) is not age-dependent anymore today. Obviously the radionuclide has largly been eliminated from the bone matrix due to the higher turnover rate of these bones.

SUMMARY

As in many other countries, examinations on the Sr-90 content of human bone have been conducted in the Federal Republic of Germany. In defined sections of the tibia and femur a maximum Sr-90 concentration was found in 1977 in persons aged 20-25 years that time. Within the course of 7 years this maximum decreased and shifted towards the older age groups. This may be explained by the fact that

the amounts of Sr-90 retained in the examined bone section
during the time of maximum fallout in 1963/64 are eliminated only at a slow rate, whereby only unimportant amounts
of this radionuclide were incorporated into the bone
during the years thereafter. For natural strontium, no
age-dependence was observed in the bone sections under
study. In examinations of a complete right femur from a
woman aged 72, the Sr-90 content was found to increase by
about 60 % from the bone centre to the epiphyses, whereby
natural strontium shows, however, an almost uniform distribution.

REFERENCES

Ku60 Kulp, J.L., Schulert, A.R. and Hodges, E.J., 1960,
      Strontium-90 in Man IV , Science, 132, 448-454.

Em82   1982 EML Procedures Manual (HASL 300) , 25th Edi-
      tion. Eds. H.L. Volchock, G. de Planque, Environmental
      Measurements Laboratory, U.S. Department of Energy, N.Y.

De84 Dehos, R., Schmier, H. and Eder, M., 1984,
      Strontium-90 Content in Human Bone of West German
      Residents. 6th International Congress of the Interna-
      tional Radiation Protection Association (IRPA) , Berlin
      (West), May 7-12, 1984.
      Compacts Vol. I, 337-340, Eds. A. Kaul, R. Neider,
      J. Peńsko, F.-E. Stieve and H. Brunner. Publ. Fachver-
      band für Strahlenschutz e.V.

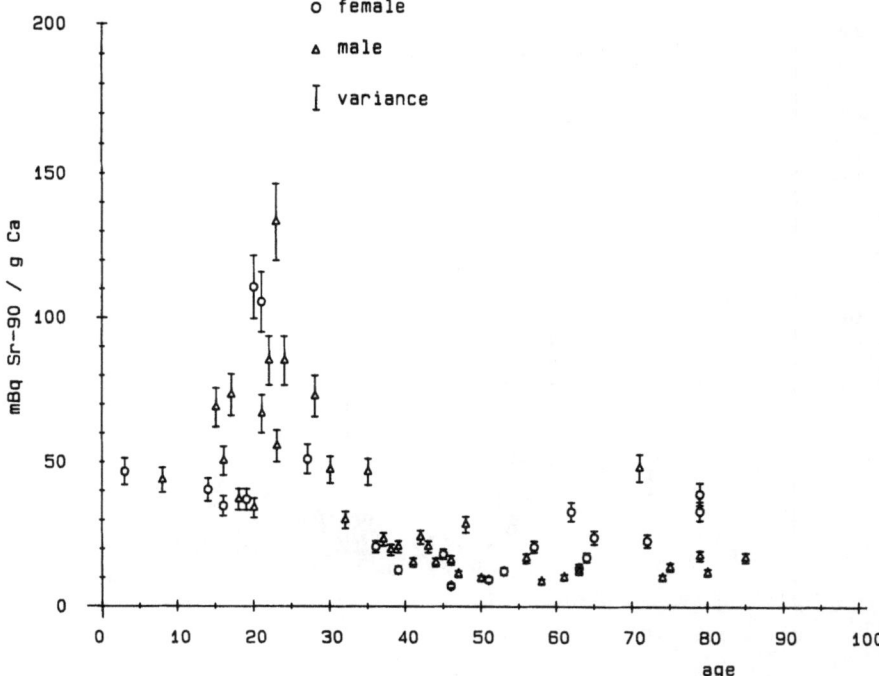

Fig. 1 :   Age dependent Sr-90 content per unit calcium in human bone (mBq Sr-90/g Ca) as assessed in West German residents in 1977

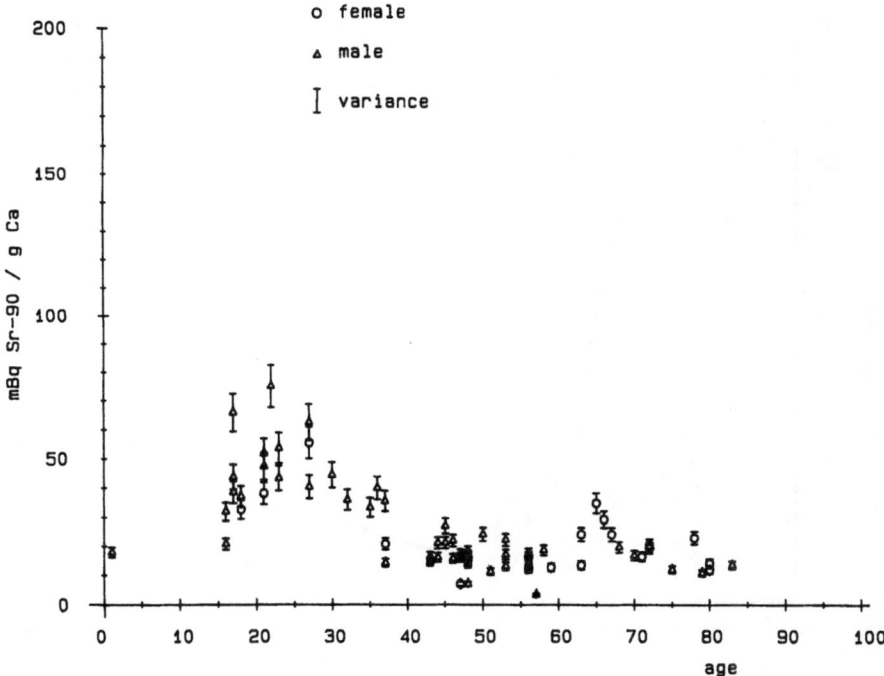

Fig. 2 :   Age dependent Sr-90 content per unit calcium in human bone (mBq Sr-90/g Ca) as assessed in West German residents in 1980

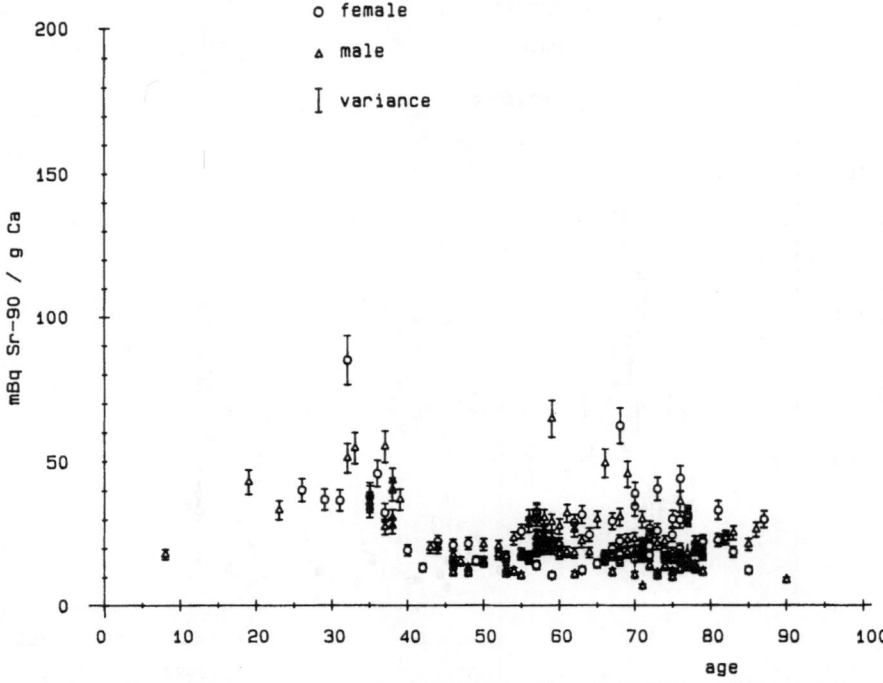

Fig. 3 :   Age dependent Sr-90 content per unit calcium in human bone (mBq Sr-90/g Ca) as assessed in West German residents in 1982

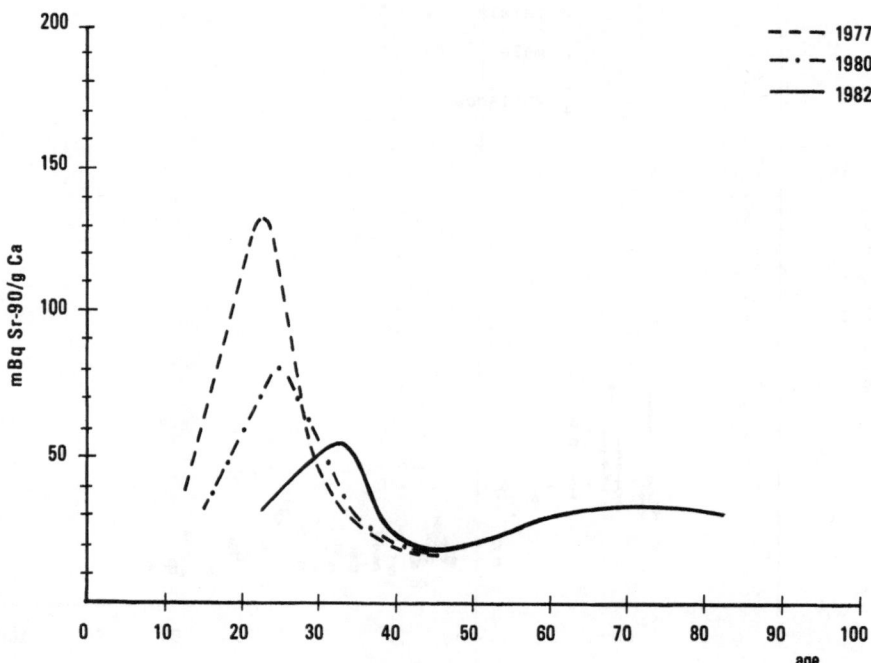

Fig. 4 :   Comparative diagram of the age-dependent Sr-90 content in human bone (based on Fig. 1–3)

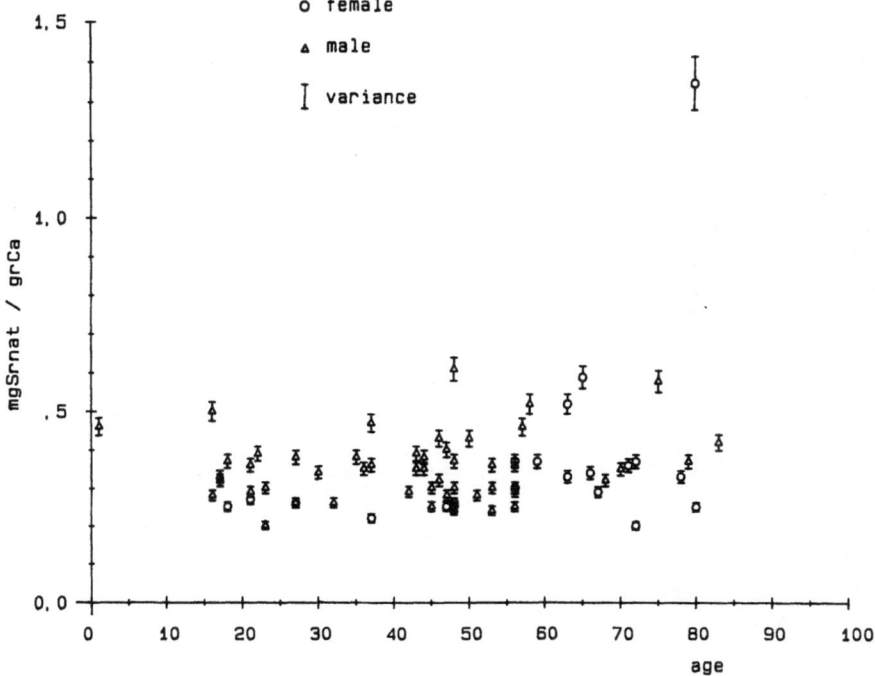

Fig. 5 :   Age dependent content of natural strontium per unit calcium in human bone (mg Sr nat/g Ca) as assessed
in West German residents in 1980

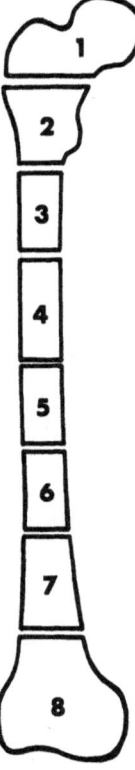

bone section	mBq Sr-90 pro g Ca	mBq Sr-90 pro mg Srnat	mg Srnat pro g Ca
1	23 ± 2	97 ± 10	0.24 ± 0.01
2	22 ± 2	98 ± 10	0.22 ± 0.01
3	16 ± 2	74 ± 7	0.21 ± 0.01
4	15 ± 2	73 ± 7	0.20 ± 0.01
5	13 ± 1	63 ± 6	0.20 ± 0.01
6	12 ± 1	56 ± 6	0.22 ± 0.01
7	13 ± 1	63 ± 6	0.21 ± 0.01
8	18 ± 2	80 ± 8	0.23 ± 0.01

Fig. 6 :   Distribution of Sr-90 and natural strontium in
a complete femur from a woman aged 72

10

Long-Term Retention and Turnover Studies with ^{85}Sr

P. N. SAMBROOK, R. HESP, J. R. GREEN, M. TELLEZ, P. J. MEUNIER and J. REEVE

INTRODUCTION

Over the last thirty years there has been considerable interest in the study of the metabolism of the radioisotopes of strontium in man. This has been stimulated by three main factors. Firstly, the need arose to quantitate the dangers arising from the contamination of the environment and of workers in the nuclear industry, by ^{90}Sr and other bone-seeking radionuclides. Secondly, it was recognised that ^{85}Sr might be a useful tracer for bone calcium; and finally, before the development of ^{99}Tc^{m} based agents, ^{87}Sr^{m} was widely used for bone scanning purposes in clinical nuclear medicine.

The main stimulus to our work has been the need to develop new atraumatic techniques for the measurement of physiological fluxes in bone. These have included bone blood flow (Wo81), bone formation rate (Re76), the exchange of calcium between the surface pools of bone and the blood stream (Re78), and the resorption rate of old bone (Re76).

METHODOLOGICAL PRINCIPLES

Kinetic methods of measuring bone turnover have a long history in clinical studies (Pe64; Bu71; He78). The principles underlying all measurements with radioisotopic tracers are fundamentally the same. Tracer is introduced into the blood stream and thereby presented to bone. The 'exposure' of the bone to the tracer is the mathematical integral of the curve of plasma tracer concentration with time. At a given time 't' the amount of tracer in bone is measured, either directly by bone biopsy or quantitative isotopic scanning; or indirectly as the difference between the injected dose and the sum of the soft tissue and excreted fractions including dermal losses (Ch83). This amount is divided by the integral of the plasma curve to time 't', giving the plasma clearance.

Bone surfaces are separated from the blood stream by

osteocytes, and autoradiographical studies showed that all such surfaces accumulate radio-activity in the two days following an injection of ^{45}Ca (Ro66). This is also true of $^*Sr$, ^{32}P and agents used currently or previously in bone scanning such as $^{99}Tc^m$-MDP and ^{18}F. At quiescent sites the tracer returns to the blood stream, but at sites of new bone formation intense uptake of ^{45}Ca is still seen four to seven days later. Kinetic methods have sought to differentiate empirically between uptake into the surface exchangeable pools (which may partially approximate to the 'bone fluid compartment') and uptake secondary to new bone formation.

If the exchangeable pools could be mathematically represented by one or more well-mixed compartments such a differentiation would, in principle, be straightforward. Unfortunately, the demonstration by Rowland (Ro66) that bone deep to blood accessible surfaces and remote from bone-forming osteoblastic surfaces becomes diffusely labelled with ^{45}Ca for considerable periods after administration of tracer made this task more complex than was originally anticipated.

The 'long-term' element of radiocalcium (and radiostrontium) exchange has been the subject of considerable interest to radiation biologists as well as bone physiologists (Ro66; Ma69; Ma73; Ca73; Re83). For those interested in the quantitation of bone turnover, the crucial practical question is whether long-term exchange, which may contribute half the accretion rate, is independent of processes regulating osteoblastic bone formation.

If long-term exchange (LTE) is an independent process with little variation between individuals, then it is reasonable to use the 'accretion' rate, generally agreed to be the sum of LTE and true bone formation, in the non-invasive study of bone formation in osteoporosis. The accretion rate may be calculated by a variety of methods, which have been critically evaluated by Jung (Ju78), from data collected for 10 to 20 days.

To investigate the physiological significance of LTE processes required that they be measured. Marshall (Ma69) had introduced the concepts of 'Augmentation' and 'Diminution', equal and opposited components of this exchange. We published a technique for their estimation based on stochastic analysis of long-term ^{85}Sr tracer data and metabolic calcium balance data (Re76), having shown that the single passage retention in bone of ^{85}Sr is indistinguishable from that of $^*Ca$ (Re76a; Re83).

Our approach to the problem of differentiating between exchange processes and true bone formation was based on deconvolution analysis, whereby we obtained distributions of transit time for ^{85}Sr through the skeleton. Figure 1 shows the results of a typical study with ^{85}Sr in a patient with osteoporosis (Re82). It will be seen that the power function of time observed by Harrison and co-workers (Ca73) to fit the whole body retention data for ^{85}Sr extended to the transit time distribution. In this example 48% of the tracer taken up into the arbitrarily defined 'fixed' bone pools ($H_F(t)$) at 20 days had been lost again by 200 days. The question then arose as to whether this calcium had been lost by bone resorption or during the course of

LTE, and this and various other questions relating to the interpretation of kinetic tracer studies with [85]Sr and [47]Ca have been addressed by comparison with results obtained on simultaneous bone biopsies (Re83a; Re81) analysed by dynamic histomorphometry (Me83).

RESULTS AND DISCUSSION

The possibility that a substantial fraction of the tracer which is lost to bone in the first 200 days had been removed by osteoclastic resorption seemed unlikely when we found no significant correlation with trabecular resorption surfaces measured in simultaneous trans-iliac 7.5 mm bone biopsies in patients with untreated osteoporosis (Re83a). Instead, we found a highly significant positive correlation between the osteoid surfaces measured as a fraction of total trabecular surfaces taking a double in $vivo$ tetracycline label (DLS) and the fraction of the accretion rate retained for 200 days. The exchange-corrected whole body bone formation rate measured in mass/time units also correlated with DLS (for both; r = 0.69, P < 0.001, n = 18) and with calcium balance (P < 0.004, n = 21) (Re82).

We have recently shown that the metabolic calcium balance may be quite well predicted by DLS and resorption surfaces (RS) in a bivariate regression (R = 0.66, P < 0.01, n = 23) (Ar84), in which DLS correlates positively with calcium balance and RS inversely with balance. However, LTE ('Augmentation'), calculated in mmol Ca/day correlated poorly with calcium balance (r = -0.17, N.S.) (Re82).

Since accretion rate (including LTE) is a less good predictor of both calcium balance and doubly labelled trabecular osteoid surfaces than indices of bone formation corrected for exchange (Re83a), it seems likely that the effects of including exchange in the simpler kinetic estimations of bone formation are a) to overestimate substantially its absolute magnitude and b) to degrade its measurement precision. Clearly, LTE rates can vary substantially between patients (Re82) and this variability bears no consistent relationship to indices of true bone formation. Thus, although the accretion rate can be derived with considerable measurement precision (Ju78) and does not appear to vary much between measurements in the same untreated individuals (La77; Re81), it is not appropriate to infer that the accretion rate can be used to estimate true bone formation with the same precision.

We have recently studied a group of 14 normal female volunteers aged 51 to 69 for comparison with patients with metabolic bone disease, using our [85]Sr technique. The results of the analysis of their skeletal [85]Sr kinetics are presented in Tables 1 and 2, with the previously published results of a study of 21 patients with crush fracture osteoporosis for comparison. Whereas each of the patients also underwent an 18-day metabolic calcium balance study as an in-patient, this was not possible with the volunteers, who are currently undergoing serial axial and peripheral bone densitometry. This should permit the determination of bone formation and resorption rates and also the range of mean transit times of accreted [85]Sr in this group of subjects.

It will be observed that the mean whole body retention time from days 0-200 appears to be higher for ^{85}Sr in the osteoporotic patients than in the controls. By the principle of indicator fractionation, when ^{85}Sr is administered intravenously, its retention time is largely determined by the ratio between the whole body excretion rate of tracer and its uptake by the skeleton. When the *single passage* data for the skeleton were similarly analysed, it was found that the mean retention time was about 12% less in the patients. Thus their increased whole body retention time reflect an increased probability of second and subsequent recyclings of tracer through the skeleton in osteoporosis compared to normals.

It has been well documented that calcium absorption is comparatively reduced in osteoporosis (Ga79), and usually urinary calcium output is reduced in parallel to a rather lesser extent. Since calcium and strontium compete for the same reabsorption sites in the renal tubule, measures tending to increase urinary calcium output (such as a high calcium diet) will tend to reduce ^{85}Sr whole body retention.

In osteoporosis the single passage long-term retention time of ^{85}Sr in the skeleton appears to be principally determined by osteoblast function, and in a state of negative calcium balance ^{85}Sr removal from the skeleton is relatively more rapid. Thus in our study of the relationship between calcium balance and ^{85}Sr retention in osteoporosis (Re82), the regression equation relating calcium balance with the exponent of time β suggested that if balance became more adverse by a mean of 5 mmol Ca/day (200 mg) the mean single passage retention time over the first 200 days after ^{85}Sr administration would be reduced by 37% as β rose from 0.194 at calcium equilibrium to 0.294. Measures that reduce osteoblast activity, such as bed rest, also tend to increase urinary calcium output and thereby reduce *Sr reabsorption by the nephron. They should therefore be useful on both counts in reducing radiation exposure in contaminated individuals and be an adjunct to existing techniques designed to inhibit absorption of radiostrontium from the GI tract and to remove longer term deposits of strontium from the skeleton (Bu83).

SUMMARY

^{85}Sr has been used as a tracer for bone mineral to investigate the pathophysiology of bone turnover in osteoporosis and in normal subjects. About half the conventionally estimated 'accretion' rate is due to long-term exchange processes, which are quite variable between subjects. This variability degrades the precision with which the 'tissue level' rate of bone formation derived from iliac histomorphometry (after double *in vivo* tetracycline labelling) may be predicted by the accretion rate in osteoporosis, but this can be corrected for by longer term measurements of ^{85}Sr.

The simultaneous study of ^{85}Sr kinetics and calcium balance in osteoporosis has suggested that measures which reduce osteoblast activity and increase urinary calcium excretion, such as bedrest, may be useful adjuncts in the management of individuals contaminated with *Sr.

Table 1. Single passage retention of ^{85}Sr in the 'fixed' bone pools fitted by the function: $H_F(t) = A e^{\beta} (t + e)^{-\beta}$ (t in days)

		Accretion rate (A) (mmol Ca/day)	$H_F(t)$ (t = 20 d)	$H_F(t)$ (t = 200 d)	β	$\sqrt{e}$
Controls	Mean	5.73	4.26	3.09	0.171	2.49
(n = 14)	S.D.	2.13	1.54	1.43	0.075	1.84
	Range	2.4-8.9	2.6-7.2	1.4-5.6	0.065-0.345	0.19-5.8
Patients	Mean	6.41	5.35	3.41	0.200	3.05
with osteo-	S.D.	1.55	1.46	0.92	0.068	1.62
porosis						
(n = 21)	Range	4.3-9.2	3.5-9.6	1.6-4.9	0.053-0.342	0.1-7.2
(Re82)						

Table 2   Parameters of the equation of Carr et al. (Ca73(for whole-body retention of ^{85}Sr;

$$R(t) = A e^{-k_1 t} + B t^{-k_2} \quad (t \text{ in days, } R \text{ \% injected dose})$$

		A (%)	B (%)	k_1	k_2	$\int_0^{200 \text{ days}} R(t)\,dt$ (days)
Controls	Mean	53.9	34.1	0.168	0.156	35.3
(n = 14)	S.D.	7.2	11.3	0.025	0.079	9.0
	Range	44.8-69.4	20.6-56.8	0.139-0.245	0.018-0.333	23.6-56.8
Osteoporotics	Mean	33.9	49.2	0.159	0.173	47.6
(n = 21)	S.D.	11.7	14.7	0.055	0.065	12.8
	Range	11.4-57.0	25.6-75.9	0.072-0.315	0.047-0.333	28.4-72.1

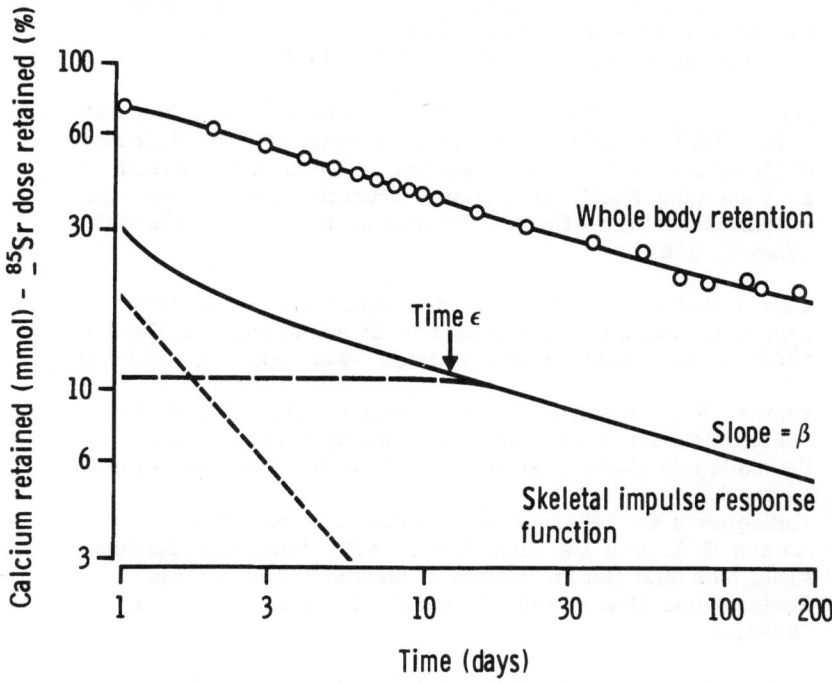

Upper curve: whole body retention of ^{85}Sr dose in a patient with osteoporosis. Data points (o) are superimposed on the fitted sum of a power function and an exponential (Ca73).

$$R(t) = 11 \, e^{-0.24t} + 65 \, t^{-0.23} \quad (\% \text{ of dose})$$

Lower curve: impulse response function of skeleton for ^{85}Sr (----- short and _____ long-term retention functions respectively (from Re82, with permission from *Clinical Science*).

REFERENCES.

Ar84   Arlot M., Edouard C., Meunier P.J., Neer R.M. and Reeve
        J., 1984, "Impaired Osteoblast Function in Osteoporosis:
        Comparison between Calcium Balance and Dynamic
        Histomorphometry", *Br. Med. J.* **289**, 517-520.

Bu71   Bullamore J.R., Nordin B.E.C., Wilkinson R. and Marshall
        D.H., 1971, "Radiocalcium Measurements of Bone Turnover
        in Disorders of Calcium Metabolism using a Model Based on
        an Expanding Pool", in: *Dynamic Studies with Radioisotopes
        in Medicine* (Proc. Symp., Rotterdam 1970), pp. 519-538
        (Vienna: IAEA).

Ca73   Carr T.E.F., Harrison G.E. and Nolan J., 1973, "The
        Long-term Excretion and Retention of an Intravenous Dose of
        ^{45}Ca in Two Healthy Men", *Calcif. Tiss. Res.* **12**, 217-226.

Ch83   Charles P., Jensen F.T., Mosekilde L. and Hansen H.H.,
        1983, "Calcium Metabolism Evaluated by ^{47}Ca Kinetics:
        Estimation of Dermal Calcium Loss", *Clin. Sci.* **65**, 415-422.

Ga79   Gallagher J.C., Riggs B.L., Eisman J., Hamstra A.,
        Arnaud S.B. and De Luca H.F., 1979, "Intestinal Calcium
        Absorption and Serum Vitamin D Metabolites in Normal
        Subjects and Osteoporotic Patients", *J. Clin. Invest.* **64**,
        729-736.

He78   Heaney R.P., Recker R.R. and Saville P.D., 1978,
        "Menopausal Changes in Bone Remodeling", *J. Lab. Clin.
        Med.* **92**, 964-970.

Ju78   Jung A., Bartholdi P., Mermillod B., Reeve J. and Neer
        R.M., 1978, "Critical Analysis of Methods for Analysing
        Human Calcium Kinetics", *J. Theoret. Biol.* **73**, 131-157.

La77   Lauffenburger T., Olah A.J., Dambacher M.A., Guncaga J.,
        Lentner C. and Haas H.G., 1977, "Bone Remodelling and
        Calcium Metabolism: A Correlated Histomorphometric, Calcium
        Kinetic, and Biochemical Study in Patients with Osteoporosis
        and Paget's Disease", *Metabolism* **26**, 589-606.

Ma69   Marshall J.H., 1969, "Measurements and Models of Skeletal
        Metabolism", in: *Mineral Metabolism*, vol. 3 (Edited by C. L.
        Comar and F. Bronner), pp. 1-122 (New York: Academic
        Press).

Ma73   Marshall J.H., Lloyd E.L., Rundo J., Liniecki J., Marotti
        G., Mays C.W., Sissons H.A. and Snyder W.S., 1973,
        "Alkaline Earth Metabolism in Adult Man" (ICRP Publication
        20), *Health Phys.* **24**, 125-221.

Me83   Meunier P.J., 1983, "Histomorphometry of the Skeleton", in:
        Bone and Mineral Research Annual I (Edited by W. A. Peck),
        pp. 191-222 (Amsterdam: Excerpta Medica.)

Pe64   Pearson O.H. and Joplin G.F. (Editors), 1964, *Dynamic Studies of Metabolic Bone Disease* (Oxford: Blackwell).

Re76   Reeve J., Hesp R. and Wootton R., 1976, "A New Tracer Method for the Calculation of Rates of Bone Formation and Breakdown in Osteoporosis and Other Generalised Skeletal Disorders", *Calcif. Tiss. Res.* 22, 191-206.

Re76a   Reeve J. and Hesp R., 1976, "A Model-Independent Comparison of the Rates of Uptake and Short Term Retention of ^{47}Ca and ^{85}Sr by the Skeleton", *Calcif. Tiss. Res.* 22, 183-189.

Re78   Reeve J., 1978, "The Turnover Time of Calcium in the Exchangeable Pools of Bone in Man and the Long-term Effect of a Parathyroid Hormone Fragment", *Clin. Endocrinol.* 8 445-455.

Re81   Reeve J., Arlot M., Bernat M., Charhon S., Edouard C., Slovik D., Vismans F.J.F.E. and Meunier P.J., 1981, "Calcium-47 Kinetic Measurements of Bone Turnover Compared to Bone Histomorphometry in Osteoporosis: the Influence of Human Parathyroid Fragment (hPTH 1-34) Therapy", *Metab. Bone Dis. Rel. Res.* 3, 23-30.

Re82   Reeve J., Green J.R., Hesp R. and Hulme P., 1982, "Rates of New Bone Formation in Patients with Crush Fracture Osteoporosis", *Clin. Sci.* 63, 153-160.

Re83   Reeve J., Green J.R., Maletskos C.J. and Neer R.M., 1983, "Skeletal Retention of ^{45}Ca and ^{85}Sr Compared: Further Studies on Intravenously Injected ^{85}Sr as a Tracer for Skeletal Calcium", *Calcif. Tiss. Int.* 35, 9-15.

Re83a   Reeve J., Arlot M., Hesp R., Tellez M. and Meunier P.J., 1983, "Tracer Measurements of Bone Remodeling and their Significance in Involutional Osteoporosis", in *Clinical Disorders of Bone and Mineral Metabolism* (Edited by B. Frame and J.T. Potts, Jr), pp. 99-104 (Amsterdam: Excerpta Medica).

Ro66   Rowland R.E., 1966, "Exchangeable Bone Calcium", *Clin. Orthop. Rel. Res.* 49, 233-248.

Wo81   Wootton R., Tellez M., Green J.R. and Reeve J., 1981, "Skeletal Blood Flow in Paget's Disease of Bone", *Metab. Bone Dis. Rel. Res.* 4 & 5, 263-270.

11

Dynamics of Lifespan Strontium-90 Distribution in Beagles with Uniformly Labelled Skeletons Acquired by Radionuclide Ingestion from *In Utero* to Adulthood

N. J. PARKS

INTRODUCTION

In a previous paper (Pa80), I reported the data from lifespan studies of intra-skeletal radionuclide distribution in radium-226 injected beagles and examined it with respect to the fundamental tenets of Marshall et al. in their theoretical model of alkaline-earth metabolism in humans (ICRP73). This was regarded as particularly important because the data acquired under controlled conditions in the long-term beagle studies is more detailed and subject to fewer confounding effects. The dog:human comparison for exposure to injected radium is the basis for predicting the effects of other radionuclides and exposure routes. Consequently, the partitioned clearance model (PCM), which was consistent with the general principles of ICRP Report 20 and also adequately described radium clearance from individual bones, must also adequately describe the clearance of Sr-90 from bones formed during continuous ingestion that have a uniform Sr:Ca ratio (Go72). Otherwise, a uniform theoretical construct for describing the flux of radioactive alkaline earths through both dog and human skeletons is still lacking and the utility of the dog as a surrogate for the study of skeletal biology and radiation biology in humans is compromised.

Supported by U.S. Department of Energy

Experimental Methods

The experimental design of this project and the experimental
methods developed to quantitate the life span variation of whole body
Sr-90 radioactivity levels have been previously reported (Pa84,
Ra81). The skeletal distribution of Sr-90 found for dogs dying at
various times after the ingestion sequence was determined. The data
fit by the model described are the percent of total body burden
represented by a given bone or bone group in 9 dogs who died at times
of 0 to 4,229 days after the cessation of Sr-90 feeding at 540 days
of age.

Analytical Methods and Results

The method employed herein to describe Sr-90 redistribution after
uniform labelling requires parameter estimates obtained by analysis
of short duration exposure to alkaline-earths such as the previously
reported radium injection study (Pa80). Clearance kinetics of radium
after injection into young adult beagles have been described with a
partitioned clearance model that includes a set of assumptions
generally congruent with those adopted by Committee 2 of the ICRP
(ICRP73) for their model of alkaline-earth metabolism in humans.
Assumption I is that the skeleton can be considered as composed of a
high surface-to-mass-ratio class of bone, generically referred to as
"cancellous", and a low surface-to-mass-ratio class of bone generically referred to as "compact." Additional assumptions were (II)
that the ratio of compact to cancellous bone in the skeleton on a
mass basis is about 4:1, and (III), that the surface area available
for radium deposition in these two bone-classes are about equal. The
fourth (IV) assumption was that radium clearance rates for thoracic
and lumbar vertebrae were representative estimators for rates applicable to cancellous bone throughout the skeleton. These assumptions
were combined into mathematical statements giving the partition of
the skeletal retention function, R_{dog}, into two functions which
estimate the mean fraction of initial dosage injected that is
retained in compact bone (F_{COM}) and cancellous bone (F_{CAN}).

The analysis of strontium distribution kinetics is dependent upon
the results of the radium study for the values of parameters that
cannot be obtained from an initially uniform tracer distribution in

skeletal mineral. The whole body retention of Sr-90 can be represented by

$$\text{Fractional retention } (R_{dog}) = d^b(t+d)^{-b} \tag{1}$$

where d and b are parameters and t is the time after the end of feeding at 540 days; representative [d;b] parameter values are [170;
0.257], for dogs. On the basis of assumption III, the value of
F_{CAN} and F_{COM} was originally set to 0.5 at t = 0, a time when
R_{dog} = 1, for injected radium. The percent-of-body-burden values
for thoracic and lumbar vertebrae, which were considered to be
effectively 100% cancellous bone in the prior treatment, were found
to be described with a decreasing exponential function. The results
of considering the strontium data have led to a current estimate for
the vertebrae of only 60 to 70% effective cancellous bone (Table 1).
However, the mean fraction of the initial dosage retained in
cancellous bone is still conveniently described by

$$F_{CAN} = R_{dog}(Ce^{-kt}) \tag{2}$$

where C is presently set at 0.46 for injected alkaline-earths
(Assumption III) and about 0.2 for uniform tracer:calcium labels
(Assumption II). The sum of F_{CAN} and F_{COM} must equal R_{dog} at
all times; therefore, F_{COM} is described by

$$F_{COM} = R_{dog} (1 - Ce^{-kt}) \tag{3}$$

The partitioned-clearance description of radionuclide metabolism
in the whole skeleton was incorporated into the descriptive functions
for the data sets such that each bone group (i) provides an estimate
of the rate constant, k. For injected radium these functions also
provide estimates for the fraction (f_{ij}) of skeletal radioactivity
initially deposited (surfaces plus volume) in compact (j=1) and
cancellous (j=2) classes of each anatomical components, and estimates
of the mass fraction (m_{ij}) for each class in each component.

The f_{ij} and m_{ij} values were obtained from a partitioning of
the t=0 intercepts (A-values) obtained from the short-term exposures
by injection. This was accomplished by relating the f_{ij} values to

Table 1. Distribution of Sr-90 in the beagle skeleton[†] as a function of time[††]; regression fit to per cent of body-burden: $(R_i/R_{dog}) = A_i[m_{i,COM}(1.25-.25e^{-kt}) + (1-m_{i,COM})e^{-kt}]$

Bone Group (i)	A_i (SE)	$m_{i,COM}$	$k \times 10^4$/day (SE)	P(k>0)
Forepaws	4.37 (0.23)	0.94	7.44 (9.90)	0.77
Rad.-Ulnae	6.22 (0.42)	0.96	5.83 (9.65)	0.73
Humeri	6.19 (0.21)	0.90	3.92 (5.93)	0.75
Scapulae	3.48 (0.23)	0.72	10.21 (25.24)	0.66
Hindpaws	6.62 (0.31)	0.98	7.21 (6.46)	0.87
Tib.-Fibulae	6.78 (0.33)	1.00	4.64 (4.28)	0.86
Femora	6.73 (0.28)	0.96	4.75 (5.02)	0.83
Pelves	4.58 (0.45)	0.76	11.96 (82.06)	0.56
Skull	13.16 (0.64)	0.89	10.91 (19.47)	0.71
Mandible	6.52 (0.20)	0.95	1.52 (2.77)	0.71
Teeth*	6.22 (0.48)	1.38	25.04 (7.30)	--
Ribs-Rib. Cart.	8.00 (0.49)	0.33	7.02 (2.92)	0.99
Sternum	0.35 (0.05)	0.00	9.87 (3.46)	1.0
Cer. Vert.	7.80 (0.21)	0.95	2.12 (2.13)	0.84
Thor. Vert.	5.72 (0.26)	0.35	4.92 (1.41)	1.0
L. Vert.	4.03 (0.17)	0.36	3.46 (0.92)	1.0
Tail	2.67 (0.37)	0.59	6.12 (14.53)	0.66

[†]Data from 9 beagles sacrificed at 31, 287, 440, 526, 552, 800, 1324, 2202, and 4229 days post the ingestion exposure period of in utero to 540 days of age. Dosage levels were 0.123 to 3.33 Ci Sr-90/g Ca.

[††]Zero time is taken as the end of feeding (540 days).

*Teeth do not undergo the mineral exchange activity of bone; the m_{ij} value is an unrestricted best fit parameter.

the A/%Ca ratios and by considering the total range of such ratios to be from 0.58 to 2.00, which corresponds to 100% compact or 100% cancellous bone, respectively. The lower limit of 0.58 and the range of 1.42 is consistent with a ratio of surface-to-mass ratios for compact and cancellous bone of 3.4:1, i.e., (46% surface/20% mass) for cancellous bone divided by (54% surface/80% mass) for compact bone. This is a relaxation of the implicit hypothesis of assumptions II and III that the initial radium concentration (μCi/gm bone mineral) in cancellous bone should be 4 times that in compact bone. In beagles, the ratio appears to be about 3.4; the value for humans may be about 4.

The appropriate expressions are

$$f_{i,j=1} = \frac{U - (A_i/\% \ Ca_i)}{U - L} \tag{4a}$$

where U=2 and L=0.58 are the upper and lower limits

$$f_{i,j=2} = 1 - f_{i,j=1} \tag{4b}$$

$$m_{i,j=1} = \frac{(U/L)f_{i,j=1}}{(U/L)f_{i,j=1} + f_{i,j=2}} \tag{4c}$$

and

$$m_{i,j=2} = 1 - m_{i,j=1}, \tag{4d}$$

where i = ith bone-group = 1,2,...17 and j = jth class = 1(COM), 2(CAN).

It is now possible to write the model retention function, $Q_{ij}(t)$, for the fraction of injected dosage retained by each class in each bone. For injected radium, and presumably other alkaline-earths, this function (where the t = 0 intercept, A_i, is taken as a fraction) is

$$Q_{ij}(t) = [f_{ij}][A_i][F_j/F_j(t = 0)], \tag{5}$$

where the f_{ij} and A_i are related by equations (4a) and (4b) and the F_j functions are described by equations (2) and (3). For uniform labelling as a function of skeletal mass, the f_{ij} values in

equation 5 are replaced by m_{ij} values predicted from the injection
data with equations 4c and 4d.

The summation of $Q_{ij}(t)$ over i and j is equal to R_{dog} and the
summation over j for each i give R_i, the model retention function
for each bone group. The data represents the experimental measurement of radioactivity in each bone group divided by whole body
radioactivity; it is described in terms of the index of functions

$$(R_i/R_{dog}) = A_i[m_{i,COM}(1.25-.25e^{-kt}) + (1-m_{i,COM})e^{-kt}]$$

(6)

derived from equation (5). Table 1 shows the mean parameter values
and associated standard errors (S.E.) derived from fitting equation
(6) to the data by least-squares regression.

If the assumptions and equations (4a-4d) are biologically meaningful, then the exponential rate constant, k, must be positive in
the sign convention used in Table 1. This derives from the
prediction of the model that a positive deviation from zero-slope
should be observed when $m_{i,COM}>0.8$ and a negative deviation when
$m_{i,COM}<0.8$. If the inverse is true, the model fails to predict
correctly the observed data trends obtained by regression analysis
and the sign of k is negative. Thus, the probability (P) that $k>0$
for each bone group (Table 1) is a measure of validity for the
hypothesized assumptions and $1-P(k>0)$ is a measure of failure
probability. Given,in Table 2,is an index of deviation, the ratio
$(R_i/R_{dog})_{t=4229}/(R_i/R_{dog})_{t=0}$, of final to initial values
of the fitted functions.

DISCUSSION

The first observation in fitting the strontium data was that
either assumption II about a 4:1 ratio of compact to cancellous mass
or assumption III about equal surface area had to be adjusted. This
conclusion stemmed from the finding that m_{ij} values obtained from
equations 4a,b,c,d with those ratios incorporated were too small to
allow equation 6 to properly fit the Sr-90 data. There is reason to
believe that the 4:1 mass ratio is about right on the basis of
recently performed skeletal surveys (Je84). Therefore, the surface

area fraction for cancellous bone (C) was adjusted downward from 0.5 to 0.46. This permitted a satisfactory fit to the radium injection data. The incorporation of a U/L value of 3.4, which follows from reducing C to 0.46, into equations 4a,b,c,d, gave m_{ij} values large enough for equation 6 to describe the strontium data also.

As determined by fits to the data, the change in the fractional contribution of individual bone groups to the total skeletal radioactivity during the time of this study ranged from a negative deviation to zero for sternum to a positive deviation of 1.22 for the tibia-fibula group (Table 2). The direction of the deviation is consistent with whether the value of $m_{i,COM}$ is greater than or less than 0.8. The t=0 intercepts (A) match the available skeletal calcium distribution fraction within 1 standard error in all cases. The k-values for all groups were positive which is consistent with the model.

The final consideration of the model is how well it describes all the data sets taken together. The median probability for k>0 and consistency of the model with each individual set is about 0.8. Because the data sets are not independent of each other, some

Table 2.   Index of functions $(R_i/R_{dog})_{t=4229}/(R_i/R_{dog})_{t=0}$

Forepaws	1.17	Mandibulae	1.08
Rad-Ulnae	1.18	Teeth*	1.73
Humeri	1.10	Ribs+cart.	0.45
Scapulae	0.90	Sternum	0.02
Hindpaws	1.22	Cer. Vert.	1.11
Tib-Fibulae	1.21	Thor. Vert.	0.51
Femora	1.18	L. Vert.	0.58
Pelves	0.95	Tail	0.76
Skull	1.08	* see note, Table 1	

internal checks for consistency of the model are available. The sum
of fractional values obtained at any time t from the fitted functions
for all the data sets is expected to be 1; it was found to be between
0.99 and 1.04 because the summation includes teeth which do not
mineralize like bone. In addition, the sum over all i of
$m_{i,COM}(A_i)$ was close to the expected value of 0.8 if teeth are
deleted and only bone groups considered. Thus the hypotheses
underlying the partitioned clearance model for the whole skeleton are
supported by the results of strontium clearance analyses for each
skeletal component.

SUMMARY

The dynamics of intra-skeletal radioactivity distribution is an
important factor in characterizing the fundamental phenomena that
governs the formation and location of tumors induced by bone-seeking
radionuclides. The distribution of Sr-90 among the bone groups of
the skeleton in 9 beagles has been measured at times of zero to 12
years after the end of feeding. These dogs ingested 0.123 to 3.33
microcuries Sr-90 per gram dietary calcium from in utero to 1.5 years
of age and acquired maximum body burdens of 1 to 20 microcuries per
kg body weight. At the end of feeding, the Sr-90 distribution among
the skeletal components of these animals closely matched the calcium
distribution. The partitioned clearance model (Pa80), first
developed to describe temporal changes in the initially non-uniform
distribution of Ra-226 with respect to skeletal Ca, has been found to
successfully describe Sr-90 dynamics in the chronic ingestion
experiment where initially uniform Sr:Ca ratios are the case. The
model is congruent with the assumptions of Committee 2 in ICRP
Publication 20 that the skeleton can be considered in terms of a
bimodal distribution of high surface-to-mass (Cancellous) and low
surface-to-mass (Compact) classes of bone; however, in the present
case, individual retention functions for each skeletal component are
produced. Combined with bone turnover measurements, these radiochemical measurements may illuminate the role of chemical exchange
and bone resorption in alkaline-earth removal and clarify the
relationship of radiation flux, cell population and tumorigenesis.

ACKNOWLEDGEMENT

I wish to thank S. Soo, L. Swartz, and F. Gielow for their assistance, and P. Carroll and C. Baty for manuscript preparation.

REFERENCES

Go72 Goldman, M., Della Rosa, R. J., and Momeni, M. H. 1972, Radiation Dose to Beagles from Continuous Sr-90 Exposure, in Biomedical Implications of Radiostrontium Exposure (Ed. M. Goldman and L. K. Bustad), AEC Symposium Series 25.

ICRP73 International Commission of Radiological Protection, 1973, Alkaline-Earth Metabolism in Adult Man, ICRP Publication 20 (Oxford: Pergamon Press).

Je84 Jee, W.S.S., Parks, N.J., Miller, S.C., and Dell, R.B., 1984 in press, Relationship of Bone Composition to the Location of Radium-Induced Bone Cancer , in The Radiobiology of Radium and Thoratrast, Symposium Proceedings, Neuherberg, W. Germany, Oct. 29-31, 1984.

Pa80 Parks, N.J., 1980, Life Span Dynamics of Intra-skeletal Radionuclide Distribution in Radium Injected Beagles , Health Phys. 38, 11.

Pa84 Parks, N.J., Book, S.A., Pool, R.R., 1984, Squamous Cell Carcinoma in the Jaws of Beagles Exposed to 90Sr Throughout Life: Beta Flux Measurements at the Mandible and Tooth Surfaces and a Hypothesis for Tumorigenesis , Radiat. Res. 100, 139-156.

Ra81 Raabe, O.G., Book, S.A., Parks, N.J., Chrisp, C.E., Goldman, M., 1981, Life-time Studies of Ra-226 and Sr-90 Toxicity in Beagles - A Status Report , Radiat. Res. 86, 515.

12

Effect of Stable Strontium on Bone Metabolism in Rats

P. J. MARIE, M.-T. GARBA, M. HOTT and L. MIRAVET

INTRODUCTION

The effects of stable strontium (Sr) on bone and mineral metabolism have been studied for many years.However,most investigations were concerned with high dosage levels of Sr and the influence of low doses of Sr on bone are yet to be determined. It is known that high doses of Sr diminish the intestinal absorption of calcium (Ca) and inhibit the renal conversion of 25 hydroxyvitamin D (25-OH D) to 1,25 dihydroxyvitamin D (1,25 $(OH)_2$ D (Co 70, Om 72). Dietary Sr supplementation at the dose of 1.5 % in the rat induces hypocalcemia (St 62) as well as defective bone mineralization which occurs in spite of adequate amounts of Ca in the diet (St 62). By contrast, low doses of Sr do not seem to generate detectable abnormalities in mineral and bone metabolism in the rat despite significant elevation of Sr levels in serum (Sk 81). Interestingly, Sr supplementation at low dosage was reported to increase bone calcification in osteoporotic patients (Sh 52, Ja 59) but it is not known whether this beneficial effect resulted from decreased bone resorption and / or increased bone formation. This study was therefore undertaken to evaluate the effects of low doses of stable Sr on mineral homeostasis, vitamin D metabolism and bone histology in the rat.

METHODS

Experimental design
Forty male Sprague Dawley rats were fed a semisynthetic diet containing

0.50 % Ca, 0.54 % phosphorus (P) and 0.16 % magnesium (Mg). The experimental groups were composed of 8 rats receiving 0 (controls), 0.19,
0.27, 0.34 or 0.40 % of $SrCl_2$ given in the drinking water from weaning
to sacrifice which occured at 12 weeks of age. Body weight and water
and food consumption were recorded throughout the study. After 4 weeks
and 9 weeks of treatment, blood and urine samples were collected under
fasting conditions. All animals were injected i.p. on days 5 and 2
before sacrifice with tetracycline, a marker of bone calcification. At
sacrifice, the right femur and tibia were removed, freed of bone marrow, dried and ashed. Bone ashes were dissolved in hydrochloric acid
and bone mineral content was determined.

Biochemistry

The concentrations of Ca, Mg and Sr were evaluated in serum, urine and
bone ash by atomic absorption spectrophotometry. Phosphate levels in
serum, urine and bone ash, and serum and urine creatinine concentrations were determined by colorimetric methods. The renal threshold for
phosphate concentration (TmP/GFR) was evaluated using the nomogram of
Walton and Bijvoet (Wa 75). Urinary cyclic AMP (cAMP) was determined
by a competitive binding assay. Serum vitamin D metabolites were determined by modified competitive binding assays (Sh 80).

Bone histology

At sacrifice, the tail was fixed in cold neutral formaldehyde, dehydra
ted and embedded undecalcified. The seventh caudal vertebra was embedded in methylmethacrylate and 5 μm longitudinal sections were stained
with toluidine blue while 15 μm thick unstained sections were used for
fluorescence microscopy. The eight caudal vertebra was embedded in
glycolmethacrylate. Longitudinal 5 μm sections were stained for acid
phosphatase (Ev 79). The number of multinucleated, acid phosphatase-
stained chondroclasts and osteoclasts actively engaged in bone resorption were recorded and expressed as number of cells per mm^2 of metaphyseal bone tissue (Ma 83). The osteoclastic surface (% endosteal
surface showing active osteoclasts) was also recorded.

The following parameters of bone formation were determined by histomorphometric methods using a Zeiss 100 point integrating eyepiece and
a semi-automatic image analyzer : the trabecular bone volume (% of

endosteal bone area occupied by bone and cartilage), the osteoid volume (% of endosteal bone area occupied by osteoid), the osteoid surface (% of endosteal surface covered by an osteoid seam), the osteoblastic surface (% of endosteal surface showing active osteoblasts) and the mean osteoid seam thickness (average width of more than 30 osteoid seams). The endosteal calcification rate was determined by dividing the mean distance between the two fluorescent tetracycline labels by the interval of time between the two labelings. The percentage of the endosteal surface showing a double fluorescent tetracycline label was also recorded. The mineralization lag time was calculated by dividing the osteoid thickness by the calcification rate.

All results were expressed as mean $\pm$ SD and probabilities of difference between means of control and experimental groups were evaluated by student's t-test.

RESULTS

Growth

The water and food consumption was similar in all groups and the calculated amount of ingested Sr rose progressively in the treated groups from 316.0 $\pm$ 97.4 to 633.7 $\pm$ 264.3 mg/kg/day at the 0.19 % and 0.40 % dosages respectively. The body weight and the growth rate were similar in treated and control animals throughout the study.

Biochemistry

All doses of Sr produced a moderate and transitory fall in serum Ca at 4 weeks of treatment (table 1).

Table 1.   Serum biochemistry in controls and treated rats.

	Ca (mg/dl)[a]	Mg (mg/dl)[a]	Sr (mg/dl)[a]	1,25(OH)2D (pg/ml)[b]
Controls	9.34 $\pm$ 0.48	2.53 $\pm$ 0.24	ND	72 $\pm$ 15
0.19 % SrCl$_2$	8.44 $\pm$ 0.51[c]	2.18 $\pm$ 0.19	2.07 $\pm$ 1.35	74 $\pm$ 21
0.27 % SrCl$_2$	8.23 $\pm$ 0.39[c]	2.01 $\pm$ 0.32	2.90 $\pm$ 0.70	51 $\pm$ 19
0.34 % SrCl$_2$	8.22 $\pm$ 0.44[c]	2.12 $\pm$ 0.14	3.19 $\pm$ 0.89	71 $\pm$ 20
0.40 % SrCl$_2$	8.37 $\pm$ 0.53[c]	2.05 $\pm$ 0.32	3.48 $\pm$ 0.73	48 $\pm$ 22

a - Four-week study, b - Nine-week study, c - significantly different from controls (p < 0.01), ND = not detectable.

Urinary Ca remained unchanged except a slight rise after 9 weeks of
treatment at the 0.27 % dosage (table 2). Serum P remained normal.
TmP/GFR and urinary cAMP were similar in the control and treated
groups throughout the study. Serum and urinary Mg concentrations tended to decrease slightly in treated animals compared to controls (tables 1 and 2).

Table 2.   Urinary biochemical levels in controls and treated rats
(nine-week study).

	Ca (mg/mg creat.)	Mg (mg/mg creat.)	Sr (mg/mg creat.)	cAMP (nM/mg creat.)
Controls	0.023 ± 0.008	0.10 ± 0.02	ND	17.1 ± 2.9
0.19 % SrCl$_2$	0.035 ± 0.017	0.11 ± 0.03	0.063 ± 0.050	20.2 ± 8.9
0.27 % SrCl$_2$	0.042 ± 0.022^a	0.07 ± 0.04	0.103 ± 0.083	14.1 ± 1.7
0.34 % SrCl$_2$	0.035 ± 0.015	0.05 ± 0.01^a	0.078 ± 0.029	16.7 ± 2.5
0.40 % SrCl$_2$	0.038 ± 0.025	0.07 ± 0.01^a	0.107 ± 0.059	19.2 ± 3.1

a - Different from controls ($p < 0.05$ or better level of significance)
ND = not detectable.

Strontium levels in serum rose in correlation with the dosage level
at both 4 and 9 weeks of treatment and the Ca : Sr ratios in serum and
urine decreased linearly with the dose given at 4 and 9 weeks of treatment. Serum 25 OH-D and 1,25(OH)$_2$D levels were not significantly different in the control and experimental groups (table 1). Bone ash was
decreased at the doses of 0.34 and 0.40 % of SrCl$_2$ (table 3).

Table 3.   Bone mineral content in controls and treated rats.

	Bone ash (% dry bone)	Mg (mg/g ash)	Sr (mg/g ash)
Controls	65.3 ± 2.9	6.81 ± 0.52	ND
0.19 % SrCl$_2$	63.6 ± 1.8	7.43 ± 0.31	41.7 ± 6.3
0.27 % SrCl$_2$	62.6 ± 2.2	7.24 ± 0.11^a	46.1 ± 4.6
0.34 % SrCl$_2$	61.6 ± 1.1^a	7.66 ± 0.26^a	55.9 ± 5.7
0.40 % SrCl$_2$	60.0 ± 1.5^a	7.61 ± 0.51^a	62.8 ± 8.3

a - $p < 0.05$ or lower compared to controls, ND = not detectable.

While bone Ca and P remained normal, bone Mg increased in treated groups. Bone Sr content increased progressively with the dose given, and the Ca : Sr ratio decreased accordingly.

Bone histology

After 9 weeks of treatment with $SrCl_2$, the tibia lenght was similar in control and treated animals, indicating normal bone growth. Treated rats showed increased osteoid volume and surface associated at the highest dose given with increased osteoblastic surface (table 4). Table 4. Histologic parameters of bone formation in controls and treated rats.

	Osteoblastic surface (% endosteal surface)	osteoid volume (% bone tissue)	osteoid surface (% endosteal surface)	osteoid thickness (μm)
Controls	13.0 ± 2.7	0.97 ± 0.20	18.8 ± 4.3	4.8 ± 0.7
0.19 % $SrCl_2$	16.2 ± 4.2	1.46 ± 0.43 [a]	25.6 ± 7.5[a]	5.4 ± 0.9
0.27 % $SrCl_2$	16.9 ± 6.1	1.65 ± 0.50[b]	26.8 ± 8.3[a]	5.2 ± 0.9
0.34 % $SrCl_2$	15.7 ± 3.1	1.75 ± 0.64[b]	25.9 ± 6.8[a]	5.3 ± 0.7
0.40 % $SrCl_2$	18.2 ± 4.7[b]	1.96 ± 0.37[b]	34.3 ± 4.5[b]	6.7 ± 1.6[b]

a,b - Different from controls (a : $p < 0.05$, b : $p < 0.02$ or better level of significance).

Individual values for the osteoblastic surface rose in correlation with the osteoid surface and volume ($r = 0.79$ and 0.69, $p < 0.001$ respectively). The percentage of endosteal surface showing a double tetra cycline labeling increased in treated animals (table 5) in correlation with the osteoblastic surface ($r = 0.84$, $p < 0.02$).

Table 5. Dynamic parameters of bone formation.

	Double-labeled surface (% endosteal surface)	Calcification rate (μm/day)	Mineralization lag time (days)
Controls	16.7 ± 3.0	1.32 ± 0.12	3.7 ± 0.8
0.19 % $SrCl_2$	21.4 ± 6.8	1.31 ± 0.05	4.1 ± 0.7
0.27 % $SrCl_2$	22.3 ± 7.2	1.25 ± 0.16	4.2 ± 0.9
0.34 % $SrCl_2$	23.1 ± 4.7 [a]	1.18 ± 0.9 [a]	4.4 ± 0.5
0.40 % $SrCl_2$	22.4 ± 3.2 [a]	1.10 ± 0.13 [a]	6.1 ± 1.6[a]

a,b - different from controls (a : $p < 0.02$ or better level of significance)

On the other hand, the calcification rate was decreased and the mineralization lag time was prolonged at the high dosage levels(table 5),
producing an elevation of the osteoid thickness (table 4). Doses lower
than 0.40 % of $SrCl_2$ induced a 10 % rise in the trabecular bone volume
(table 6).

Table 6.   Bone density and bone resorption parameters.

	Trabecular bone volume (% bone tissue)	Osteoclastic surface (% endosteal surface)	Active bone resorbing cells (No/mm²)
Controls	20.1 ± 2.1	3.4 ± 0.5	26.1 ± 3.4
0.19 % $SrCl_2$	24.2 ± 3.5[a]	3.2 ± 0.5	22.6 ± 4.3
0.27 % $SrCl_2$	23.4 ± 3.3[a]	3.5 ± 0.7	23.3 ± 7.2
0.34 % $SrCl_2$	24.6 ± 2.7[a]	3.3 ± 0.8	25.1 ± 5.1
0.40 % $SrCl_2$	19.6 ± 2.3	3.5 ± 0.6	23.9 ± 3.2

a - different from controls ($p < 0.02$ or better level of significance)

Increased trabecular bone density did not result from decreased bone
resorption since the number of active bone resorbing cells and the
osteoclastic surface were not altered by the treatment (table 6).

DISCUSSION

As evidenced by the normal body and bone growth in treated animals,
the small oral doses of Sr used in this study did not produce deleterious effect on growth rate. Serum levels of Sr rose according to the
Sr dosage and a major fraction of the element was progressively incorporated into bone. In accordance with a previous study (St 68),
low doses of Sr produced a transitory drop in serum Ca during the
period of rapid growth of the animals. Hypocalcemia could have resulted from reduced intestinal Ca absorption in presence of Sr salts
but we did not observe a fall in Ca excretion that would have resulted from decreased Ca intake. We found normal levels of 25 OH D and
$1,25(OH)_2D$ in serum indicating that low doses of Sr did not affect
the production of vitamin D metabolites. We surmised that the slight

hypocalcemia resulted from the observed stimulated bone formation
that was more intense at the time the animals were growing rapidly.
Displacement of bone Ca by Sr during calcification could probably
account for the observed late hypercalciuria (Wa 81). It is also likely that the increased bone Mg content resulted from substitution of
both Mg and Sr for Ca ions during the process of calcification (Wa 81).
Using quantitative dynamic bone histology we were able to evaluate the
dosage level at which Sr produced toxic effects on bone calcification.
Defective bone mineralization was documented at the 0.40 % dosage
level by excessive osteoid thickness, decreased calcification rate and
prolonged mineralization lag time. Inhibition of bone mineralization
is likely to result from competition of Ca and Sr at sites of calcification (Wa 81). At $SrCl_2$ dosage levels lower than 0.34 % , the
amount of osteoid was increased in parallel with both the osteoblastic
surface and the double tetracycline labeled surface, indicating that
the number of active bone forming centers was increased or that the
period of activity of each forming site was prolonged. This effect does
not appear to result from a rise in PTH production since indices of
PTH activity on kidney or bone, namely urinary cAMP, TmP/GFR, serum 1,25
$(OH)_2D$ levels and bone resorption, remained normal. Strontium may
have influenced directly the osteoblastic activity through a protective effect on the cellular elements (Ka 65) or the ionic transport
mechanisms (Ca 65).
In parallel with the increased bone matrix production, we found that
low doses of $SrCl_2$ increased the trabecular bone density at doses that
did not inhibit bone mineralization. The positive trabecular bone
balance resulted from increased bone formation since the histomorphometric parameters of bone resorption remained normal. Our finding that
low doses of Sr can increase the trabecular bone formation in rats is
in accordance with the recent report showing that high local concentration of Sr stimulates the formation of alveolar bone in rats(Fe 83).

The beneficial effect of Sr on bone formation demonstrated experimentally could be of possible interest in the treatment of metabolic bone
diseases characterized by decreased trabecular bone formation. Further
studies are necessary to elucidate more precisely the effect of stable
strontium on bone cell metabolism.

SUMMARY

The effects of low doses of oral stable Sr (0.19 - 0.40 % $SrCl_2$) on
mineral and bone metabolism have been examined in rats using biochemical and histomorphometrical methods. Serum and bone levels of Sr rose
according to the intake of the element.
Oral Sr supplementation did not produce deleterious effects on body
growth or on mineral homeostasis except a transitory slight fall in
serum calcium. A slight defective bone mineralization was also observed at the dosage level of 0.40 % $SrCl_2$. At lower levels, strontium
supplementation stimulated bone matrix production while bone mineralization and the histochemical parameters of bone resorption remained
normal. Stimulation of bone formation without change in bone resorption
resulted in a 10 % increase in trabecular bone density. Increased
trabecular bone formation was not associated with changes in $1,25(OH)_2D$
production or parathyroid hormone effects. While the precise influence
of Sr on bone cells remains to be elucidated, this study indicates
that Sr can stimulate bone formation without altering bone resorption
in the rat.

Acknowledgments

The authors wish to thank Ms D. Modrowski and Mr A. Barbara for their
technical assistance and Ms B. Treillard for her secretarial work.

REFERENCES

Ca65 - CARAFOLI E., 1965, Active accumulation of Sr^{2+} by rat liver
mitochondria. II. Competition between Ca^{2+} and Sr^{2+}. Biophys.
Acta 97, 99-106.

Co70 - CORRADINO R.A., WASSERMAN R.H., 1970, Strontium inhibition of
vitamin D_3- induced calcium-binding protein (Ca-BP) and calcium
absorption in chick intestine. Proc. Soc. Exp. Biol. Med. 133,
960-963.

Ev79 - EVANS R.A., DUNSTAN C.R., BAYLINK D.J., 1979, Histochemical
identification of osteoclasts in undecalcified sections of
human bone. Mineral Electrolyte Metab. 2, 179-185.

Fe83 - FERRARO E.F., CARR R., ZIMMERMAN K., 1983, A comparison of the effects of strontium chloride and calcium chloride on alveolar bone. Calcif. Tissue Int. 35, 258-260.

Ja59 - JANES J.M., Mc CASLIN F., 1959, The effect of strontium lactate in the treatment of osteoporosis. Proc. Mayo Clin. 34, 329-334.

Ka65 - KAPLAN A.I., CARAFOLI E., 1965, Effect of Sr^{2+} + on swelling and ATP linked contraction of mitochondria. Biochem. Biophys. Acta 104, 317-329.

Ma83 - MARIE P.J., TRAVERS R., 1983, Effects of magnesium and lactose supplementation on bone metabolism in the X-linked hypophosphatemic mouse. Metabolism 32,2, 165-171.

Om72 - OMDAHL J.L., DELUCA H.F., 1972, Rachitogenic activity of dietary strontium. I-inhibition of intestinal calcium absorption and 1,25-dihydroxycholecalciferol synthesis. J. Biol. Chem. 247, 5520-5525.

Sh80 - SHEPARD R.M., DE LUCA H.F., 1980, Determination of vitamin D and its metabolites in plasma. In D.B.Mc Cormick, L.D. Wright ed. Methods in Enzymology 393-414, Academic Press, New York.

Sh52 - SHORR E., CARTER A.C., 1952, The usefulness of strontium as an adjuvant to calcium in the remineralization of the skeleton in osteoporosis in man. Bull. Hosp. for Joint Diseases. 13, 59-66.

Sk81 - SKORYNA S.C., FUSKOVA M., 1981, Effects of stable strontium supplementation.In Skoryna S.C. ed : Handbook of Stable Strontium, 593-617, Plenum Press, New York.

St62 - STOREY E., 1962, Intermittent bone changes and multiple cartilage defects in chronic strontium tickets in rats. J. Bone Joint Surg. 443, 194-208.

St68 - STOREY E., 1968, Calcium and strontium changes in bone associated with continuous administration of stable strontium to rats. Arch. Biochem. Biophys. 124, 575-581.

Wa81 - WADKINS C.L., PENG C.F., 1981, Strontium metabolism and mechanism of interaction with mineralized tissues. In : Skoryna S.C. ed : Handbook of Stable Strontium 545-561, Plenum Press, New York.

Wa75 - WALTON R.J., BIJVOET O.L.M., 1975, Nomogram for derivation of renal threshold phosphate concentration. Lancet 2,309-310.

13

The Distribution of Radium and Plutonium in Human Bone

R. A. SCHLENKER

INTRODUCTION

The dosimetry of radionuclides in bone provides information essential
to the interpretation of radiation effects data. The relative
biological effectiveness of different radiations is expressed as a
ratio of absorbed doses, and dose or dose equivalent are the
intermediaries through which the risk from one radionuclide is
estimated from risk data on another. Because of the wealth of
information on the skeletal effects of radiation in humans
accumulated in the study of radium poisoning, bone dosimetry has
played an important role in radiation protection. Historically,
energy deposition in the whole skeleton was the quantity first used
in radiation protection calculations for internal emitters, but
recently the International Commission on Radiological Protection
(ICRP) shifted to bone surface tissue dose (In78). For the alpha
emitters, the experimental study of dosimetry is difficult because it
must be carried out on a microscopic scale, and therefore methodology
is an important aspect of the work. Traditionally, the necessary
data have been collected from autoradiographs, but alpha spectrometry
is being developed as a tool. This paper presents aspects of current
and recent work conducted in my laboratory on the distribution of
radium and plutonium near the surfaces of human bone and applications

This work was supported by the U.S. Department of Energy under
Contract No. W-31-109-ENG-38.

of the data. There are sections on methods, surface deposit thickness, radium distribution near the endosteal surface, the use of alpha spectrometry in conjunction with autoradiography, radium distribution in the mastoid, and factors affecting plutonium specific activity. Much emphasis is placed on the alpha spectrometry technique because of its usefulness and its recent application to problems of local dosimetry.

METHODS

(a) Alpha Spectrometry

Because the energy loss of alpha particles in matter is well understood, it is possible to extract information on the spatial distribution of an alpha emitter within the effective sample volume* from the alpha energy spectrum, dn/dE, of a thick embedded or unembedded bone sample. By the chain rule of differential calculus, $dn/dx = (dn/dE)(dE/dx)$, where dn/dE is the number of alpha particles reaching the detector with energies between E and $E + dE$, dn/dx is the number which travels distances in bone between x and $x + dx$ before escaping into the vacuum between the sample and the detector (Sc75), and dE/dx is the stopping power. The distance spectrum, dn/dx, is closely related to the spatial distribution of the alpha emitter. For plane samples measured with a sample-to-detector distance that is much greater than the largest sample dimension, dn/dx is directly proportional to the average concentration of emitter as a function of depth beneath the surface. Because the energy resolution of surface barrier detectors is so great, typically 40 to 50 keV for alphas of 3 to 9 MeV, the resolution of the distance spectrum is also high, less than 1 μm under optimum conditions (Sc75).

By the use of stripping techniques, energy spectra of radionuclide mixtures can be resolved into separate components and the relative abundances of the nuclides established. It is also possible to obtain a quantitative calibration which permits the estimation of radionuclide concentration.

---

*The effective sample volume is the surface layer of bone to a depth of one alpha particle range.

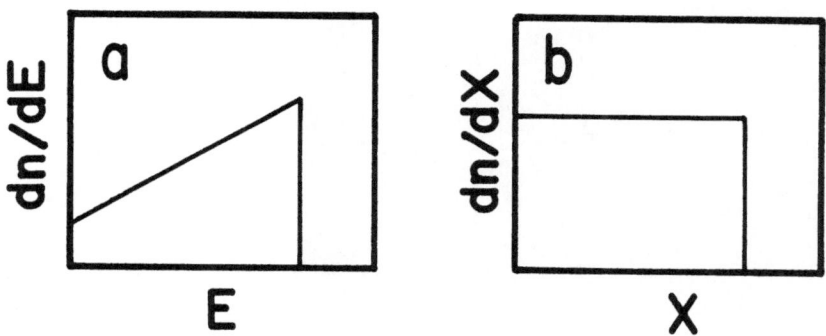

FIGURE 1 Schematic representations of (a) energy and (b) distance
spectra.

Figure 1 illustrates the duality between energy and distance
spectra. An energy spectrum with the shape of a linear ramp is shown
to the left and beside it is the corresponding distance spectrum. In
practical situations, a rectangular, i.e. constant, distance spectrum
indicates a uniform spatial distribution of nuclide within the
effective sample volume. It is not difficult to imagine that if the
energy spectrum were concave upward, the distance spectrum would be
also and if the energy spectrum were concave downward, the distance
spectrum would be also. Hence, energy spectra that are concave
upward, linear ramps, or concave downward strongly suggest the
existence of distributions within the effective sample volume, that
decrease with depth, are constant, or increase with depth,
respectively.

(b) <u>Autoradiography</u>

For alpha detection, we use Eastman Kodak NTA emulsion plates in
tight contact with 100-μm thick bone sections. Emulsion allows a
faint shadow of the section (Figure 2) to be recorded on the
autoradiograph as a guide to establishing registration when the
autoradiograph and section are viewed simultaneously through a single
set of eyepieces connected to a pair of microscopes (Mar75). The
section is stained with methyl green to increase its opacity for the
shadow-casting process.

For fission fragment detection, a 100-μm thick bone section laden
with ^{239}Pu is placed in tight contact with a 300-μm thick sheet of
Lexan plastic and the combination is exposed to thermal neutrons.
Tracks are etched by floating the Lexan on 6N NaOH at temperatures

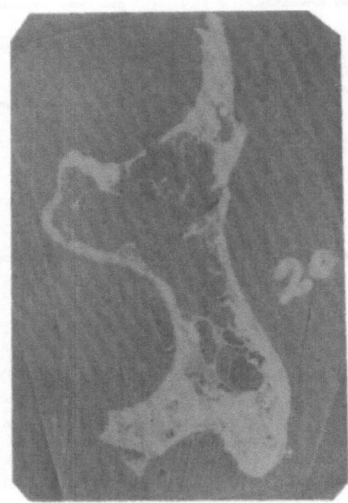

FIGURE 2   An example of shadowing on NTA emulsion. Because the
photographic image is negative, the shadow is light.

between 40 and 90°C, to avoid the introduction of visible artifacts
on the underside of the Lexan sheet. The bone image (Je72) assures
registration between the pattern of tracks and the outline of the
section.

(c) Spatial Resolution

Of the three methods, alpha spectrometry has the greatest spatial
resolution.   Fission   track autoradiography is second.   When
autoradiographs are carefully developed and viewed, the position of
the track entry point in Lexan relative to the bone surface can be
determined with an accuracy better than 5 μm.   Since the fission
fragments can originate at any depth in the bone section within range
of the Lexan, the actual spatial resolution is somewhat poorer than
5 μm. With alpha track autoradiography, the difficulty of achieving
truly precise registration limits the resolution greatly. The shadow
edge is not always easy to detect and may not correspond precisely to
the outline of the section because of penumbra and non-zero section
thickness.   Entry points are not easy to determine, especially for
short tracks that lie nearly parallel to the emulsion surface with
high grain density along their full length.   The best resolution
achievable is probably 20-30 μm except in extremely favorable
circumstances.

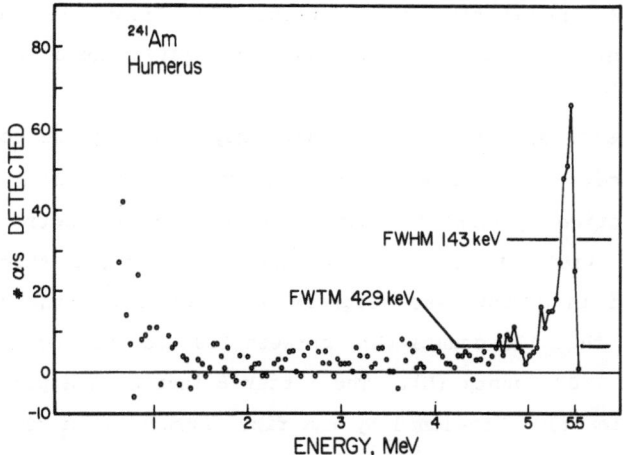

FIGURE 3   Endosteal surface alpha spectrum of ^{241}Am in human bone.

SURFACE DEPOSIT THICKNESS

Figure 3 shows the endosteal surface alpha spectrum of cortical bone
from a person accidentally exposed to ^{241}Am (sample supplied by the
U.S. Transuranium Registry).   The spectrum peak is confined to a
narrow range close to 5.49 MeV, the average energy of alpha particles
emitted by disintegrating ^{241}Am. The alphas that created the peak,
therefore, lost little energy and traveled only a short distance
through bone before being detected and could only have originated in
deposits at or near the surface. The full width at half maximum of
the peak (FWHM), divided by the alpha stopping power in bone provides
an index of deposit thickness, which here equals 143 keV $\div$ 134 keV/μm
= 1.1 μm.   Although the relationship between them is unknown, the
index and the deposit thickness cannot differ greatly in value.

The width of the peak at its base, divided by the stopping power,
provides an upper limit on deposit thickness. Non-flatness of the
bone surface, small sample-detector separation, and electronic noise
from the pulse amplifiers in the data collection system widen the
peak and guarantee that this quotient exceeds the deposit
thickness. Since the spectrum tail obscures the base of the peak,
the full width at one-tenth maximum (FWTM) is used as a practical
alternative to the base width. All but a negligible fraction of the
peak area is included within this energy interval and the ratio of
FWTM to stopping power defines a distance which is equal to, or
greater than, the distance traveled by all but a negligible fraction

of the particles contributing to the peak. For Figure 3, the full width at one-tenth maximum is 429 keV and the equivalent distance is 3.2 μm.

Table 1 presents data for radionuclides deposited on the cortical endosteal surface. The data were obtained from spectra which varied widely in statistical precision. Since a more precise spectrum would be expected to yield a more precise index of deposit thickness, letters included in parentheses signify peaks in which the highest point was less than 100 counts (L), between 100 and 1000 counts (M), or in excess of 1000 counts (H). The letter B indicates a peak width that was significantly broadened by the fine structure of the alpha

Table 1. Surface deposit thickness index

Species	Nuclide	FWHM,[a] keV	Index, μm
Dog	^{212}Pb[b]	140(M)[c]	1.5
	^{224}Ra	133(H)	1.0
	^{226}Ra	178(H)	1.2
	^{228}Th	246(M,B)	1.8
Human	^{239}Pu	122(M)	0.87
	^{241}Am	143(L)	1.1

[a] Full width at half maximum.
[b] Based on the ^{212}Po daughter product.
[c] See text for explanation of letters in parentheses.

particle spectrum; for ^{228}Th, the principal emission energies are 5.42 and 5.34 MeV. Thus, the FWHM may be 0.08 MeV (80 keV) wider than if particles of a single energy were emitted in the decay of ^{228}Th. Fine structure is present with ^{239}Pu and ^{241}Am, but its effect is probably less pronounced. Because ^{212}Pb is a beta emitter, the thickness index and FWHM are based on observations of its alpha emitting daughter, ^{212}Po.

The similarity in values for the different nuclides suggests the existence of a single anatomical compartment in human and dog bone capable of binding all radionuclides at bone surfaces regardless of their chemical properties. This compartment may be the boundary zone, represented by the lamina limitans (Mi80) in electron micrographs, between the thin layer of collagenous tissue which occurs at bone surfaces and the mineralized matrix.

RADIUM DISTRIBUTION NEAR THE ENDOSTEAL SURFACE

In the radiation protection literature, endosteal tissue dose values for bone volume seekers are calculated by assuming the radionuclide to be uniformly distributed throughout bone (In78). Advantage has been taken of the high spatial resolution of alpha spectrometry to test this assumption. In the three subjects examined so far, the radium distribution near the bone surface has been quite nonuniform, with a pronounced tendency to rise to a maximum at the surface. Figure 4 shows a spectrum from this group. Although peaks reminiscent of those found for surface seekers are prominent (compare to ^{241}Am, Figure 3), this spectrum was recorded 39 years after first exposure, at a time when radium would be classified as a volume seeker. For contrast, the spectrum of a spatially uniform source, made by grinding ashed bone to a powder and mixing it thoroughly, is shown in Figure 5 (Mau78).

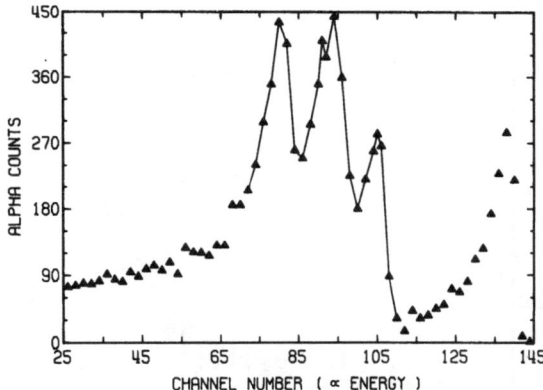

FIGURE 4   Endosteal surface alpha spectrum of ^{226}Ra and its daughters in human bone 39 years after injection (Case 01-302). From the left, the peaks correspond to ^{226}Ra, ^{210}Po, ^{222}Rn, ^{218}Po, and ^{214}Po.

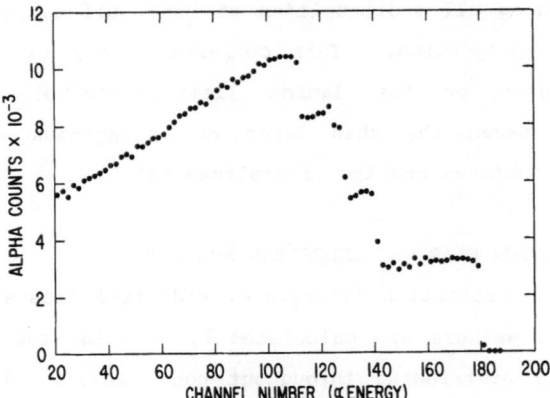

FIGURE 5   Alpha spectrum of ^{226}Ra and its daughters uniformly
distributed in ashed bone. From the left, the
discontinuities correspond to ^{226}Ra, ^{210}Po, ^{222}Rn, ^{218}Po,
and ^{214}Po.

Radium daughter product concentrations are usually different in
vitro than in vivo due to the delay between death and measurement,
and to the fact that ^{222}Rn retention is affected by changes in the
water content of bone.   The daughter product contributions must,
therefore, be separated from the total spectrum.   This can be
performed electronically with alpha-gamma coincidence spectrometry or
mathematically by stripping away the daughter product contributions
(Mau79). Figure 6 compares the results of the two methods.

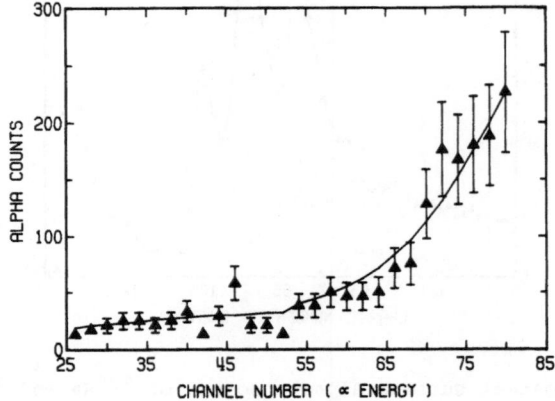

FIGURE 6   The ^{226}Ra component from Figure 4 determined by
coincidence counting (points) and independently by
mathematical deconvolution (solid curve).

The sample-detector geometry can be calibrated through the use of standardized solutions. A gold foil cover is molded to the sample surface. A known quantity of solution is then spread over the foil and dried and an alpha count is made to determine the fraction (g) of particle emission from the foil which is detected. For accuracy, the angular distributions of alpha particles from the foil and bone surface should be the same. This requirement is met sufficiently well when the sample-to-detector distance exceeds the detector radius and the largest sample dimension is less than the detector radius. If N_{226} is the number of ^{226}Ra alpha particles detected, N_{226}/g is the number of alphas emitted within the effective sample volume during the data collection period.

For dose-rate calculation, the endosteal tissue mass and $(dn/dx)/g$, the spatial distribution corrected for sample-detector calibration are required. The latter can be computed from the distance spectrum, an example of which is given in Figure 7 for the ^{226}Ra component of Figure 6. The former may be determined from the

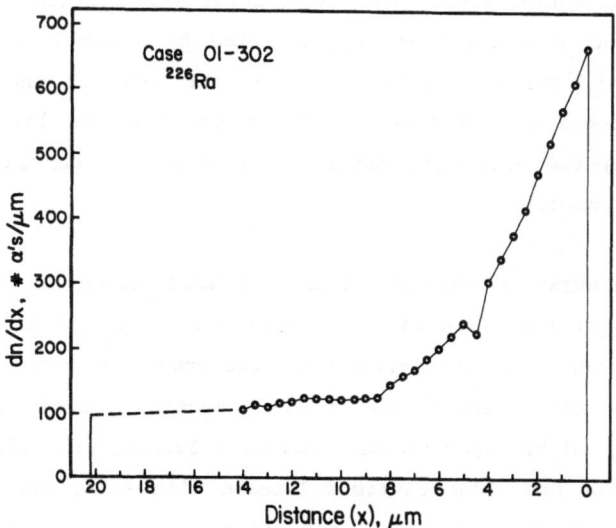

FIGURE 7   The distance spectrum for the solid curve of Figure 6. The dashed portion is an extrapolation.

sample surface area, which can be estimated from a photograph of the sample surface or calculated from the three-dimensional coordinates of the surface measured with a light section microscope. A photograph gives the sample area projected onto a plane and,

therefore, always underestimates the total area. Figure 8 shows a
computer reconstruction of the sample surface from light section
data. The area measured this way is 0.253 cm^2 and that measured from
a photograph is 0.241 cm^2, a 5% difference.

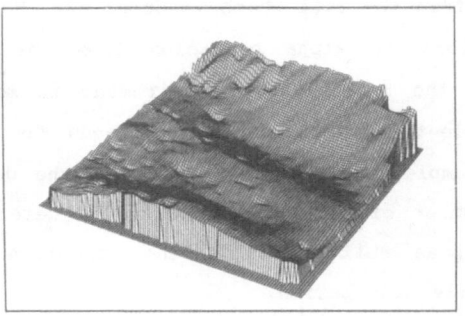

FIGURE 8   Computer reconstruction of the cortical endosteal surface
of the sample used to obtain the spectrum of Figure 4.

The dose is calculated assuming a plane bone surface because the
short range of the alpha particles makes the dose quite insensitive
to surface irregularities. For the spatial distribution of Figure 7
and reciprocal stopping power approximated by a linear function of
energy (Sc75), the dose rate, based on the calculations of Thorne
(Th77), averaged over a 10-μm thick endosteal tissue layer is 0.49
rad/day, compared with 0.34 rad/day when a uniform concentration of
radium is assumed.

ALPHA SPECTROMETRY IN CONJUNCTION WITH AUTORADIOGRAPHY
The analysis of track lengths and angles can be used to determine the
relative abundances of different radionuclides when mixtures
(Fe83,Ro56) are present in tissue sections used for autoradiography. Alpha spectrometry offers a labor-saving alternative.

The spectra from bone sections labeled with ^{226}Ra are similar to
the spectrum shown in Figure 5 but often with an additional narrow
^{210}Po peak attributable to the fallout of airborne short-lived radon
daughters during the storage of sections in closed containers or
other environments from which radon released by the sections cannot
readily escape. The long-lived beta emitter, ^{210}Pb, thus accumulates
in thin deposits on the section surface and its daughter, ^{210}Po,
produces a peak in alpha spectra. An example is shown in Figure 9.

The composite spectrum can be easily stripped because the nuclides within bone are uniformly concentrated as a function of depth in the effective sample volume and, therefore, all contribute linear ramp

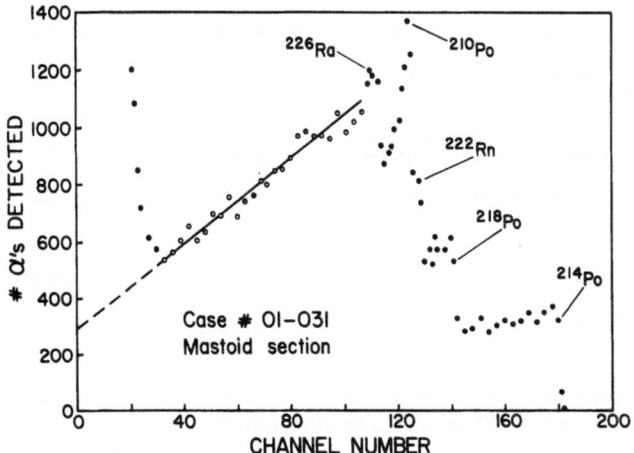

FIGURE 9   Alpha spectrum of a mastoid bone section. The straight line is used in spectrum stripping.

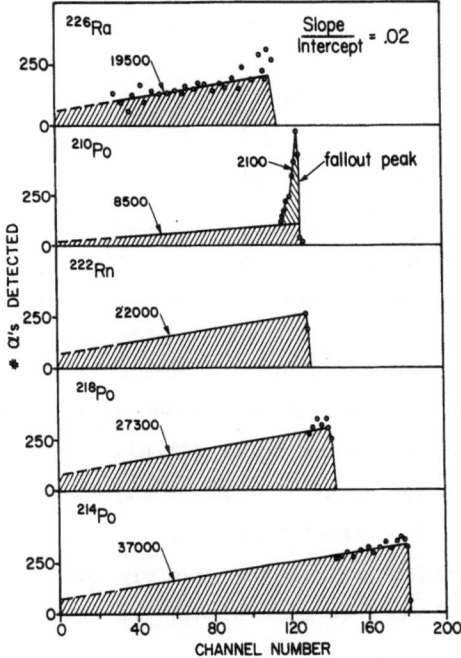

FIGURE 10   The component spectra of Figure 9, obtained by spectrum stripping as described in the text.

components with the same ratio of line slope to y-axis intercept. This ratio can be determined by fitting a straight line to the linear portion of the composite as shown in Figure 9. Linear ramps with the same ratio of slope to intercept can be fitted to the high energy ends of the components, and the components can be subtracted out one by one. The components thus obtained for Figure 9 are shown in Figure 10.

The area beneath each component (Figure 10) gives the number of alpha particles contributing to the composite spectrum, and the ratio of component area to composite area gives, with reasonable accuracy, the fraction of tracks in an autoradiograph attributable to each nuclide (Table 2).

Table 2. Percentages of alpha tracks in NTA emulsion expected to be produced by ^{226}Ra and its daughters

Nuclide	Best estimate	Ratio of areas
^{226}Ra	14	17
^{222}Rn	17	19
^{218}Po	23	23
^{214}Po	37	32
^{210}Po - total	9	9
- fallout	3	2

RADIUM DISTRIBUTION IN THE MASTOID

The mastoid, middle ear, and sinuses have been prominent sites for carcinoma induction in radium cases (Ev66). By a combination of autoradiographic measurement, bone morphometry, quantitative histology, and modeling (Ha81,Sc80,Sc83), it appears possible to determine the terminal dose rate and possibly the total lifetime dose to the epithelial tissues at risk within the mastoid and middle ear mucosa.

The epithelial cell dose is thought to be delivered by alpha particles emitted from the bone and air space (Ev66) as illustrated for a single sinus cavity in Figure 11. The presence of radioactivity in the air space results from the production of radon gas by radium deposits in bone and the subsequent translocation of most of the radon by atomic diffusion.

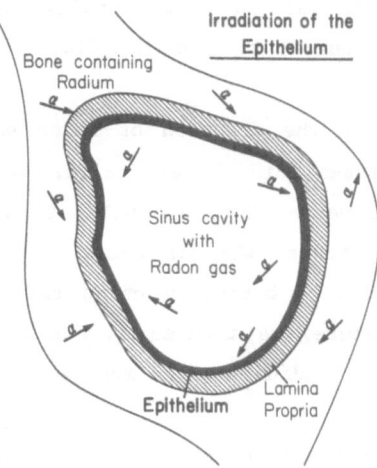

FIGURE 11   Schematic representation of a sinus showing epithelial irradiation by alpha particles from bone and from the air space.

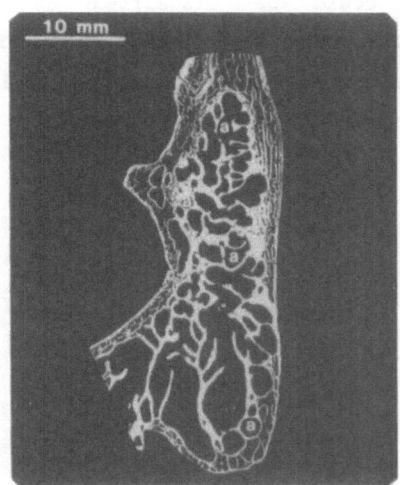

FIGURE 12   A mastoid bone section viewed by microradiography. Some air cells are identified by labels (a).

The mastoid consists of a honeycomb of air cells (Figure 12), each irradiated similarly to the sinus.   There are two morphologically distinct regions, the thin trabeculae-like bony septa that separate the air cells and the envelope of compact or cancellous bone that surrounds the air cell honeycomb. These regions differ also in their circulation. The envelope is liberally penetrated by blood vessels while the bony septa are almost totally devoid of internal circulation. Their nutrients are supplied from vessels in the mucosa.

These factors affect the fraction of radon generated within the two regions that diffuses into the air cells. Nearly all free radon will diffuse from the septa, but only half of the free radon in the envelope will diffuse toward the air cells, and much of it will be cleared by the circulation before reaching the air cells. The two regions should, therefore, be treated as distinct sources of radon and the partitioning of radium between the regions is quite important dosimetrically.

Low-resolution autoradiographs have revealed the radium distribution pattern exemplified by Figure 13, in which the radioactivity concentration appears to be lower in the septa than in the envelope. Examinations of many autoradiographs from 15 subjects showed 12 that could be classified as having low septal concentrations. This phenomenon has been examined by quantitative autoradiographic measurements at randomly selected sites within mastoid bone sections.

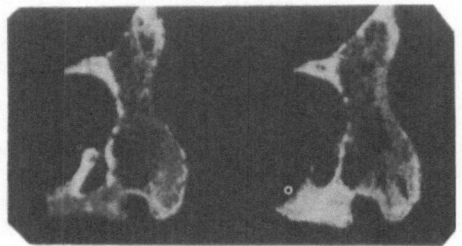

FIGURE 13 Autoradiographs of mastoid sections showing low septal and high envelope concentrations of ^{226}Ra and its daughters.

Radium specific activities estimated from track count data using an expression presented by Schlenker and Farnham (Sc76a) are given in Table 3 and verify the conclusions drawn from the visual assessment of autoradiographs, although 14 of the 15 cases, rather than 12 of 15, show lower septal than envelope concentrations. The reason for the persistent difference between concentrations is unknown. One possibility is that blood perfusion of the envelope was much higher than of the mucosal membranes lining the septa. Another possibility is that bone formation activity was greater in the envelope, at the ages of exposure (first exposure occurred between 14 and 57 years).

Whatever the explanation, it is clear that the difference in concentrations affects the assessment of radiation dose, which, in the absence of direct observations, would be computed on the assumption that the specific activity in both regions was the same and equal to the average measured in the skeletons of these subjects. This would lead to a large error in most cases.

Table 3. ^{226}Ra specific activities in mastoid septa and envelopes measured by autoradiography and the skeletal average measured by gamma-ray detection

Case Number	^{226}Ra, pCi/g wet bone		
	Septa	Envelope	Skeletal Average
00–006	590	790	920
00–009	390	1100	720
00–027	610	840	630
01–011	320	620	2200
01–014	150	360	630
01–031	120	190	310
01–046	140	200	240
01–145	110	1400	2000
01–562	940	1800	3500
01–613	70	200	210
03–209	30	130	240
03–240	320	1200	1600
10–644	1700	1600	1700
10–831	60	150	150
10–840	80	94	130

FACTORS AFFECTING PLUTONIUM SPECIFIC ACTIVITY

Substantial differences in plutonium specific activity have been observed between different parts of the skeleton (La78) in a subject from the Langham et al. injection series (Du72) for which there are autoradiographic data (Sc76b,Sc81). Because plutonium is a surface seeker, variation in the bone surface area per gram would be expected to affect specific activity. Other important factors would be the amount of buried bone surface labeled by plutonium, and the surface concentration.

Figure 14 shows a fission track autoradiograph from the subject in question verifying the surface deposition of plutonium. The arrow points to a plutonium-labeled buried bone surface near an existing surface.

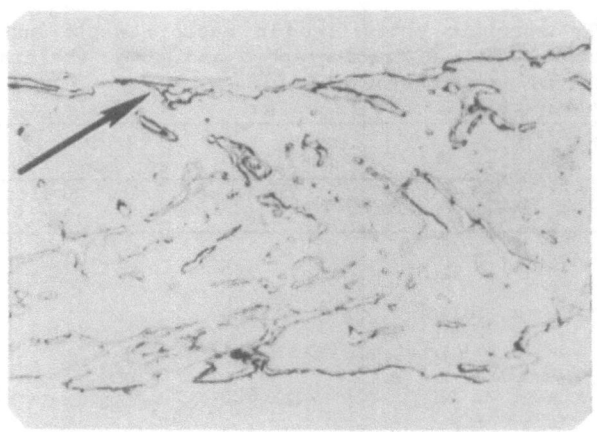

FIGURE 14   Autoradiograph of ^{239}Pu in the iliac crest. The arrow points to a plutonium laden buried bone surface.

Larsen found the plutonium specific activity in bone pieces analyzed radiochemically to be an order of magnitude higher in parts of the axial skeleton than in parts of the appendicular skeleton (La78). To determine how surface area, buried surface area and surface concentration conspire to produce such a difference, the specific activity must be expressed in terms of these quantities. The amount of plutonium on the surfaces and buried surfaces of bone is approximately S(1 + f)C where S is the surface area, f times S is the area of plutonium labeled buried surface, and C is the surface concentration. The amount of bone ash is $\rho_{ash}V$ where V is the bone volume and ρ_{ash} is the ash content per unit volume. The specific activity is, therefore, $(S/V)(1 + f)(C/\rho_{ash})$. The ratio of specific activities between two parts of the skeleton would be $[(S/V)_2/(S/V)_1][(1 + f_2)/(1 + f_1)][C_2/C_1]$.

The surface-to-volume ratio, S/V, is calculated from the perimeter to area ratio (P/A) measured from the bone section image on the autoradiograph. For cancellous bone, $S/V = (4/\pi)(P/A)$ and for compact bone, $S/V = P/A$. The ratio, f, of buried to existing surface is measured by scanning across the autoradiograph and counting the number of times a surface or a plutonium labeled buried surface is encountered. Concentration is determined by fission track counts and calibration factors.

Average values for S/V, 1 + f, and C for three anatomical regions are presented in Table 4. Specific activity ratios calculated as indicated above and those based on Larsen's radiochemical data (La78) are compared in Table 5.

Table 4. Surface-to-volume ratio, ratio of buried to existing surface, and surface plutonium concentration in Case 40-010

Region	S/V, cm^{-1}	1 + f	C, pCi/cm^2
Axial skeleton	213	1.41	1.0
Proximal femur	161	1.10	0.36
Long bone midshafts	35	1.09	0.25

Table 5. Ratios of specific activity in different regions of the skeleton, based on autoradiographic and radiochemical data

Regions	Autoradiographic	Radiochemical
Axial/femur	4.7	3.6
Axial/midshaft	31	31
Femur/midshaft	6.7	8.6

The agreement between the autoradiographic and radiochemical observations is good, verifying that S/V, f, and C are the principal determinants of specific activity in this subject.

By considering the ratios of individual factors, i.e., $(S/V)_2/(S/V)_1$, $(1 + f_2)/(1 + f_1)$ and C_2/C_1, the relative importance of each in determining the specific activity ratio can be established. These are presented in Table 6. Clearly, the difference in surface concentration is the most important determinant of the difference in specific activities between the axial skeleton and proximal femur. The difference in surface-to-volume ratios is the most important determinant of the difference in specific activities between the axial skeleton and long bone midshafts and between the proximal femur and long bone midshafts. Overall, the differences in surface-to-volume ratios and in concentrations are more important than the difference in the amount of buried bone surface.

Table 6. Ratios of the principal factors that affect the plutonium concentration in bone

Regions	$\dfrac{(S/V)_2}{(S/V)_1}$	$\dfrac{1 + f_2}{1 + f_1}$	$\dfrac{C_2}{C_1}$
Axial/femur	1.32	1.28	2.78
Axial/midshaft	6.09	1.29	4.00
Femur/midshaft	4.60	1.01	1.44

SUMMARY

This review of work at Argonne National Laboratory has dealt with the microdistribution of radium and plutonium in human bone with emphases on the alpha spectrometry method of measurement, the determination of deposit thickness for bone-surface seekers, the establishment of radium concentration close to the endosteal surface, the use of alpha spectrometry as a labor-saving method for determining the relative abundance of radionuclides in bone sections used for autoradiography, the measurement of radium concentration within different portions of the mastoid bone, and the explanation of why differences occur in plutonium specific activity within different portions of the skeleton.

Some of the findings reported are that alpha spectrometry offers particularly high spatial resolution and is therefore especially well suited to the measurement of radionuclide concentrations at, and adjacent to, the endosteal surfaces. Surface deposits for isotopes of lead, radium, and the actinides are of the order of 1 μm thick. Volume deposits of ^{226}Ra can be quite nonuniform near bone surfaces and this leads to endosteal tissue dose rates that are higher than expected under the assumption of uniform volume concentration normally used for radiation protection calculations. The bony septa of the mastoid air cell system in high-dose radium cases tend to be depleted in radium relative to the envelope of the mastoid bone surrounding them, and this is expected to have a significant influence on the dosimetry of the mastoid epithelia. A combination of autoradiographic and morphometric measurements indicates that plutonium specific activities are higher in the axial than in the appendicular skeleton primarily because the axial skeleton has higher bone surface-to-volume ratios and higher bone surface concentrations of plutonium.

REFERENCES

Du72   Durbin P. W., 1972, "Plutonium in Man: A New Look at the Old Data", in Radiobiology of Plutonium (Stover B. J. and Jee W. S. S., eds.), J. W. Press, University of Utah, Salt Lake City, pp. 469-537.

Ev66   Evans R. D., "The Effect of Skeletally Deposited Alpha-Ray Emitters in Man", 1966, Brit. J. Radiol. 39, 881-895.

Fe83   Fews A. P. and Henshaw D. L., 1983, "Alpha-particle Autoradiography in CR-39: A Technique for Quantitative Assessment of Alpha Emitters in Biological Tissue", Phys. Med. Biol. 28, 459-474.

Ha81   Harris M. J. and Schlenker R. A., 1981, "Quantitative Histology of the Mucous Membrane of the Accessary Nasal Sinus and Mastoid Cavities", Ann Otol., Rhinol., Laryngol., 90, 33-37.

In78   International Commission on Radiological Protection, 1978, "Limits for Intakes of Radionuclides by Workers", ICRP Publication 30, Part 1, Pergamon Press, Oxford, 1978, p. 37.

Je72   Jee W. S. S., 1972, "239Pu in Bones as Visualized by Photographic and Neutron-Induced Autoradiography", in Radiobiology of Plutonium (Stover B. J. and Jee W. S. S., eds.), J. W. Press, University of Utah, Salt Lake City, pp. 171-193.

La78   Larsen R. P., Oldham R. D., Cacic C. G., Farnham J. E. and Schneider J. R., 1978, "Distribution of Injected Plutonium in the Skeleton and Certain Soft Tissues", in Radiological and Environmental Research Division Annual Report, Center for Human Radiobiology, Argonne National Laboratory Report Number ANL-78-65, Part II, pp. 145-153.

Mar75   Marshall J. H., Groer P. G., Selman R. F., Keefe D. J. and Paul J. M., 1975, "The Microanalyzer", J. Nucl. Med. Biol. 2, 67-72. See also Radiological and Environmental Research Division Annual Report, Center for Human Radiobiology, July 1972-June 1973, Argonne National Laboratory Report Number ANL-8060, Part II, pp. 242-255.

Mau78   Mausner L. F. and Schlenker R. A., 1978, "Analysis of Thick Source Alpha Particle Spectrum from Radium and its Daughters in Bone", in Radiological and Environmental Research Division Annual Report, Center for Human Radiobiology, Argonne National Laboratory Report Number ANL-78-65, Part II, pp. 80-94.

Mau79   Mausner L. F. and Schlenker R. A., 1979, "Stripping of the Alpha Spectrum from a Bone with a Non-Uniform Depth Distribution of Radium", in Radiological and Environmental Research Division Annual Report, Center for Human Radiobiology, Argonne National Laboratory Report Number ANL-79-65, Part II, pp. 66-69.

Mi80   Miller S. C., Bowman B. M., Smith J. M. and Jee W. S. S., 1980, "Characterization of Endosteal Bone-Lining Cells from Fatty Marrow Bone Sites in Adult Beagles", Anat. Rec. 198, 163-173.

Ro56   Rotblatt J. and Ward G. B., 1956, "Analysis of the Radioactive Content of Tissues by α-Track Autoradiography", Phys. Med. Biol. 1, 57-70.

Sc75   Schlenker R. A. and Marshall J. H., 1975, "Thicknesses of the Deposits of Plutonium and Radium at Bone Surfaces in the Beagle", Health Phys. 29, 649-654.

Sc76a   Schlenker R. A. and Farnham J. E., 1976, "Microscopic Distribution of 226Ra in the Bones of Radium Cases: A Comparison Between Diffuse and Average 226Ra Concentrations", in The Health Effects of Plutonium and Radium (Jee W. S. S., ed.), J. W. Press, University of Utah, Salt Lake City, pp. 437-449.

Sc76b   Schlenker R. A., Oltman B. G. and Cummins H. T., 1976, "Microscopic Distribution of ^{239}Pu Deposited in Bone from a Human Injection Case", in The Health Effects of Plutonium and Radium (Jee W. S. S., ed.), J. W. Press, University of Utah, Salt Lake City, pp. 321-328.

Sc80   Schlenker R. A., 1980, "Dosimetry of Paranasal Sinus and Mastoid Epithelia in Radium-Exposed Humans", in Radiological and Environmental Research Division Annual Report, Center for Human Radiobiology, Argonne National Laboratory Report Number ANL-80-115, Part II, pp. 1-21.

Sc81   Schlenker R. A. and Oltman B. G., 1981, "Plutonium Microdistribution in Human Bone", in Actinides in Man and Animals (Wrenn M. E., ed.), R. D. Press, University of Utah, Salt Lake City, pp. 199-206.

Sc83   Schlenker R. A., 1983, "Mucosal Structure and Radon in Head Carcinoma Dosimetry", Health Phys. 44, 556-562.

Th77   Thorne M. C., 1977, "Aspects of the Dosimetry of Alpha-emitting Radionuclides in Bone with Particular Emphasis on ^{226}Ra and ^{239}Pu", Phys. Med. Biol. 22, 36-46.

14

Skeletal Distribution of Stable Strontium and its Incorporation into Bone Mineral *In Vivo*

S. BANG, C. A. BAUD, H. J. TOCHON-DANGUY, and J. –M. VERY

Twenty-one-day-old mice were maintained on a high strontium (Sr) diet up to 16 months. The femurs were analysed for the incorporation of stable strontium into the bone tissue and its effects on bone mineral substance, by means of X-ray emission, absorption, and diffraction, and of infra-red (IR) spectrophotometry.

Sr $L\alpha_1$ characteristic X-ray images and the line scan profiles (Fig.1) show the topographical distribution pattern of Sr in the bone sections. The Sr is highly deposited in the bone layers formed during the period of the Sr diet, whereas a small amount of Sr is found in the bone tissue existing before the Sr administration (Ba72).

The microdensitometric analysis of the microradiographs indicates a low degree of mineralization in the Sr-laden bones (1.35g. min/cm^3) comparing with those of control animals (1.50g. min/cm^3).

The X-ray diffraction analysis of powdered bone samples reveals a lengthening of the parameter a of the unit cell as a function of increasing Sr-content: +0.04 Å for Sr/Ca molar ratio 0.1/1. These observations indicate that systemically ingested stable strontium incorporates into the crystalline structure as an isomorphous exchange of Sr for

Ca in the bone apatite.

Infra-red spectra of bone mineral deposited under the
influence of Sr-diet are consistent with a partial Sr substitution in the apatite structure, and show a lower
crystallinity index than that of control animals. Crystal
size and/or perfection, evaluated by measuring the width
of the X-ray diffraction lines, is also low (Ba77).

REFERENCES

Ba72   Bang S. and Baud C.A., 1972, Topographic distribution of strontium and its incorporation into bone
  mineral substance *in vivo* , in: Shinoda G., Kohra K. and
  Ichinokawa T. (eds.), Proc.6th Int.Conf.X-ray Optics and
  Microanalysis, pp. 835-840 (Univ. of Tokyo Press).

Ba77   Baud C.A., Bang S. and Very J.M., 1977, Minor elements in bone mineral and their effects on its solubility,
  J. Biol. Buccale **5**, 195-202.

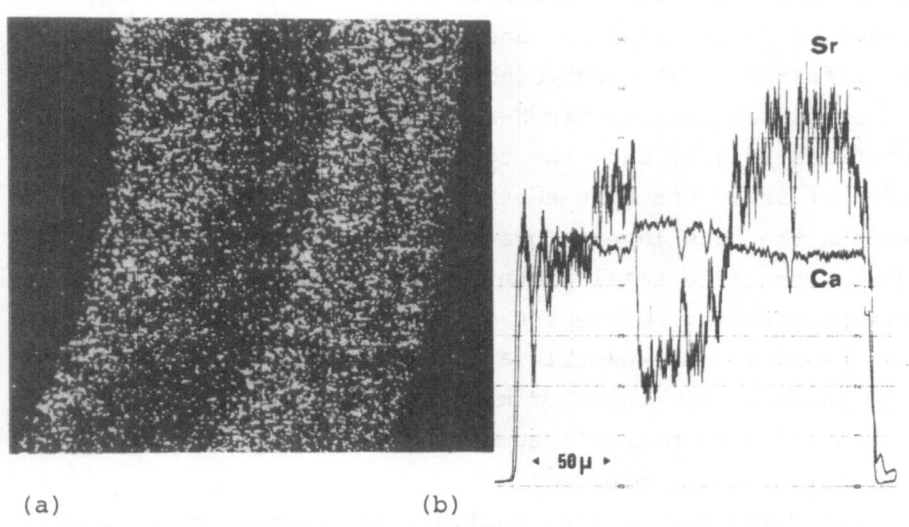

(a)   (b)

FIGURE 1   Sr $L\alpha_1$ X-ray image (a) and line scan profile of
           Ca and Sr (b) of femoral bone section of a mouse
           kept on a Sr-diet for 5 months. Sr is predomi-
           nantly deposited in the bone layers formed
           during the Sr-diet.

15

Convolution Analysis Applied to Skeletal Uptake of ^{47}Ca and ^{85}Sr Measured by External Counting

V. JOVANOVIĆ

V. JOVANOVIĆ

INTRODUCTION

Convolution methods have been applied to analyse the
relationship between serum radioactivity (S(t)) and the skeletal
retention (R(t)) of Ca* and Sr*:

$$R(t) = F \int_o^t S(x) \cdot W(t-x)dx$$

where W(t) is the impulse response function of the skeleton for
tracer. It has been postulated that the retention of the tracer in
the bone could be expressed by the following equation (Re 76):

$$R(t) = 100 - CS(t) - k \int_o^t S(t)dt$$

where C represents the space of the extracellular Ca (C=13-15% of the
body weight) and k is the whole body clearance of the tracer.

The aim of this work was to proceed with the investigation of
the application of the deconvolution method to the retention data
measured by external counting of the arm and leg radioactivities.
For this purpose we analysed data taken from literature (ICRP 72) and
our own data for subjects who received ^{47}Ca orally and ^{85}Sr i.v.
(Jo 79).

RESULTS & DISCUSSION

The impulse function of the bone (W(t)) declines as a power
function during the first day and after that on about 3rd day W(t)
has a constant value (c. 400 mgCa/d). Within the experimental error

W(t)s for Ca* and Sr* are not different. The radioactivities of Ca* and Sr* in blood are controlled by W(t) and urinary clearance of the tracer.

The "regional" impulse functions wr(t) are similar to W(t) but not identical. The wr(t) describes transfer of Ca between blood/soft tissues and bone in proportion depending on the region of the measurements and "field of view" of the instrument. The deconvolution analyses of the retention data measured by external counting showed that wr(t)s in the first few hours differ depending on whether the tracer was given orally or i.v. However it is not clear whether this fact is connected with faulty theoretical/model assumption or with errors involved in the calculations. In the period between the 3rd and 5th day after application of tracer, wr(t)s are nearly constant (about 7 mg Ca/d).

Comparison of regional wr(t)s with W-bone suggested that the W-bone in the first few hours reflects the equilibration of the tracer with soft tissues. After about one day wr(t) correlates with W-bone, and this fact gives opportunity to determine the accretion rate of bone calcium after oral administration of Ca* (Jo 81).

The results of this work indicate that deconvolution analysis will find application for better understanding of bone/tracer exchange and bone physiology.

REFERENCES

ICRP 72   ICRP Publication 20. (1972). Alkaline Earth Metabolism in Adult Man. Report of Task Group of Committee 2.

Jo 79   Jovanovic, V and Peric, M (1979). Determination of the rate of radiocalcium intestinal absorption on the basis of ^{85}Sr and ^{47}Ca radioactivities measured by external counting. Calcif. Tiss. Int. Suppl., A19 (Abstracts)

Jo 81   Jovanovic, V and Harmut, M (1981). Determination of the accretion rate of the bone calcium after single oral administration of ^{47}Ca. Coll. Antropol., 5, 59-71

Re 76   Reeve, J and Hesp, R (1976). Comparison of uptake and short term retention of ^{47}Ca and ^{85}Sr. Calcif. Tiss. Res., 22, 183-189.

Part 4
Actinide Metals and Bone

16

Toxicity of Plutonium and Americium: Relationship of Bone Composition to Location of ^{226}Ra, ^{239}Pu and ^{241}Am-Induced Bone Sarcomas

W. S. S. JEE, R. B. DELL, N. J. PARKS, S. C. MILLER and M. E. WRENN

INTRODUCTION

Young adult beagles were injected with a single injection of graded doses of ^{226}Ra, ^{239}Pu and ^{241}Am and were followed throughout their lifespan. Bone sarcoma was the principal radiation-induced endpoint and the risk associated with average skeletal doses of ^{239}Pu and ^{241}Am (relative to ^{226}Ra = 1) were ^{239}Pu = 19 and ^{241}Am = 5.

More ^{226}Ra-induced bone sarcoma were located in the highly corticalized appendicular skeleton, while ^{239}Pu- and ^{241}Am-induced tumors preferred the highly trabecularized axial skeleton sites (especially the vertebral bodies). The number of ^{226}Ra-induced tumors was linearly related to the corresponding percentage of cortical bone with a moderate value of the correlation coefficient. A consistent negative correlation was found for all three radionuclides for the number of tumor and corresponding trabecular bone calcium and surface area. Further analysis of the spine data alone indicated that bone sarcoma induction in dogs occurred in parts of bones containing about 55% trabecular bone. Between 10% and 55% trabecular bone, there were an increasing number of tumors with increasing percentage of trabecular bone.

In 1950, the Radiobiology Laboratory at the University of Utah was established for the purpose of determining the long-term biological effects of ^{226}Ra and ^{239}Pu in adult beagles. The program was later expanded to include other bone-seeking radionuclides such as ^{241}Am. These studies involved single intravenous injection of radionuclides to small groups of beagles in graded doses, from levels at which no effects were expected up to levels where a 100% incidence of bone tumors was detected. This report will summarize the status of the chronic toxicity studies for ^{226}Ra, ^{239}Pu and ^{241}Am in adult beagles as well as present information on the skeletal locations of ^{226}Ra, ^{239}Pu and ^{241}Am-induced bone sarcoma. The skeletal location data are compared with measured cortical and trabecular masses in the beagle skeleton, determined in a collaborative project with the Laboratory for Energy-Related Health Research, University of California at Davis.

Long Term Effects of ^{226}Ra, ^{239}Pu and ^{241}Am in Young Adult Beagle Studies

Background

The University of Utah studies were based on the concept that the relative toxicity of two bone-seeking radionuclides may be independent of species, even though the absolute toxicity is known to be species-dependent (Ma84). Results of animal experiments giving the ratio of the toxicity of ^{239}Pu to ^{226}Ra could be used to infer the human sensitivity to ^{239}Pu-induced bone tumor according to the relationship:

$$\frac{^{239}Pu \text{ dog}}{^{226}Ra \text{ dog}} \approx \frac{^{239}Pu \text{ man}}{^{226}Ra \text{ man}}$$

Information from the radium dial painter and patient studies (Mar81; Au52; Lo55; Ev66,67,69; Fi69; Ro78,83), establishes the toxicity of ^{226}Ra (a bone volume seeker) in man, the animal studies established the relative toxicity of ^{239}Pu to ^{226}Ra and from these data the toxicity of ^{239}Pu in humans can then be inferred. Mays et al. (Ma84) recently reviewed the rationale and utility of the toxicity ratio approach.

The basic plan for the study of radium, plutonium and americium was formulated with assistance from scientific consultants (Do62a,b; St72; Je76). Briefly, a single intravenous injection of radionuclide was given to young adult beagles (about 17 months of age) to allow a long period of observation, but with the requirement that the skeleton be mature. The injected dose and number of dogs in the ^{226}Ra, ^{239}Pu and ^{241}Am parts of the study are summarized in Table I. The lowest levels of ^{239}Pu and ^{226}Ra resulted in retained radionuclide concentrations that corresponded closely to those of the maximum permissible occupational burdens of 0.04 µCi ^{239}Pu and 0.1 µCi ^{226}Ra. Bone tumors were detected radiographically and histologically. Emphasis was placed on metabolic and autoradiographic studies on long-lived laboratory animals with skeletons more similar to those of man than that of rodents.

Table 1. Injected dosages and number of dogs

Dose Level	Injected Dosages (µCi/kg) and Number of Dogs (No.)					
	^{226}Ra	No.	^{239}Pu	No.	^{241}Am	No
5	10	9	2.8	9	3.0	2
4	3.2	12	0.9	12	0.9	12
3	1.1	12	0.3	12	0.3	13
2	0.34	12	0.096	12	0.1	12
1.7	0.17	12	0.048	13	0.048	23
1	0.057	22	0.016	25	0.016	25
0.7	-	-	0.01	38	-	-
0.5	0.02	25	0.006	41	0.006	14
0.2	0.007	10	0.0018	41	0.002	14
0.1	-	-	0.0007	28	-	-
0	0.000	44	0.0000	46	0.000	-
		158		282		115

The effectiveness for induction of bone tumors, the chief cause of death, is based on the classically used average skeletal dose in rads at death. Detailed dosimetry for the three radionuclides in beagles has been described (Ll70,76; St77). Another dose parameter is local endosteal dose, defined as dose to cells or volumes adjacent to endosteal surface. Insufficient local endosteal dose data have been generated to date (Po84) to use this dose parameter in dose-response studies for predicting the level at which bone tumors can be expected. The estimate of the toxicity ratio for each bone-seeking radionuclide was calculated by dividing its linear risk coefficient (bone sarcoma per 10^6 average skeletal rad) by the linear coefficient for ^{226}Ra (Ma76; Wre84).

Status of ^{226}Ra, ^{239}Pu and ^{241}Am Studies

All dogs in the ^{226}Ra study have died. Forty eight dogs injected with low doses of ^{239}Pu (4 controls, 6 at 0.0007 µCi/kg; 5 at 0.0018 µCi/kg; 9 at 0.006 µCi/kg; 21 at 0.01 µCi/kg and 2 at 0.016 µCi/kg), and 20 with low doses of ^{241}Am (2 at 0.006 µCi/kg; 12 at 0.016 µCi/kg and 6 at 0.048 µCi/kg) are alive (Table 2)

Table 2. Status of ^{226}Ra, ^{239}Pu and ^{241}Am Lifetime Toxicity Studies in Beagles (August, 1984)

		Beagles		Range of Ave.
Nuclide	No.	Living	With one Bone Sarcoma	Skeletal Dose (rads)
^{226}Ra	158	0	42	35 - 19,000
^{239}Pu	191	48	70	3 - 726
^{241}Am	115	20	35	10 - 2,200

Recently, Wrenn et al. (Wre84) summarized the on-going experiments by plotting the cumulative bone sarcoma incidence versus average skeletal dose for dogs injected with ^{226}Ra, ^{239}Pu and ^{241}Am (Fig. 1). Radium is less toxic than ^{241}Am which in turn is less toxic than ^{239}Pu. The preliminary estimate of the toxicity ratios for bone sarcoma induction (relative to ^{226}Ra = 1) are ^{239}Pu = 19 and ^{241}Am = 5 (Fig. 2). Previously Taylor and colleagues (Ta83) reported toxicity ratios of ^{239}Pu = 15.3 ± 3.9 and ^{241}Am = 4.9 ± 1.4 for bone sarcoma induction in C57Bl/Do (combined black and albino mice). The toxicity ratios are similar between these 2 species, and varied much less than the variation in relative sensitivities of ^{239}Pu by a factor of 150 (Ma76,84).

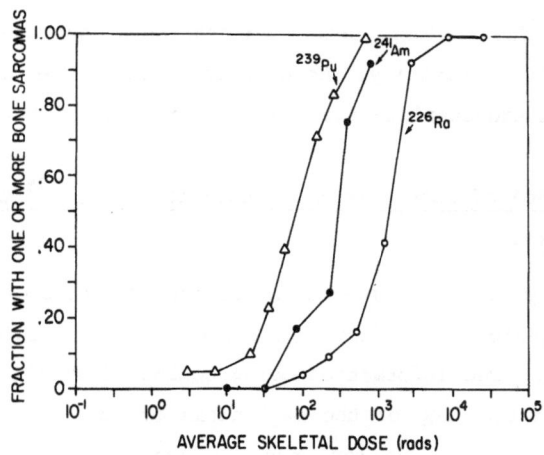

Figure 1 Cumulative bone sarcoma incidence versus average skeletal dose plotted for dogs injected with ^{239}Pu, ^{241}Am and ^{226}Ra.

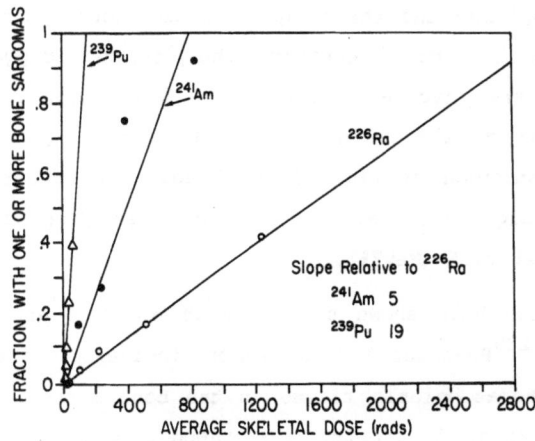

Figure 2 Linear dose response plot of fraction of animals with bone sarcomas in the low dose region for ^{239}Pu, ^{241}Am and ^{226}Ra.

The difference in the relative toxicity of ^{239}Pu and ^{241}Am can be attributed to the slight difference in their microdistribution (L172) and lower initial uptake or a combination of both. The higher deposition of ^{241}Am than ^{239}Pu on periosteal surfaces and the burial of ^{241}Am due to lower uptake on trabecular surfaces can contribute to its lower toxicity. More information on the microdistribution and local endosteal surface dose would be helpful (Po84).

Sites of Incidence of Bone Sarcoma Induced in ^{226}Ra, ^{239}Pu and ^{241}Am Injected Beagles

This report is part of a program to define the tissue characteristics of osteogenic tumor incidence sites in beagles injected with ^{226}Ra and ^{239}Pu. The information being collected should contribute to a better understanding of the mechanisms of α-radiation-induced osteogenic sarcomas. A similar study in man will help to predict the risk of α-radiation-induced osteogenic sarcoma to man.

Background

Among bone radiobiologists, it has been recognized for some time that endosteal tissues are the principal sites for bone sarcomas in man (Lo67). Spiers et al. (Sp77) were able to demonstrate a linear relationship between the frequency of tumor occurrence at sites in the long bones of man and the beagle and the corresponding trabecular surface area. More recently, they further suggested that surface tissues are involved and that the bone tumor induction by radiation depends on the number of cells at risk (Sp83); in the interspecies comparison of man and the beagle, it appears that the fraction of the organ irradiated is more important than the absolute number of cells at risk (May75).

Studies at Utah have shown that certain features are characteristic of high ^{239}Pu-induced bone tumor incidence sites (Wro80; Mi84): 1) more hematopoietic tissue in the bone marrow; 2) greater trabecular bone mass; 3) greater bone remodeling rates; 4) greater mineral apposition rates;, 5) greater density and activity of bone surface cells; 6) greater density of putative bone cell precursors; 7) greater initial uptake of ^{239}Pu on bone surfaces; and 8) greater marrow vascular volumes. While most of these studies are not yet complete, the information being collected should contribute to our understanding of the mechanisms of α-irradiation-induced bone sarcomas.

Relationship of Cortical and Trabecular Bone Mass to Tumor Incidence.

Recently, we turned to study the relationship of ^{226}Ra , ^{239}Pu and ^{241}Am-induced bone tumor location relative to cortical and trabecular bone distribution. Unfortunately, before any such effort could begin, more detailed data on the actual amount and distribution of trabecular and cortical bone in the beagle was required (Go64; Sp77,83). Dr. Norris J. Parks, University of California at Davis, Dr. George E. Miller, University of California at Irvine, and I made a total skeletal survey of parts of bones of a beagle by neutron activation analysis and dissection, which allowed a more thorough examination of the relationship of bone structure to tumor site distribution for the entire dog skeleton rather than for long bones only (Sp77,83).

The techniques used to perform the total skeletal survey of trabecular and cortical bone by neutron activation analysis and dissection have been reported (Pa84). Briefly, the skeleton of a 1985 day old female beagle was dissected into 400 one cm-thick pieces and assayed for ^{49}Ca produced in the University of California, Irvine, TRIGA reactor. Trabecular bone and marrow were removed and samples were reassayed. In Table 3, examples of the distribution of trabecular and cortical bone in g of activated calcium and the percentage of cortical bone for parts of lumbar vertebrae, pelvis and humerus are given.

Our values for percentage of trabecular bone are higher than those listed by Gong, Arnold and Cohn (Go64). For example, in the three bones listed in Table 1, we list higher percentage of trabecular bone values (lumbar vertebrae 35.3 vs. 15.7%, pelvis 26 vs. 21.4% and humerus 31.9 vs 24.1%).

Data on Bone Sarcoma Location

Table 3 Distribution of Trabecular and Cortical Bone and Percent
Cortical Bone in Select Bones

Bony Parts	gm Ca		Cortical Bone %
	Trabecular	Cortical	
Lumbar Vertebrae	1.87	3.44	64.7
body	0.99	1.46	59.5
arch	0.64	1.03	61.7
spine	0.18	0.52	74.3
transverse process	0.07	0.42	85.7
Innominate	0.74	2.11	74.0
ilium	0.44	1.06	70.7
pubis	0.12	0.22	64.7
ischium	0.18	0.83	82.1
Humerus	1.08	2.31	68.1
proximal	0.57	0.54	53.5
proximal shaft	0.07	0.49	87.5
distal shaft	0.11	0.69	86.3
distal	0.33	0.59	64.1

Information on the sites of occurrence of ^{226}Ra-induced bone tumors
in beagles has already been assembled and analyzed (Th83; Wre84) and
the results will be used in this paper. Wrenn et al. (Wre84) reported the completed ^{226}Ra portion of an experiment to determine the
relative radiotoxicity of injected ^{226}Ra and ^{239}Pu. Bone sarcomas
were identified radiographically or clinically, with subsequent
histopathological confirmation and classification. Furthermore, we
worked from available in vivo radiographs to determine as accurately
as possible the location of the bone sarcomas in our 400 bone
parts.

Table 4 lists the bone sarcoma location and distribution in the
axial and appendicular skeleton of dogs given ^{226}Ra, ^{239}Pu and
^{241}Am. Table 5 gives a partial listing of the tumor locations with
the corresponding (percentage of cortical bone, activated cortical
and trabecular calcium (GCA)) data base used to perform the linear
regression analysis for all tumors. Table 6 summarizes our linear
regression analyses; Table 7 digests the significant findings.

Table 4. Distribution of ^{226}Ra, ^{239}Pu and ^{241}Am-induced bone
sarcoma

Location	% Distribution		
	^{226}Ra	^{239}Pu	^{241}Am
Axial Skeleton			
jaws	33.3	11.8	0
ribs	0	8.8	18.5
vertebral column	57.1	79.4	59.3
vertebral bodies	28.6	61.7	59.3
Appendicular Skeleton			
proximal/distal	52.9	77.3	66.7
mid-shaft	47.0	18.2	33.3
innominate	12.8	21.9	16.7
scapula	0	9.4	16.7

Table 5. Select tumor location with their corresponding % cortical
bone, activated cortical and trabecular bone calcium (GCA)

Animal No.	Location	Code	Cortical Bone %	GCA Cortical (g)	GCA Trabecular (g)
M1R5	Lumbar Arch	LV6A	73.2	0.202	0.074
M5R5	Prox. Femur	LF3	88.8	0.318	0.040
F3R4A	Thoracic Vert.	LV3B	43.9	0.065	0.083
F9R5	Dist. Tibia	RT8	94.1	0.239	0.015
F6R3	Humeral Shaft	RH7	96.7	0.236	0.0084

Numerous relationships with negative slope (more bone with less
tumors) were found. Most surprising is the consistent negative
slopes with all 3 radionuclides for trabecular bone calcium, percentage of trabecular bone calcium, trabecular bone calcium per
post-injection days and trabecular surface area parameters. The
only positive slopes were for percentage of cortical bone in ^{226}Ra-
induced tumors and for trabecular surface to volume ratios and
trabecular turnover in ^{239}Pu-treated dogs (Tables 6 and 7).

Table 6. Percentage ^{226}Ra, ^{239}Pu and ^{241}Am tumor occurrence and regression line data as a function dose, post-injection days and bone morphometry

Parameters	Linear				Log			
	a	b	r	F	a	b	r	F
Days Post-Injection of Radionuclide								
Ra-226	26.1	-.006	-.65	5.92*	114.5	-30.7	-.63	5.15*
Am-241	31.3	-.001	-.59	2.63	134.6	-35.3	-.59	2.62
Pu-239	35.2	-.008	-.88	21.31**	178.1	-48.1	-.91	30.32**
Skeletal Dose								
Ra-226	29.5	-.001	-.76	7.03*	125.4	-28.4	-.89	19.12**
Am-241	31.3	-.012	-.75	7.61*	137.6	-40.0	-.88	20.87**
Pu-239	16.0	-.002	-.59	9.01**	83.3	-22.0	-.84	40.71**
Dose Rate								
Ra-226	31.4	-1.96	-.62	3.09	41.4	-32.7	-.74	6.12*
Am-241	29.3	-17.2	-.62	3.11	8.93	-31.5	-.81	9.88*
Pu-239	35.4	-8.19	-.66	4.73	28.2	-47.3	-.88	20.21**
Cortical Bone GCA								
Ra-226	13.9	-19.8	-.30	.97	5.67	-4.26	-.13	.16
Am-241	17.8	-31.8	-.59	4.85	3.4	-8.4	-.38	1.49
Pu-239	16.2	-25.7	-.45	2.26	6.1	-4.3	-.18	.31
Trabecular Bone GCA								
Ra-226	35.0	-140.9	-.72	6.49*	-28.1	-44.6	-.91	30.70**
Am-241	26.5	-97.4	-.73	5.58	-10.4	-24.5	-.90	20.40**
Pu-239	25.2	-60.6	-.85	20.15**	-6.9	-23.5	-.86	23.08**
Cortical Bone GCA + Trabecular Bone GCA (Total Bone)								
Ra-226	11.9	-8.58	-.18	.29	9.97	1.46	.06	.03
Am-241	18.5	-21.7	-.62	4.31	7.44	-6.31	-.34	.91
Pu-239	16.9	-17.9	-.45	2.27	6.40	-5.64	-.21	.43
Cortical Bone GCA/(Cortical Bone GCA + Trabecular Bone GCA)								
Ra-226	-15.4	38.7	.71	6.16*	21.6	58.0	.67	5.01
Am-241	11.0	2.16	.07	.03	13.4	4.72	.10	.06
Pu-239	9.18	5.10	.16	.16	14.6	9.5	.22	.32
Trabecular Bone GCA/(Cortical Bone GCA + Trabecular Bone GCA)								
Ra-226	29.6	-53.6	-.83	12.80*	-6.08	-30.5	-.94	45.21**
Am-241	21.1	-19.5	-.54	2.02	6.91	-13.0	-.64	3.52
Pu-239	19.8	-18.3	-.58	3.03	6.90	-10.9	-.55	2.64
Cortical Bone GCA/Trabecular Bone GCA								
Ra-226	28.5	-.17	-.56	4.46	95.5	-44.5	-.82	20.79**
Am-241	26.8	-1.35	.57	10.41**	41.0	-31.7	.86	50.57**
Pu-239	29.4	-1.43	-.66	6.78*	54.4	-43.2	-.87	27.86**

Table 6 (cont.)

Parameters	Linear				Log			
	a	b	r	F	a	b	r	F
Trabecular Bone GCA/Cortical Bone GCA								
Ra-226	36.1	−29.6	−.67	4.93	2.21	−48.6	−.88	21.54**
Am-241	31.1	−15.5	−.71	6.15*	11.2	−35.0	−.86	16.53**
Pu-239	26.4	−13.8	−.79	8.27*	10.6	−21.9	−.90	20.99**
Cortical Bone GCA/Days Post-Injection								
Ra-226	18.9	−.43	−.51	2.41	17.0	−5.16	−.22	.35
Am-241	21.1	−.73	−.80	15.89**	25.1	−14.6	−.64	6.35*
Pu-239	18.7	−.57	−.79	16.71**	21.3	−11.5	−.59	5.23*
Trabecular Bone GCA/Days Post-Injection								
Ra-226	29.4	−1.23	−.66	7.04*	54.4	−41.2	−.89	35.01**
Am-241	32.4	−2.00	−.86	17.66**	43.8	−35.4	−.98	175.15**
Pu-239	21.9	−.70	−.79	19.32**	38.9	−26.5	−.96	133.29**
Surface/Volume Ratio[+]								
Ra-226	−4.48	.07	.29	.98	−59.8	30.2	.32	1.24
Am-241	−11.2	.12	.59	4.28	−93.9	46.6	.59	4.25
Pu-239	−19.4	.15	.68	7.68*	−136.3	64.3	.68	7.74*
Trabecular Surface Area								
Ra-226	20.76	−.19	−.69	10.61**	54.4	−26.3	−.90	53.34**
Am-241	25.5	−.22	−.66	4.67	55.9	−26.1	−.85	15.71**
Pu-239	24.4	−.15	−.73	7.83*	52.4	−22.5	−.80	12.14*
Trabecular Turnover Rate[+]								
Ra-226	16.25	−.02	−.08	.03	16.1	−.92	−.02	.00
Am-241	9.23	.03	.18	.19	.35	5.83	.15	.14
Pu-239	−19.4	.15	.68	7.68*	−136.3	64.3	.68	7.74*

* $p < .05$;   ** $p < .01$;   [+] Values obtained from Kimmel and Jee (Ki82)

Increasing evidence suggests that radium-induced bone tumors have a high probability of originating in cortical bone sites in dogs and man: 1) about half of the ^{226}Ra-induced bone sarcomas of the axial skeleton occurring in 38 beagles in the University of California at Davis study originated from mid-shaft cortical lesions of long bones (Po83); 2) no bone tumors were observed in the spine of human radium cases despite the fact that the vertebral column is a major skeletal mass of trabecular bone (Ke71); and 3) ^{226}Ra-induced bone tumors occur much less frequently in areas with large amounts of spongy bone than has been observed for plutonium-induced bone sarcomas in beagles in the University of Utah long-term toxicity studies (Wre). Furthermore, when the distributions of ^{226}Ra , ^{239}Pu and ^{241}Am-induced bone tumors were compared, it was apparent that more ^{226}Ra-induced than ^{239}Pu and ^{241}Am-induced bone sarcomas occurred in bones with high cortical bone content such as mandible and maxilla (jaws) and long-bone mid-shafts (Table 4). The more highly trabecularized skeleton showed fewer bone sarcomas induced by ^{226}Ra (35%) than by ^{239}Pu (51%) and ^{241}Am (60%). This is most apparent in the comparison of tumor frequency in vertebral bodies: ^{226}Ra - 28.6%, ^{239}Pu - 61.7% and ^{241}Am - 59.3% (Table 4). Furthermore, if it is arbitrarily assumed that a 70% cortical bone content is comparable in composition to a typical long bone midshaft, 72.7% of the ^{226}Ra vertebral tumors will fit into this category; thus, most of the spine tumors take their origin from other than the highly trabecularized vertebral body (Table 9).

Table 7. Summary of significant linear regression analyses* of percentage tumor occurrence in beagles given ^{226}Ra, ^{239}Pu and ^{241}Am with their corresponding dose, post-injection times and bone morphometry

Parameters	^{226}Ra	^{239}Pu	^{241}Am
Trabecular Ca	−	−	−
Cortical Ca/total Ca	+	−	−
Trab. Ca/Cort. Ca	−	−	−
Cort. Ca/P.I. days**	0	−	−
Trab. Ca/P.I. days	−	−	−
Trab. Surface/Volume	0	+	0
Trab. Surface Area	−	−	0
Trabecular Turnover	0	+	0

*Slopes = 0 - none, - negative; + positive.
**P.I. Days - post-injection days.

Ample radiographic data demonstrate that ^{226}Ra-induced bone sarcomas occurring in the ends of long bone may arise from the cortical fraction. Inspection of sequential radiographs shows that the earliest lesions occurred in the cortical bone portion of the ends of long bones.

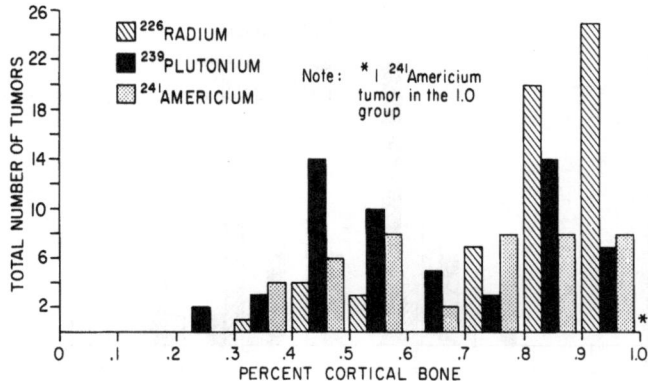

Figure 3   Total number of bone sarcomas versus percent cortical bone
for dogs injected with ^{239}Pu, ^{241}Am and ^{226}Ra.

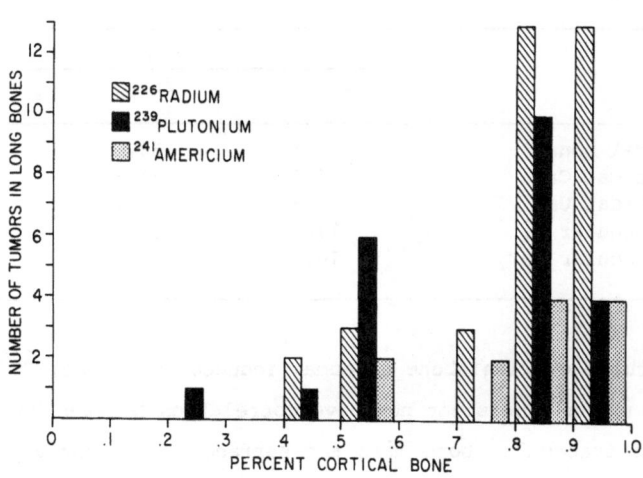

Figure 4   Numbers of long bone sarcomas versus percent cortical bone
for dogs injected with ^{239}Pu, ^{241}Am and ^{226}Ra.

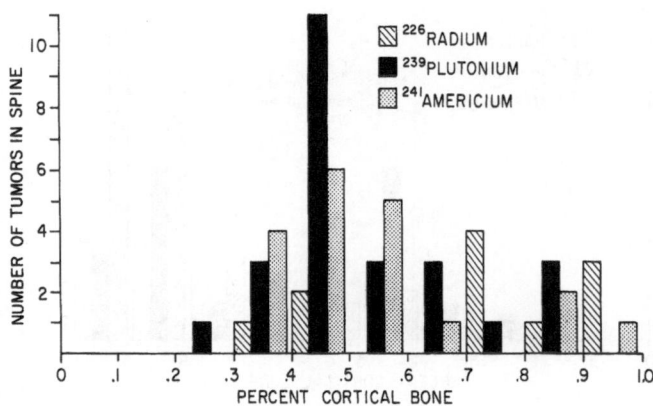

Figure 5 Number of spine bone sarcomas versus percent cortical bone for dogs injected with ^{239}Pu, ^{241}Am and ^{226}Ra.

Table 8. Relationship of % cortical bone, trabecular and cortical calcium to the frequency of ^{226}Ra, ^{239}Pu and ^{241}Am-induced long bone sarcomas

Parameters	Percent		
	^{226}Ra	^{239}Pu	^{241}Am
> 70% Cortical bone	85.3	63.6	83.3
>0.2 gm Cortical Ca	72.7	81.8	50.0
>0.1 gm Cortical Ca	96.9	100.0	100.0
>0.2 gm Trabecular Ca	14.7	36.4	8.3
>0.1 gm Trabecular Ca	14.7	36.4	16.6

In all the dogs with bone sarcoma induced by ^{226}Ra, ^{239}Pu and ^{241}Am there was a consistent negative correlation between bone tumor location and trabecular bone mass and surface area, contrary to the observation of Spiers and colleagues (Sp77,83) who reported a strong positive linear relationship between the frequency of tumor occurrence at sites in the long bones of man and beagle and the corresponding trabecular area. We recently reported a shaky relationship between ^{239}Pu-induced bone sarcoma and trabecular bone ash (Mi84). Our linear regression analysis showed a correlation coefficient of 0.52 and r_s = 0.74, p < 0.02 for the Spearman's rank test.

Table 9. Relationship of % cortical bone, trabecular and cortical calcium to the frequency of ^{226}Ra, ^{239}Pu and ^{241}Am-induced vertebral bone sarcomas

Parameters	Percent		
	^{226}Ra	^{239}Pu	^{241}Am
> 70% Cortical Bone	72.7	16.0	16.7
> .2 g Cortical Ca	45.5	56.0	50.0
> .1 g Cortical Ca	72.7	80.0	72.2
> .2 g Trabecular Ca	0	32.0	33.3
> .1 g Trabecular Ca	36.4	76.0	72.2

The locations of ^{239}Pu- and ^{241}Am-induced bone sarcomas differ from those induced by ^{226}Ra. The latter prefer more trabecularized sites, such as vertebral bodies, ends of long bone and the pelvis (Table 4). There are more ^{239}Pu than ^{226}Ra-induced bone sarcomas in long bone and vertebral sites containing greater than 0.1 g trabecular calcium (Tables 8 and 9). We analyzed our data further by dividing them into 3 groups: long bones, spine and others (Sp83); (Figs. 3, 4, and 5). In the long bones, we found the negative correlation withstood the subdivision of the skeleton, but in the spine we noted there were a large number of tumors sequestered in about 45% cortical or 55% trabecular bone, and fewer tumors when the percentage of cortical bone or trabecular bone becomes higher or lower, respectively (Fig. 5). This strongly suggests that, especially in the ^{239}Pu-induced vertebral tumor, between 10% and 55% trabecular bone there is an increasing number of tumors with increasing trabecular bone.

CONCLUDING REMARKS

The current study generated more questions than answers. Listed below are areas needing attention.

1. Why are the toxicity ratios of ^{239}Pu and ^{241}Am so dissimilar? Will more microdistribution and localized dosimetry of ^{241}Am shed some light?

2. Why do ^{226}Ra-induced bone sarcomas predominantely involve bones with high cortical bone content?

3. Although there is a negative relationship between tumor location and trabecular mass and surface, the weak positive correlation coefficient for trabecular surface to volume ratio and turnover must not be neglected. Will high surface to volume ratio and turnover improve or change the relationship of cortical bone sarcoma in ^{226}Ra-injected dogs?

4. Why do more long bone mid-shaft tumors occur in beagles given ^{226}Ra than occur in man? Will the answer be found in comparative static and dynamic bone morphometry and local dosimetry data?

5. Is the explanation of the complete lack of ^{226}Ra-induced bone sarcomas in human vertebral columns, while only a few have been observed in beagles, to be found in more detailed information on comparative bone morphometry and bone surface dosimetry?

6. It is possible the relationships between tumor location and bone morphometry will change with increasing numbers of dogs. We have included only long-term toxicity dogs in this preliminary study. It appears that with the meager data available, it may be wise to characterize the high versus low or no tumor occurrence sites to gain information on mechanisms and local dosimetry (Wro80;Mi84).

7. The difference in locations of bone sarcomas in ^{226}Ra versus ^{239}Pu and ^{241}Am injected dogs is disconcerting. This does not appear to be species specific but radionuclide specific. Will this invalidate the use of the toxicity ratio concept? It will be reassuring if the toxicity ratio for ^{224}Ra is similar to that of ^{226}Ra. The dose-response study for beagles injected with ^{224}Ra is still in its infancy. Ten more years of research are needed to settle this issue.

8. Lastly an important part of the puzzle is missing. There is a need for more and better local endosteal dose data. Until such

information is generated, it will be most difficult to draw any realistic conclusions.

ACKNOWLEDGMENT

This work was supported by U.S. Department of Energy contracts No. DE-AC02-76EV-00119 and DE-AM03-76SF00472. The authors wish to thank Mary Rieben for typing, Diane Fouts and Dawn Buster for editing this manuscript and Drs. Lowell A. Woodbury and Gerry H. Kenner for their statistical assistance.

REFERENCES

Au52   Aub J.C., Evans R.D., Hempelman L.H., and Martland H.S., 1952, The Late Effects of Internally Deposited Radioactive Materials in Man , Medicine 31, 221-329.

Do62a   Dougherty T.F., Jee W.S.S., Mays C.W., and Stover B.J., (eds.), 1962, Some Aspects of Internal Irradiation, 529 pages, (Oxford: Pergamon Press).

Do62b   Dougherty T.F., Stover B.J., Dougherty J.H., Jee W.S.S., Mays C.W., Rehfeld C.E., Christensen W.R., and Goldthorpe H.C., 1962, Studies of the Biological Effects of Ra^{226}, Pu^{239}, Ra^{228} (MsTh), Th^{228} (RdTh) and Sr^{90} in Adult Beagles , Radiat. Res. 17, 625-681.

Ev66   Evans R.D., 1966, The Effect of Skeletally Deposited Alpha-Ray Emitters in Man , Brit. J. Radiol. 39, 881-895.

Ev67   Evans R.D., 1967, The Radium Standard for Boneseekers-- Evaluation of the Data on Radium Patients and Dial Painters , Health Phys. 13, 267-278.

Ev69   Evans R.D., Keane A.T., Kolenkow R.J., Neal W.R., and Shanahan M.M., 1969, Radiogenic Tumors in the Radium and Meso-thorium Cases Studied at M.I.T. , in Delayed Effects of Bone Seeking Radionuclides, (Edited by Mays C.W., Jee W.S.S., and Lloyd R.D.), pp. 157-194, (Salt Lake City: University of Utah Press).

Fi69   Finkel A.J., Miller C.E., and Hasterlik R.J., 1969, Radium-induced Malignant Tumors in Man , in Delayed Effects of Bone-- Seeking Radionuclides, (Edited by Mays C.W., et al.), pp. 195-226, (Salt Lake City: University of Utah Press).

Go64   Gong J.K., Arnold J.S. and Cohn S.H., 1964, Composition of Trabecular and Cortical Bone , Anat. Rec. 149, 325-332.

Je76   Jee W.S.S., Atherton D.R., Bruenger F.W., Dougherty T.F., Lloyd R.D., Mays C.W., Nabors C.J., Stevens W., Stover B.J., Taylor G.N., and Woodbury L.A., 1976, Current Status of Utah Long-Term ^{239}Pu Studies , in Biological and Environmental Effects of Low-Level Radiation, ST1/Pub/409, II: 79-82, (Vienna;IAEA).

Ke71   Keane A.T., 1971, Skeletal Location of Primary Bone Tumors in the Radium Cases , Radiological Physics Division Annual Report, Center for Human Radiobiology, Argonne National Laboratory, Rep. ANL-7860, Part II, 59-66.

Ki82   Kimmel D.B., and Jee W.S.S., 1982, A Quantitative Histologic Study of Bone Turnover in Young Adult Beagles , Anat. Rec. 203, 31-45.

L170   Lloyd R.D., 1970, Retention and Dosimetry of Some Injected Radionuclides in Beagles , University of Utah Radiobiology Division Annual Progress Report, COO-119-241.

L172   Lloyd R.D., Jee W.S.S., Atherton D.R., Taylor G.N. and Mays C.W., 1972, Americium-241 in Beagles: Biological Effects and Skeletal Distribution , in Radiobiology of Plutonium (Edited by Stover, B.J.and Jee W.S.S.) pp 141-148 (Salt Lake City: J.W. Press).

L176   Lloyd R.D., Mays C.W., Atherton D.R., Taylor G.N., and Van Dilla M.A., 1976, Retention and Skeletal Dosimetry of Injected ^{226}Ra, ^{228}Ra, and ^{90}Sr in Beagles , Radiat. Res. 66, 274-287.

Lo55   Looney W.B., Hasterlik R.J., Brues A.M., and Skirmont E., 1955, A Clinical Investigation of the Chronic Effects of Radium Salts Administered Intravenously , Am. J. Roentgenol. Radium Therapy Nuclear Med. 73, 1006-1037.

Lo67   Loutit J.F., Brues A.M. Marinelli L.D., Spiers F.W. and Vaughan J.M., 1967, A Review of the Radiosensitivity of the Tissues in Bone, ICRP Publication II, (Oxford: Pergamon Press).

Mar81   Martland H.S., 1931, The Occurrence of Malignancy in Radioactive Persons , Am. J. Cancer 15, 2435-2516.

May75   Mayneord W.V. and Clarke R.H., 1975, Carcinogenesis and Radiation Risk. A Biomathematical Reconnaisance , Brit. J. Radiol. Suppl. 12, Ch.1.

Ma76   Mays C.W., Spiess H., Taylor G.N., Lloyd R.D., Jee W.S.S., McFarland S.S., Taysum D.H., Brammer T.W., Brammer D., and Pollard T.A., 1976, Estimated risk to human bone from ^{239}Pu , in The Health Effects of Plutonium and Radium, (Edited by Jee W.S.S.), pp. 343-362, (Salt Lake City: J.W. Press).

Ma84   Mays C.W., Taylor G.N. and Lloyd R.D., 1984, Toxicity Ratios: Their Use and Abuse in Predicting the Risk from Induced Cancer , in Life Span Radiation Effects Studies in Animals: What Can They Tell Us? (Edited by Thompson R.D. and McHaffey J.A.) (Oak Ridge: U.S. Department of Energy Technical Information).

Mi84   Miller S.C., Jee W.S.S., Smith J.M. and Wronski T.J., 1984, Tissue Characteristics of High and Low Incidence Pu-induced Osteogenic Sarcoma Sities in Life Span Beagles , in Life Span Radiation Effects Studies in Animals: What Can They Tell Us? (Edited by Thompson R.D. and McHaffey J.A.), (Oak Ridge: U.S. Department of Energy Technical Information Center).

Pa84   Parks N.J., Jee W.S.S. and Miller G.E., 1984, Assessment of Cancellous and Cortical Bone Distribution in the Beagle Skeleton , Laboratory of Energy-Related Health Research 1983 Annual Report, University of California at Davis, UCD 472-129, 77-81.

Po84   Polig E., Smith J.M. and Jee W.S.S., (in press), Microdistribution and Localized Dosimetry of ^{241}Am in Bones of Beagle Dogs , Intl. J. Radiat. Res.

Po83   Pool R.R., Morgan J.P. and Parks N.J., 1983, Comparative Pathogenesis of Radium-induced Intracortical Bone Lesions in Humans and Beagles , Health Physics 44, Suppl. 1, 155-177.

Ro78   Rowland R.E., Stehney A.F., and Lucas H.F. Jr., 1978, Dose Response Relationships for Female Radium Dial Workers , Radiat. Res. 76, 368-383.

Ro83   Rowland R.E., Stehney A.S. and Lucas H.F., 1983, Dose Response Reationships for Radium-Induced Bone Sarcomas , Health Phys. 44, Supp. No. 1, 15-31.

Sp77　　Spiers F.W., Wright S.D., and Beddoe A.H, 1977, Measurements of Endosteal Surface Areas in Human Long Bones: Relation
ship to Sites of Occurrence of Osteosarcoma , Brit. J. Radiol.
50, 769-776.

Sp83　　Spiers F.W. and Beddoe A.H., 1983, Sites of Incidence of
Osteosarcoma in the Long Bones of Man and the Beagle , Health
Phys. 44, Suppl 1, 49-64.

St72　　Stover B.J., and Stover C.N., 1972, The Laboratory for
Radiobiology at the University of Utah , in Radiobiology of
Plutonium, (Edited by Stover B.J., and Jee W.S.S.), pp. 29-46,
(Salt Lake City: J.W. Press).

St77　　Stover B.J., Atherton D.R., Stevens W., Buster D.S., and
Bruenger F.W., 1977, Effect of Dose Level on Skeletal Retention
of ^{239}Pu(IV) in the Beagle , Radiat. Res. 69, 442-458.

Ta83　　Taylor G.N., Mays C.W., Lloyd R.D., Gardner P.A., Talbot
L.R., McFarland S.S., Pollard T.A., Atherton D.R., VanMoorhem
D., Brammer D., Brammer T.W., Ayoroa G., and Taysum D.H., 1983,
Comparative Toxicity of ^{226}Ra, ^{239}Pu, ^{241}Am, ^{249}Cf, and ^{252}Cf
in C57BL/Do Black and Albino Mice , Radiat. Res. 95, 584-601.

Th73　　Thurman G.B., Mays C.W., Taylor G.N., Keane A.T. and Sissons
H.A., 1973, Skeletal Location of Radiation-induced and Naturally Occurring Osteosarcomas in Man and Dog , Cancer Res., 33,
1604-1607.

Wre84　　Wrenn M.E., Taylor G.N., Stevens W., Mays C.W., Jee W.S.S.,
Lloyd R.D., Atherton D.R., Bruenger F.W., Miller S.C., Smith
J.M., Shabestari L.R., Woodbury L. and Stover B.J., 1984, DOE
Lifespan Radiation Effects Studies in Experimental Animals at
University of Utah Division of Radiobiology , in Life Span
Radiation Studies in Animals: What Can They Tell Us? (Edited by
Thompson R. and McHaffey J.A.) (Oak Ridge: U.S. Department of
Energy Technical Information).

Wro80　　Wronski T.J., Smith J.M., and Jee W.S.S., 1980, The Microdistribution and Retention of Injected Pu-239 on Trabecular Bone
Surfaces of the Beagle: Implications for Induction of Osteosarcomas , Radiat. Res. 83, 74-89.

17

Initial Deposition Pattern of Actinides 91 to 96 in the Skeleton of the Rat

N. D. PRIEST, G. R. HOWELLS, D. GREEN and J. W. HAINES

INTRODUCTION.

Within the skeleton the ions of osteophilic metals mostly deposit on bone surfaces. Subsequently, many are rapidly redistributed within bone (Ma62) while others are retained either at or close to their site of deposition. For the purposes of radiation protection dosimetry the radioisotopes of those metals which become redistributed, including those of the alkaline earth elements, have been termed bone-volume seeking radionuclides, whereas those that remain on bone surfaces are described as bone-surface seekers (Ma69 Va73). This distinction is important in radiological protection because the burial of a radioactive metal in the bone matrix effectively shields the radiation sensitive cells, found close to bone surfaces and throughout the bone marrow, from the effects of its decay (ICRP67 ICRP79). Consequently, it is a consistent finding that bone-volume seeking radionuclides are much less toxic, with regard to the production of bone surface related late-effects of radiation including osteosarcomas, than similarly radioactive bone-surface seekers (Va73 May83).

Other differences between the toxicities of different radionuclides can be attributed to variations in the radionuclide distribution pattern within each of the above broad categories. For example, plutonium seems to be up to three times more toxic than americium for equal mean radiation doses to the skeleton despite the fact that both are bone-surface seeking elements (Ta83 Tay83). Such findings suggest that all bone surfaces are not equally radiation sensitive.

Studies of the microdistribution of bone-seeking radionuclides were first completed on a large scale by Hamilton and his colleagues at the University of California, Berekley (Ha47 Ha48). These studies were undertaken in the late 1940s - only about a decade after the extent of the damaging effects of radium on the skeletons of dial painters had become fully realised - using the wide range of fission and activation products made available by the recent discovery of nuclear fission. They were of rather low resolution by modern standards, but showed that of the metals, (mostly transition elements), studied most were bone-surface seekers. These became distributed in bone with one of two basic patterns. The tetravalent ions' Pu^4+, Th^4+, Zr^4+ and Nb^4+, were shown to share a common distribution pattern with a greater uptake of radionuclide by endosteal surfaces than by periosteal surfaces and with little uptake by the surfaces of vascular cavities in coritcal bone. In contrast, the trivalent ions' Ce^3+, Am^3+, Ac^3+ and Pm^3+, were more evenly distributed on all types of surface. These early studies have since been complemented by many later studies of higher resolution (see reviews Va73b Je72 Du73 Pr81) and by others on the microdistribution of additional radionuclides.

When comparing the distribution patterns of radionuclides obtained in different laboratories difficulty arises because of the uncertain effects on distribution of: differences in the radionuclide preparation used; the species, strain, sex and age of the experimental animals used, and of the multiplicity of the analytical techniques employed. These variables often conspire to make direct quantitative comparisons between the distribution patterns of different radionuclides impossible. The present paper describes some of the results of a number of experiments conducted, jointly by NRPB and MRC Radiobiology Unit, on rats using the actinide elements with atomic numbers 91 to 96. The experiments, some of which have been described in full elsewhere (Pr82 Pr83), were conducted under identical conditions so as to isolate differences in the behaviour of different radionuclides from effects caused by inconsistent experimental conditions. The actinide elements were chosen because of their different valencies (Table 1) and because of their importance in radiological protection. However, as may be deduced from the work of Hamilton (Ha47 Ha48) it is likely that the results produced will be of value in predicting the deposition patterns and toxicity of other radioactive and stable elements with similar chemical properties.

Valency	Pa	U	Np	Pu	Am	Cm
+3		·	·	·	X	X
+4	·	X	·	X	·	·
+5	X	·	X	·	·	
+6		X	·	·	·	
+7			·	·		

Table 1. The known (.) and most common (X) valency states for the actinide elements 91 - 96 (Co75). Two common valency states of similar stability have been described for uranium. It is assumed that the most common states are likely to be the most stable in the body.

METHODS.

Female, Wistar (HMT) strain rats, aged 50 - 60 days were used for all the experiments. Most of these were anaesthetized and injected via the saphenous vein with 0.2 ml of a 1% tri-sodium citrate solution, pH 6.5, containing an actinide citrate complex. The actinide isotopes used were protactinium-231, uranium-233, neptunium-237, plutonium-239, americium-241 and curium-244. Injections containing neptunium were administered intra-peritoneally to minimise both actinide polymerisation in the blood and toxic effects. All the injection solutions were filtered, immediately prior to injection, using membrane filters with a pore size of 25 nm. Animals used to study the whole-body distribution of the actinides and their macro-distribution within the skeleton were given injections containing about 90 Bq of actinide ml^{-1}. More concentrated solutions containing about 500 kBq ml^{-1} were given to animals used in the autoradiographic study.

Whole-Body Distribution Studies

Groups of five rats were killed at 1 day post-injection. They were dissected and tissues and organs were removed for analysis. Concentrations of protactinium-231, neptunium-237 and americium-241 were determined either in fresh samples or in ashed samples by gamma-counting (Pr83). Samples containing all other radionuclides were ashed and counted using liquid scintillation techniques (Ke70 Pr80 Pr82).

Gross Distribution in Skeleton

The gross distribution of the actinides in the skeleton was determined at 1 day after injection in groups of five rats. The skeletons were stripped of surrounding soft tissues by Dermestid beetles (Dermestes maculatus). The skeletons were disarticulated and analysed for their radionuclide content using the techniques employed for the whole-body distribution study. The amount of actinide in each bone/group of bones was calculated and the relative concentration (RC) of the actinides in each was determined:

$$RC = \frac{\% \text{ IA } / \text{ g ash for bone}}{\% \text{ IA } / \text{ g ash for skeleton}}$$

Additionally, the inhomogeneity factor (So84) for each radionuclide was determined

$$IF = \sqrt{\Sigma n \ Wn \ (1 - Cn)^2}$$

where Wn is a weighting function which is equal to the relative mass of the individual bones/bone group and Cn is the corresponding value for the RC. This factor (IF) is a function of variation of the RCs in the different bones of the skeleton.

Microdistribution Studies

Rats were killed at about 1 day after injection. The distal 10 - 15 mm of the posterior right ribs, the mandibular condyles and the femora were removed for examination by autoradiography. Two auto-radiographic techniques were used. The radionuclide distribution in 1 µm thick sections of the rib and condyle were determined using photographic emulsion - Kodak AR10 stripping film - and their distribution in 5 µm thick sections of the femora was determined by either alpha track autoradiography, using CR39 plastic or with AR10 as described above. These techniques and the others used have been described previously (Gr78 Fe83 Pr80 Pr82).

RESULTS & CONCLUSIONS.

Whole-Body Distribution Data

Table 2 shows the distribution of the actinide isotopes in rat tissues at 1 day after injection. The skeleton - as indicated by the carcass sample - generally contained the largest fraction of the body content. The exception was americium where more radionuclide was concentrated by the liver. The liver also concentrated appreciable quantities of curium and plutonium, but generally failed to concentrate uranium, protactinium and neptunium. All of the radio-nuclides were deposited in the kidneys to some extent, but as expected these deposits were particularly large for uranium. The levels of actinide excretion as indicated by the total radionuclide recovered for each element after 24 hours decreased in the order: uranium (~ 60%), neptunium (~23%), protactinium (~ 20%), curium (~13%), americium (~9%), plutonium (~6%).

These results may be compared with those of Durbin (Du62) who used rats of a similar age to show the dependence of the fractional deposition of radioisotopes in the skeleton and liver on ion size. While the present results conform to the same general pattern, the liver burdens are somewhat lower than those found by Durbin and the

Sample	^{231}Pa	^{233}U	^{237}Np	^{239}Pu	^{241}Am	^{244}Cm
Liver	2.5	.27	3.4	18	49	36
	±.2	±.02	±.02	±1	±.8	±.6
Kidney	2.9	7.2	2.0	.93	1.2	1.2
	±.13	±.65	±.02	±.04	±.04	±.10
Spleen	.42	.001	.14	.15	.06	.09
	.03	±.003	±.01	±.01	±.01	±.01
Femur	3.3	1.7	3.6	3.6	1.9	2.1
	±.30	±.09	±.07	±.07	±.03	±.07
G.I.T.	2.4	4.2	1.6	2.7	1.8	2.0
	±.12	±.44	±.12	±.23	±.23	±.08
Ovary	.05	ND	.05	.06	.02	.03
	±.01	–	±.01	±.01	±.01	±.003
Muscle*	~ 4.0	~ 0.9	~ 5.1	~ 5.9	~ 1.7	~ 3.3
Carcass	69	31	67	69	36	45
	±8.2	±1.3	±0.8	±1.5	±.98	±.85

Table 2. The distribution of different actinide elements in rat tissues and organs at 1 day after the injection of soluble actinide citrate complexes. *Value estimated from skeletal muscle sample. Mean ± SE of mean, n = 5.

skeletal burdens are correspondingly higher. Consequently, our findings would, at least at first sight, seem to support the relationship described by Durbin. However, Durbin was unable to explain the apparently anomalous position of some radionuclides such as thorium and did not try to fit data for uranium. Our data for uranium confirms the aberrant behaviour of this element; even when a correction is attempted for the high levels of uranium excretion.

Gross Skeletal Distribution

Table 3 shows the distribution pattern of the actinides (excluding curium) in rat skeletons at 24 hours after injection. It can be seen that, in general, all the actinides deposited preferentially in the main body of the spine, limb girdles and ribs, with least concentrated by the paw bones and caudal vertebrae. This basic pattern has been described on many occasions (Sto69 St74 Rod77 So83 So84 Pr82 Pr83 Pr83b) and probably reflects either differences in the blood supply to different anatomical regions of the skeleton (Sm84 Hu80 (To85) or, in the case of the head bones, to the presence of teeth

	^{231}Pa	^{233}U	^{237}Np	^{239}Pu	^{241}Am
RELATIVE CONCENTRATIONS					
Skull	0.6	0.7	0.6	0.5	0.8
Mandibles	0.5	0.6	0.6	0.3	0.8
Cerv/thor. v.	1.4	1.2	1.3	1.6	1.1
Lumb/sac. v.	1.5	1.3	1.4	1.7	1.3
Caudal v.	1.0	1.0	0.7	0.6	0.9
Ribs	1.3	1.1	1.2	1.2	1.1
Scapulae	1.4	1.3	1.3	1.2	1.2
Clavicles	-	1.4	1.2	1.2	1.1
Pelvis	1.3	1.2	1.3	1.3	1.1
Humeri	1.3	1.2	1.2	1.4	1.2
Fermoa	1.3	1.2	1.2	1.5	0.9
Ulnae	0.7	0.8	0.8	0.7	0.9
Radii	0.7	0.9	0.9	0.7	1.0
Tibiae/fib.	1.2	1.3	1.3	1.2	1.3
Paws	0.5	0.6	0.5	0.3	0.6
INHOMOGENEITY FUNCTION					
	0.40	0.27	0.37	0.57	0.25

Table 3. The relative concentrations and inhomogeneity functions calculated for actinides in the rat skeleton at one day after injection.

which add greatly to the ash weight of the bone/tooth complex, but add little to their radionuclide content (Pr82).

It can also be seen that the variations in the concentration of actinide in the different bones of the skeleton were greatest for plutonium (see also Rod77 So83 So84). For example, the concentration of plutonium in the lumbar and sacral vertebrae was about six times greater than that in the paw bones and mandibles. In contrast, the degree of variation exhibited by americium and uranium was much lower; the maximum value being about 2 for both radionuclides. Protactinium and neptunium showed intermediate levels of variability.

It is noteworthy that the relative concentrations calculated for americium and uranium were very close to those found for radium-226 in identical animals (Pr83b). This may be predicted for uranium as it exists in the body in the form of the divalent uranyl ion (UO_2^{2+}) (Ste80 Ne58) and may be expected to behave similarly to the divalent radium ion. In the case of americium their similar distributions more likely reflect a similar availability of americuim and radium for binding to all types of bone surface. Why plutonium and to a lesser extent some of the other actinides studied should behave differently is unclear. However, it may be related to their different binding characteristics to different types of bone surface.

Microdistribution

All actinides were found to deposit on bone surfaces. Histogrames constructed to show the distribution of plutonium and uranium about bone surfaces clearly indicated that less than about 10% of these were deposited below bone surfaces in the volume of the mineralised bone matrix (Gr78 GR79 Pr80 Pr82). This was a consistent finding for all actinides studied in this way. Also, whereas actinides were deposited on resting and resorbing bone surfaces as a very thin band, on growing surfaces this band was often much thicker (Pr80). This at least in part, must reflect the effects of protracted actinide deposition on a bone surface which is constantly repositioning. On

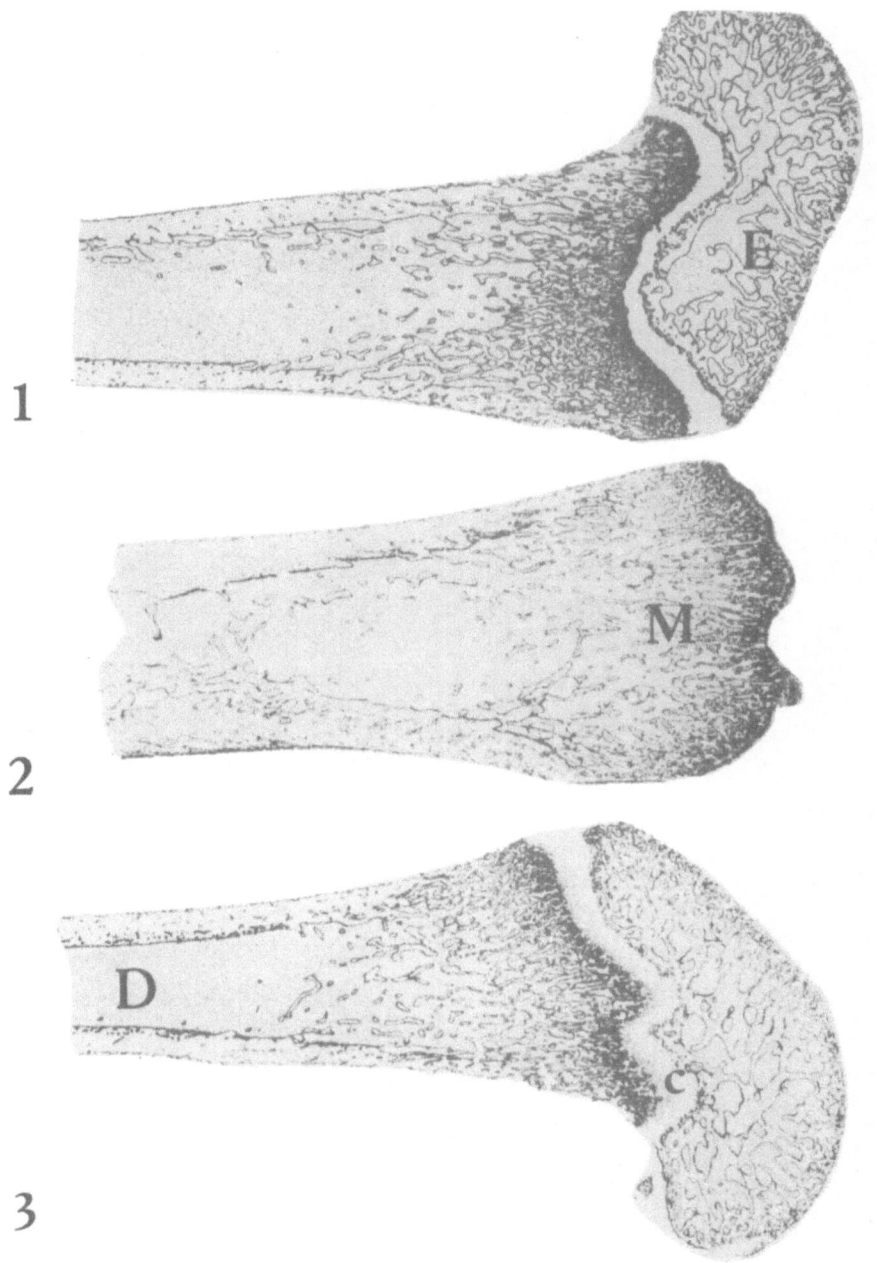

Figures 1 - 3. Autoradiographs of 5 μm sections of the distal femur made with CR39 plastic detectors. These show the distribution of protactinium-231 (Fig. 1), uranium-233 (Fig 2), and neptunium-237 (Fig 3) at 1 day after injection. Note the ephiphysis is missing for the bone containing uranium. E = epiphysis, M = metaphysis, D = diaphysis, c = epiphyseal plate cartilage, p = periosteum and e = endosteum.

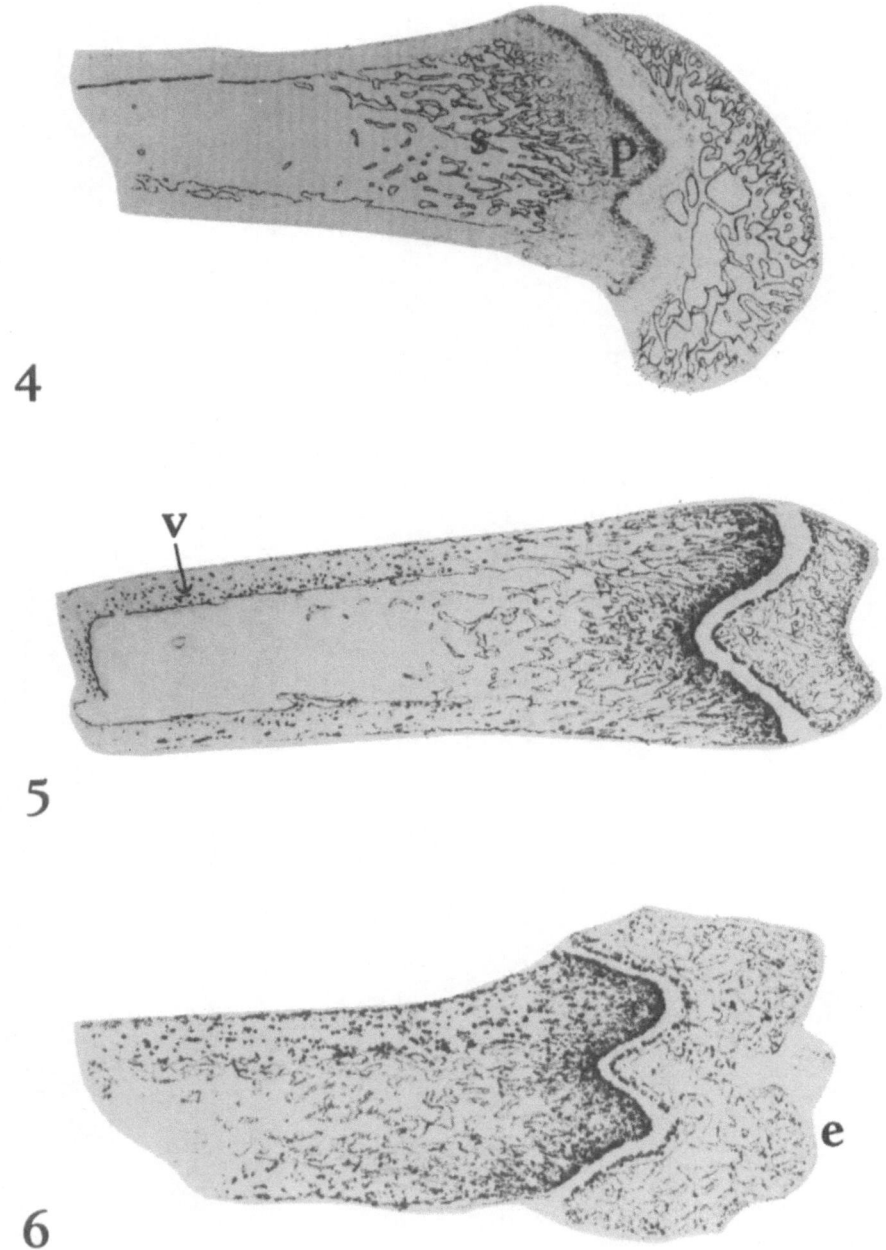

Figures 4 - 6. Autoradiographs of 5 μm sections of the distal femur made with CR39 plastic detectors showing the deposition patterns of plutonium-239 (Fig 4), americium-241 (Fig 5), and curium-244 (Fig 6) as seen at 1 day post injection.   p = primary and s = secondary spongiosa of the metaphysis, v = vascular cavities of cortical bone, e = position of epiphyseal articular cartilage.

growing surfaces the actinides were not deposited at the surface itself, but at the interface of the mineralised bone and unmineralised prebone or osteoid (Figure 7). This behaviour seems to be common for many metals and may indicate that they are bound either to the bone mineral or to a component of the organic bone matrix which is absent or otherwise unavailable for binding in osteoid. Finally, while all the radionuclides were present in the bone marrow at a low level a few more concentrated deposits associated with macrophages and osteoclasts near resorbing bone surfaces were sometimes seen (Je72 Va73b Pr80). Such deposits of uranium have never been found in the bone marrow at any time after its administration (Ste80 Pr82).

The initial deposition patterns of protactinium, uranium, neptunium, plutonium, americium and curium in the distal portion of the rat femur, as demonstrated in alpha track autoradiographs of 5 μm tissue sections with CR39, are shown in Figures 1 to 6, respectively. More detailed selected photomicrographs of autoradiographs, prepared mostly from 1 μm thick tissue sections and the photographic emulsion AR10, are presented in Figures 7 to 14.

Deposition Patterns of Americium and Curium

The deposition patterns of americium and curium in the rat femur (Figures 5 & 6) were characterised by the similar concentrations of radionuclide on the periosteal and endosteal bone surfaces and by their uptake on the bone surfaces of the vascular canals in the cortical bone of the femur shaft. In addition, both americium and curium were characteristically concentrated on the surfaces of the vascular cavities which form a band across the epiphyseal surface of the epiphyseal plate cartilages (Figure 8) (see also Nen72). The high resolution autoradiographs of 1 μm thick sections also showed that these elements are concentrated more by non-growing than by growing surfaces. Moreover, on the non-growing surfaces they were distributed unevely with many focal concentrations at specific loci. In the spongiosa of metaphyseal regions of bone, including that below the mandibular condylar cartilage, these concentrations were

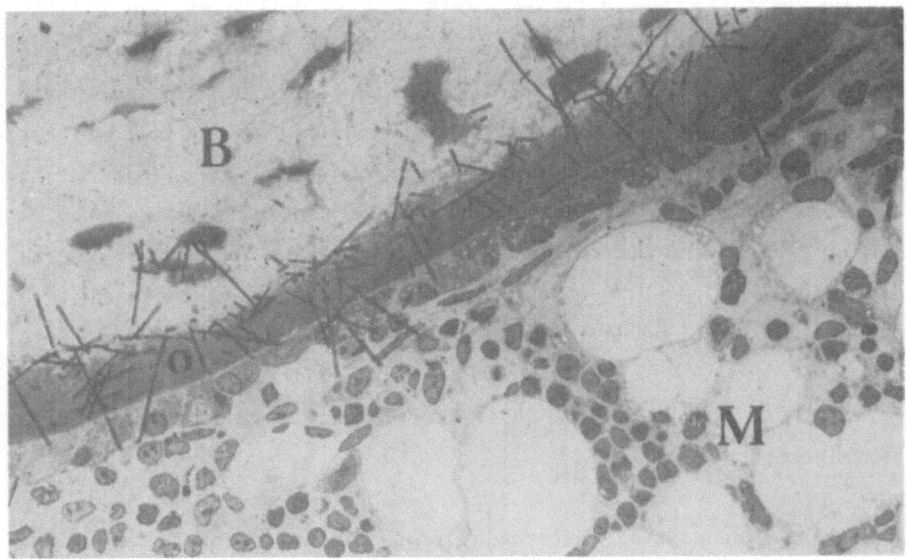

Figure 7.   Autoradiograph (1 μm section, AR10 emulsion, stained with pyronin Y) showing the deposition of plutonium at the osteoid (o)/bone (B) interface.   M = red bone marrow.

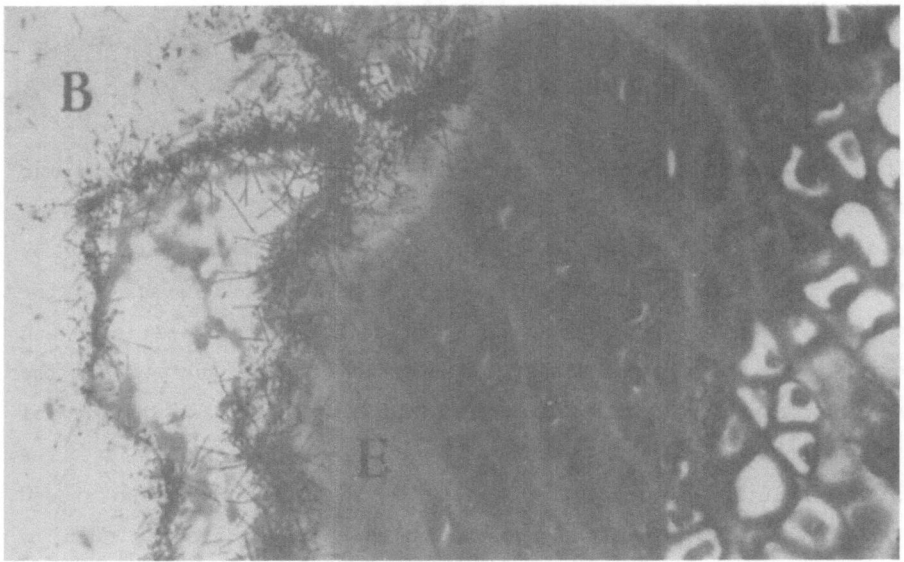

Figure 8.   Autoradiograph.   (5 μm section, AR10 emulsion, stained with azure 11) showing the heavy uptake of americium on the walls of the vascular cavities overlying the epiphyseal plate cartliage (E). B = bone of epiphsis.

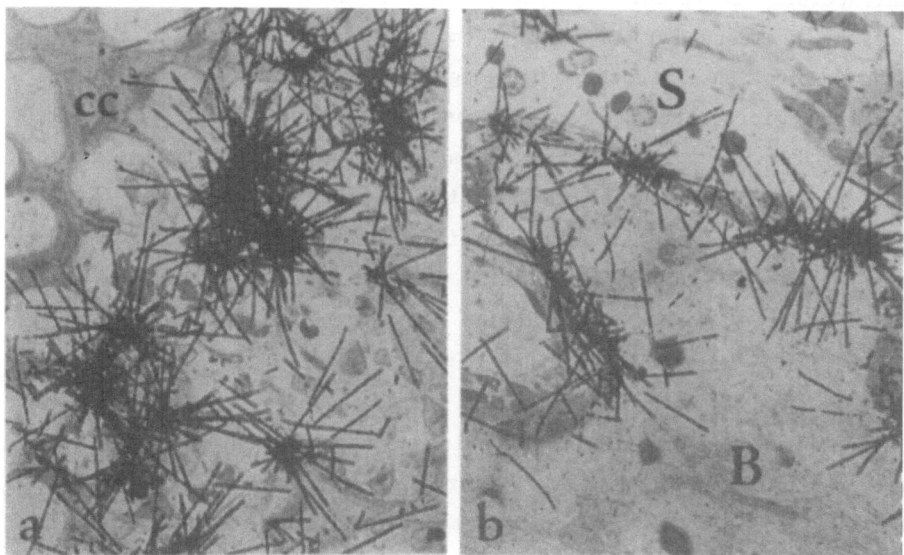

Figure 9. Autoradiographs (1 μm sections, AR10 emulsion pyronin Y) showing the focalization of americium deposits along trabeular surfaces in the primary (9a) and secondary (9b) spongiosa. cc = condylar cartilage, B = bone, S = blood sinusoid.

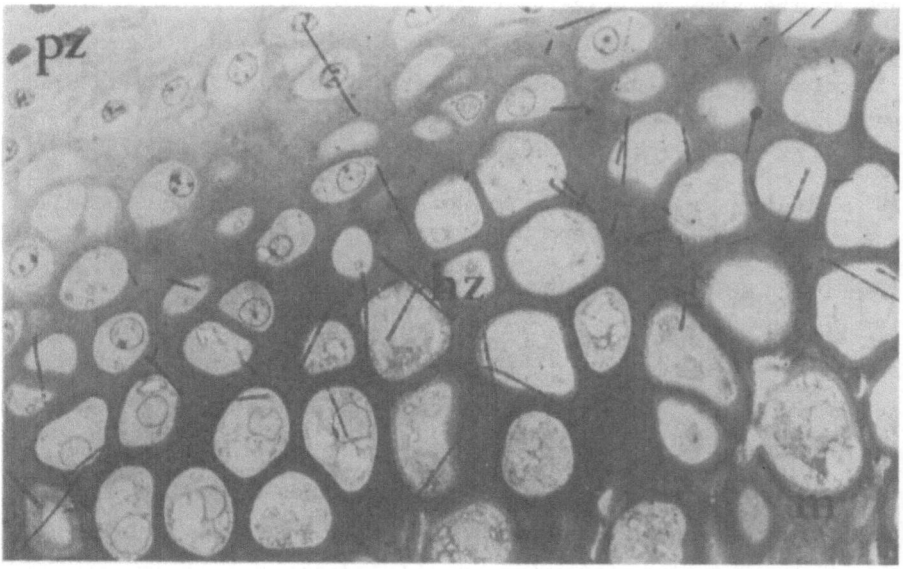

Figure 10. Autoradiograph (1 μm section AR10 emulusion, pyronin Y stain) showing deposits of curium in the hypertrophic zone (hz) of the mandibular condylar cartilage. pz = proliferating zone, m = zone of matrix mineralisation.

particularly conspicuous (Figure 9). The nature of these loci is at present unclear, but they all seem to be associated with areas of bone resorption. Further investigations of these areas using the electron microscope are in progress. In addition to the above, curium, but not americium, was conspicuously bound to the matrix of the hypertrophic zone of the mandibular condylar cartilage (Figure 10) and epiphyseal articular cartilages. No explanation for this binding is put forward.

Deposition Pattern of Plutonium

Unlike americium and curium plutonium deposited much more heavily on the endosteal surfaces of the femur than on the periosteal surfaces (Figure 4). Also, little plutonium deposited on the surfaces of the cortical vascular canals or on the walls of the vascular cavities laying along the top of the epiphyseal plate cartilages. The surfaces of the trabeculae which form a band across the deeper regions of the primary spongiosa of the metaphysis were also depleted in plutonium. Plutonium was evenly deposited along all bone surfaces and at the same anatomical location was concentrated to a similar extent by surfaces exhibiting all growth activities (Figure 11). Plutonium did not appear to be concentrated to any significant extent by any skeletal cartilages.

As plutonium is about three times more toxic than the trivalent actinides (Ta83 Tay83) it would seem that the bone surfaces irradiated preferentially by plutonium are the most radiosensitive. If so, then the surfaces of the cortical bone cavities and periosteal surfaces that are heavily irradiated by the trivalent actinides, but not by plutonium, are likely to be much less radiation sensitive than the metabolically more active surfaces of trabecular bone which are preferentially irradiated by plutonium. Moreover, as plutonium deposition is highest on bone surfaces adjacent to the bone marrow, the risk of tumour induction in this tissue may be greater for plutonium than for the trivalent actinides. Although the total risk of leukaemia is likely to be small for all bone seeking radionuclides.

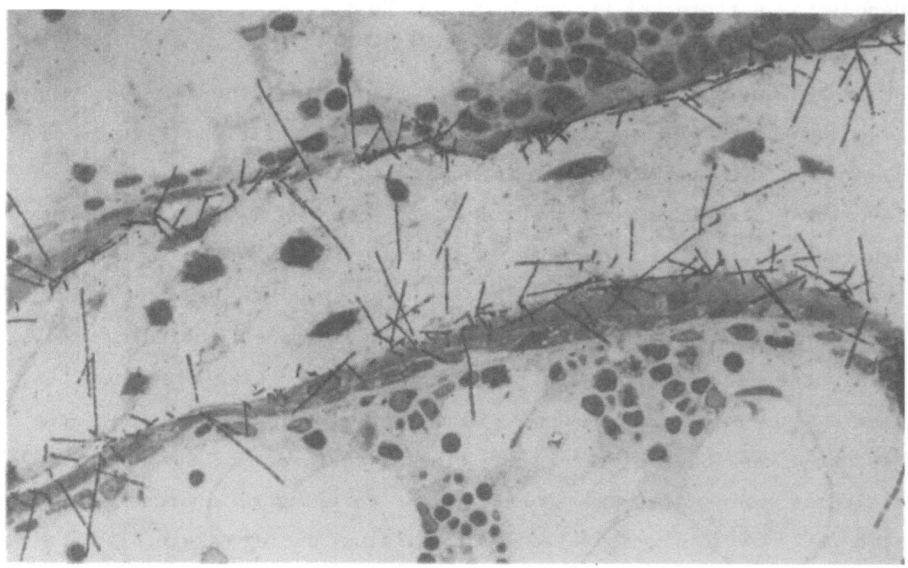

Figure 11. Shows the similar levels of plutonium uptake by bone surfaces of different growth activity at the same anatomical location. (1 μm section, AR10 emulsion, pyronin Y stain).

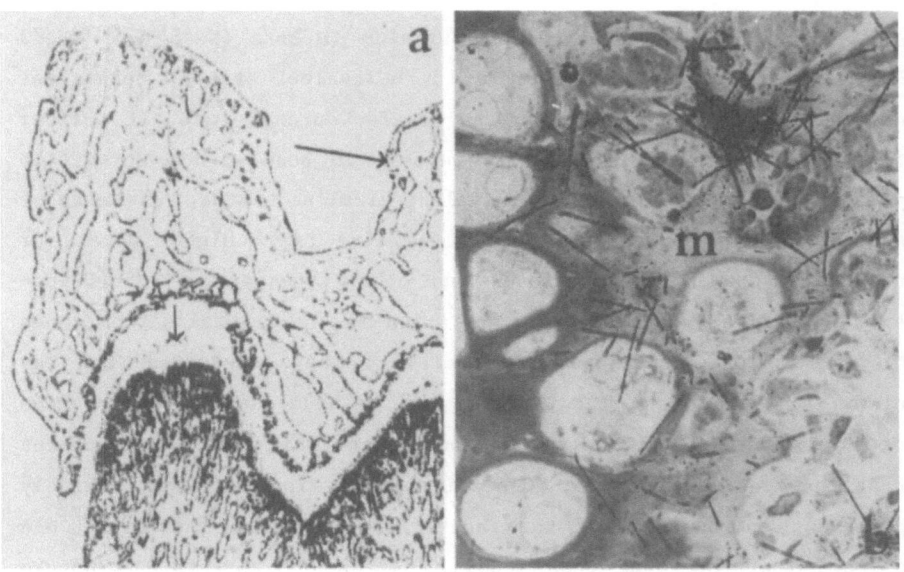

Figure 12. Neptunium deposition in the mineralising zones of the mandibular condylar cartilage (12b), epiphyseal plate cartilage (12a, short arrow) and epiphyseal articular cartilage (12a, long arrow). m = mineralised cartilage. (5 μm section, CR39 (a); 1 μm section, AR10 emulsion, pyronin Y stain (b).)

Deposition Patterns of Protactinium and Neptunium

Protactinium and neptunium are typically pentavelent (Co75). They also seemed to share a similar pattern of deposition (Figures 1 & 3) in the skeleton which was in some ways intermediate between that described for trivalent actinides and for tetravalent plutonium; consequently, these elements may prove to be of intermediate toxicity. Like the trivalent actinides, neptunium and protactinium were concentrated by all types of bone surface, including those within the cortical bone and primary spongiosa. Like plutonium they seemed to be fairly evenly concentrated along bone surfaces. Neptunium was concentrated in the mineralising zone of the epiphyseal articular and epiphyseal growth plate cartilages, indicating that some may be co-precipitated with calcium during skeletal matrix mineralisation (Figure 12). Protactinium also deposited in this zone but to a much lower extent.

Deposition Pattern of Uranium

All studies of the deposition of uranium in bone (Ne48 Ro69 Ste80 Pr82) have used this actinide in its hexavalent state. Hexavalent uranium exists in the body as the divalent uranyl ion. It follows that uranium may be expected to deposit in bone with a deposition pattern similar to that of the divalent alkaline earths. Evidence of such similarities was provided by the five times higher uptake of uranium by growing bone surfaces than other types of surface (Figure 13) and by its substantial concentration in the mineralisation zones of the skeletal cartilages (Figure 14). These suggested that the uranyl ion is being co-precipitated with calcium during the formation of bone mineral. It is perhaps because of this mode of deposition that the fractional uptake of uranium by the rat skeleton is highly dependent on the rate of bone accretion and is much lower in old animals than in young ones (So83). In other respects the uptake pattern of uranium by bone surfaces was unexceptional with deposition on all types of surface, including those within cortical bone (Figure 3), and with an even dispersion along surfaces.

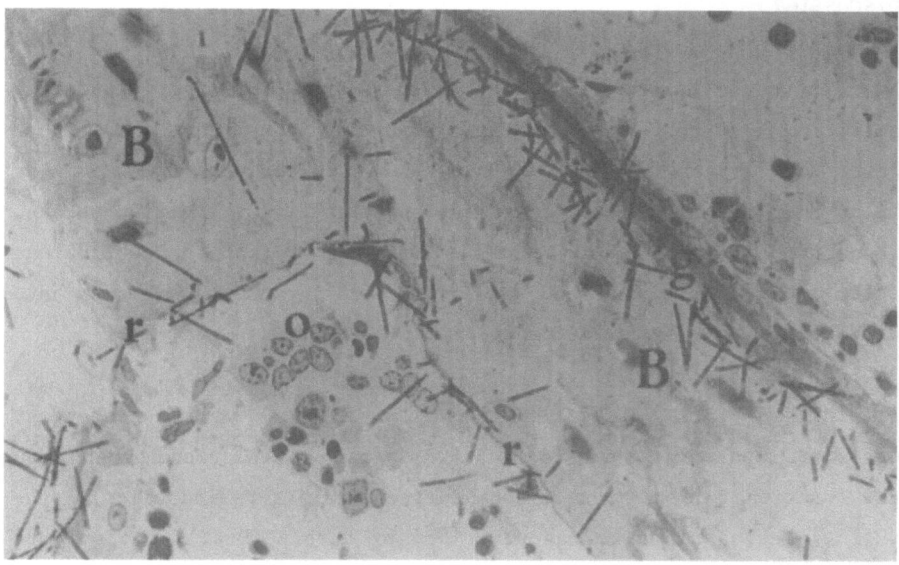

Figure 13.   Differential uranium uptake by growing (g) and resting/resorbing (r) bone surfaces. (1 μm section AR10 emulsion, pyronin Y stain.) o = osteoclast, B = trabecular bone.

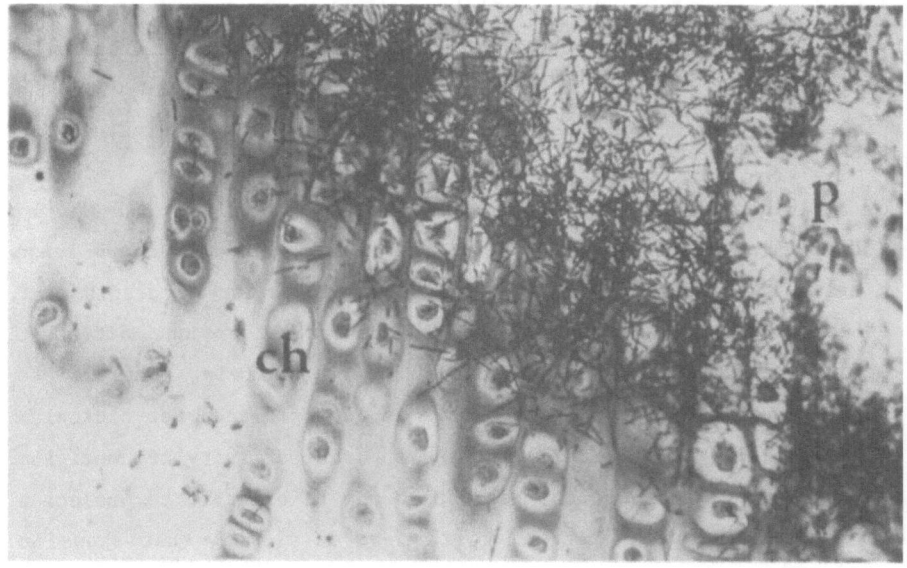

Figure 14. Autoradiograph, (5 μm section, AR10 emulsion, azure II stain), showing the heavy uptake of uranium in the mineralising zones of the epiphyseal plate cartilage. ch = chondroyctes, p = primary spongosa of metaphysis.

DISCUSSION

In general, the deposition patterns described for plutonium, americium and curium in this paper are consistent with those described 40 years ago by Hamilton and his colleagues (Ha47 Ha48) as being characteristic for tetravalent and trivalent transition metals, respectively. In addition, the results suggest that the pentavalent actinides, protactinium and neptunium, and hexavalent uranium have different and characteristic deposition patterns.

If further studies confirm the existence of valency dependent deposition patterns then it is likely that the relationship between the fractional deposition of bone-surface seeking radionuclide in the skeleton and ionic size, as described by Durbin (Du62), may only be appropriate for elements of one valency such as the trivalent actinides and rare earth elements. This is because it is unlikely that the same relationship should be appropriate when different mechanisms of actinide uptake by the skeleton are involved. It follows that it is possible that the apparent consistency of plutonium, neptunium and protactinium with the relationship described by Durbin (mostly for the trivalent elements) is coincidental. Similarly, the failure of thorium and uranium to comply with the relationship may be a consequence of their aberrant valencies.

Why actinides should deposit in bone with different patterns may be explained, at least in part, by their various methods of deposition in bone. For example, the apparent co-precipitation of uranium and neptunium with bone mineral may be expected to produce different patterns of skeletal uptake than if the ion was being complexed to components of the organic bone matrix as is postulated for plutonium and americium (Wi63). Similarly, the apparent affinity of americium and curium for areas of bone resorption may be expected to produce a different distribution pattern to that of an element that shows no such affinity. However, it would seem highly unlikely that differences such as exist between the radionuclide concentrations in different   bones   can   be   explained   in   such   ways.

Instead it is likely that these relate to the blood supply to bone surfaces in different anatomical regions.

The actual relationship between the blood supply to bone and the corresponding level of radionuclide uptake is complex and probably depends upon many factors including the flow rate, the diffusibility of the radionuclide, the diameter of the blood vessels and the permeability of the blood vessel walls. With regard to blood flow rate, Humphries (Hu77 Hu82), Smith (Sm84), Tothill (To80 To84 To85) and others have shown that the blood flow to an area will influence the availability of the bone seeker for deposition. In this way variations in the concentrations of radium, which is probably absorbed on to bone surfaces by a non-specific ion exchange process and which is likely to be freely diffusable (Nu58), may be explained: high uptakes in areas favouring the exchange of radium from blood to bone such as under the epiphyseal plate cartilage and in bones with a generous blood supply, and lower uptakes in areas of poorer vascularisation such as in long bone epiphyses and in the caudal vertebrae and paws. Consequently, it is likely that such mechanisms shape the distribution patterns of the trivalent and pentavlent actnides and uranium, but are probably less important for tetravelent plutonium. It would seem that plutonium is not freely available to deposit in the manner described above and that the basic deposition pattern has been extensively modified by other factors. One of these factors may be the way in which plutonium binds to components of the blood and the permeability of the blood vessels walls. This may be inferred from the high uptake of plutonium by bone surfaces adjacent to the blood sinusoids of the red bone marrow and its failure to deposit to the same extent on those adjacent to blood capillaries, such as those which exist in periosteal regions, in the primary spongiosa and in cortical bone (Br61). This may be explained if plutonium is more strongly bound to proteins in the blood, and if blood vessel walls are much less permeable to such protein complexes than the often ill-defined walls of sinusoidal blood cavities.

SUMMARY

Each actinide has its own characteristic distribution pattern in the soft tissues and skeleton.

The deposition patterns described are consistent with the suggestion that the transition metals deposit in bone with valency dependent patterns.

The deposition pattern of each actinide are likely to depend upon their ability to bind to different components of the bone surface, including both mineral and organic components of the bone matrix, as well as the bone surface blood supply and the growth activity of the bone.

For some elements such as plutonium the deposition pattern may be strongly influenced by the presence or absence of a sinusoidal blood supply.

To some extent the differences in distribution described may explain the variations in their toxicity.

REFERENCES

Br61 Brookes, M., Elkin, A.C., Harrison, R.G. and Heald, C.B., 1961, A new concept of capillary circulation in bone cortex, Lancet 1, 1078-1081.

Co75 Cotton, S.A. and Hart, F.A., 1975, The Heavy Transition Elements. (London: Macmillan).

Du62 Durbin, P.A. 1962, Distribution of the transuranic elements in mammals, Health Phys. 8, 665-671.

Du73 Durbin, P.A., 1973, Metabolism and biological effects of the transplutonium elements, In: Uranium Plutonium Transplutonic Elements, Eds: Hodge, H.C., Stannard, J.N. and Hursh, J.B., (Berlin: Springer-Verlag).

Fe83 Fews, A.P. and Henshaw, D.L., 1983, Alpha-particle autoradiography in CR39: A technique for quantitative assessment of alpha emitters in biological tissues, Phys Med. Biol. 28, 459-474.

Gr78 Green, D., Howells, G.R. and Thorne, M.C., 1978, Plutonium-239 deposition in the skeleton of the mouse, Int. J. Radiat. Biol. 1, 27-36.

Gr79 Green, D. Howells, G.R. and Thorne, M.C., 1979, Quantitative microscopic studies of the distribution and retention of Pu-239 in the illium of the female mouse. Int. J. Radiat. Biol. 36, 499-511.

Ha47 Hamilton, J.D., 1947, The metabolism of fission products and the heaviest elements, Radiology 49, 325-343.

Ha48 Hamilton, J.D., 1948, The metabolic properties of the fission products and actinide elements. Rev. Mod. Phys. 20, 718-728.

Hu77 Humphries, E.R., Fisher, G. and Thorne, M.C., 1977, The measurement of blood flow in the mouse femur and its correlation with 239-Pu deposition. Calcif. Tiss. Res. 23, 141-145.

Hu82 Humphries, E.R., Green, D., Howells, G.R. and Thorne, M.C., 1982. Relationships between blood flow, bone structure and Pu-239 deposition in the mouse skeleton, Calcif. Tiss. Intl. 34, 416-421.

ICRP67 A review of the radiosensitivity of the tissues in bone. ICRP Publication 11, 1967, (Oxford: Pergamon).

ICRP79 Limits for intakes of radionuclides by workers, 1979, ICRP Publication 30, Part 1, Ann. ICRP, No. 3/4.

Je72 Jee, W.S.S., 1972. Distribution and toxicity of plutonium-239 in bone, Health Pys. 2, 583-595.

Ke70 Keough, R.F. and Powers, J.G., 1970, Determination of plutonium in biological materials by extraction and liquid scintillation counting. Analyt. Chem., 42, 419-421.

Ma62 Marshall, J.H., 1962, Radioactive hotspots, bone growth and bone cancer; Self burial of calcium like hotspots, In: Radioisotopes and Bone, Eds: Lacroix, P and Budy, A.M. (Oxford: Blackwell).

Ma69 Marshall, H.H., The retention of radionuclides in bone, In: Delayed Effects of Bone-Seeking Radionuclides, Eds: Mays, C.W., Jee, W.S.S., Lloyd, R.D., Stover, B.J., Dougherty, J.H. and Taylor, G.N., 1969 (Salt Lake City: University of Utah Press).

May83 Mays, C.W., Taylor, G.N. and Lloyd, R.D., 1983, Toxicity ratios: Their uses and abuse in predicting the risk from induced cancer. Proc. 22nd Handford Life Sciences Symposium 27-29 Sept., Radiation Effects Studies in Animals: What Can They Tell Us?

Ne48 Neuman, N.W., Neuman, W.F. and Mulryan, B.J., 1948, The deposition of uranium in bone, J. Biol. Chem., 1975, 705-719.

Ne58 Neuman, W.F. and Neuman, N.W., 1958, The Chemical Dynamics of Bone Mineral (Chicago: University of Chicago Press).

Nen72 Nenot, JC., Masse, R., Morin, M. and Lafuma, J., 1972, An experimental comparative study of the behaviour of ^{237}Np, ^{238}Pu, ^{239}Pu, ^{241}Am and ^{242}Cm in bone. Hlth. Phys. 22, 657-665.

Pr80 Priest, N.D. and Giannola, S.J., 1980, 241-Plutonium deposition and redistribution in the rat rib, Int. J. Radiat. Biol., 37, 281-298.

Pr81 Priest, N.D., 1981, Plutonium in bone: The effects of bone remodelling, In: Bone and Bone-Seeking Radionuclides - Physiology, Dosimetry and Effects, Ed: Volf, V. EUR 7168 EN.

Pr82 Priest, N.D., Howells, G.R., Green, D. and Haines, J.W., 1982, Uranium in bone: Metabolic and autoradiographic studies in the rat, Human Toxicol. 1, 97-114.

Pr83 Priest, N.D., Howells, G.R., Green, D. and Haines, J.W.., 1983, The uptake of americium-241 by the rat skeleton and its subsequent redistribution and retention, Human Toxicol., 2, 101-120.

Pr83b Priest, N.D., Howells, G.R., Green, D. and Haines, J.W., 1983, Autoradiographic studies of the distribution of radium-226 in rat bone: Their implications for human radiation dosimetry and toxicity, Human Toxicol., 3, 479-496.

Ro69 Rowland, R.E. and Farnham, J.E., 1969, The deposition of uranium in bone, Health Phys., 17, 139-144.

Rod77 Rodwell, P. and Stather, J.W., 1977, The distribution of plutonium-239 and americium-241 in the syrian hamster following its intravenous adminstration as citrate. NRPB R&D/2, 11-14.

Sm84 Smith, J.M. Miller, S.C. and Jee, W.S.S., 1984, The relationship of bone marrow type and microvasculature to the mirco-distribution and local dosimetry of plutonium in the adult skeleton. Radiat. Res., 99, 324-335.

So83 Sontag, W., 1983, The early distribution of Pu-239, Am-241 and U-233 in the soft tissues and skeleton of old rats: A comparative study, Human Toxicol., 2, 91-100.

St74 Stather, J.W., 1974, Distributions of ^{32}P, ^{45}Ca, ^{85}Sr and ^{133}Ba as a function of age in the mouse skeleton, Hlth Phys. 26, 71-79.

Ste80 Stevens, W., Bruenger, F.W., Atherton, D.R., Smith, J.M. and Taylor, G.N., 1980, The distribution and retention of hexavalent U-233 in the beagle, Radiat. Res., 83, 109-126.

Sto69 Stover, B., Atherton, D.R. Brunegen, F.W. and Buster, D.S., 1969, Pu(IV): its distribution in the beagle, In: Delayed Effects of Bone-Seeking Radionuclides, Eds: Mays, C.W., Jee, W.S.S., Lloyd, R.D. Stover, B.J., Dougherty, J.H. and Taylor, G.N., (Salt Lake City: University of Utah Press).

Ta83 Taylor, D.M., 1983, The comparative carcinogenicity of Pu-239, Am-241 and Cm-244 in the rat. In: Proc 22nd Hanford Symposium, Sept 1983, Life Span Radiation Effect Studies in Animals: What Have They Told Us?

Tay83 Taylor, G.N., Mays, C.W., Lloyd, R.D., Gardner, P.A., Talbot, L.R. and McFarland, S., 1983, Comparative toxicity of radium-226, plutonium-239, americium-241, californium-249 and californium-252 in C57Bl/Do black and albino mic, Radiat. Res., 95, 584-601.

To80 Tothill, P. and MacPherson, J.N., 1980, Limitations of microspheres as tracers for bone blood flow and extraction ratio studies, Calcif. Tiss. Int., 31, 261-265.

To84 Tothill, P. and Hooper, G., 1984, Bone blood flow and extraction ratios: microspheres and bone seekers, In: Proc. 3rd Int. Symposium on Circulation in Bone, Ed: Hungerford, D.S. and Arlet, J., (Baltimore: Williams and Wilkins).

To85 Tothill, P. and Hooper, G. McCarthy, I.D. and Hughes, S.P.F., 1985, The variation with flow rate of the extraction of bone seeking tracers in recirculation experiments.   This publication.

Va73 Vaughan, J., 1973, The Effects of Irradiation on the Skeleton (Oxford: Clarendon Press).

Va73b Vaughan, J., Bleaney, B. and Taylor, D.M., 1973, Distribution, excretion and effects of plutonium as a bone-seeker, In: Uranium Plutonium Transplutonic Elements, Eds: Hodge, H.C., Stannard, J.N. and Hursh, J.B., (Berlin: Springer-Verlag).

Wi63 Williamson, M. and Vaughan, J., 1963, A preliminary report on the sites of deposition of Y, Am and Pu in cortical bone and in the region of the epiphyseal cartilage plate. In: Proc. 1st European Symposium of the Bone and Tooth Society, April 193, Oxford, Ed: Blackwood, H.J.J.

18

Pu Microdistribution Study in Cortical Bones of Beagle Dogs

G. INGRAO and W. S. S. JEE

INTRODUCTION

In cases of plutonium contamination, performance of a microdosimetric
evaluation is important from the radiation protection point of view
because of the short range of the emitted alpha particles. This
makes it necessary to obtain accurate data on the microdistribution
of plutonium at various times after intake. Since plutonium is
essentially a bone surface seeker, most of the data available in the
literature refer to the plutonium microdistribution near endosteal
and periosteal bone surfaces (1,2,3,4,5,6,7,8,9,10,11,12) considered
the critical tissues for the induction of bone osteosarcomas. There
is a paucity of data on plutonium microdistribution in adult cortical
bone. The purpose of this study was to obtain data on plutonium
microdistribution in cortical bone, which consists of a mineralized
component and a soft tissue component, lining the forming and resorbing cavities and the Haversian and Volkmann's canals. The soft
tissue consists of various bone cells (13,14) considered to be at
risk from radiation-induced osteosarcomas including bone lining cells
and "osteoprogenitor" cells. Cortical bone is a dynamic structure
subject to continuous remodeling: the removal of compact bone is
followed by the replacement of a new Haversian system or osteon.
Alpha irradiation of the remodeling units could promote pathological
alterations in the skeleton (radiation osteodystrophy) as well as the
induction of osteosarcomas (15,13,7,16).

MATERIALS AND METHODS

Table 1 shows details concerning the experimental animals. Cross
sections from samples from the mid-ulnar shaft and the dorsal
spine of the thoracic vertebrae of dogs injected with about
0.3 µCi/kg ^{239}Pu monomeric citrate were fixed, dehydrated in
acetone of increasing concentrations, and embedded in methylmethacrylate. Two sections from each block were ground to a thickness
of about 100 µm, placed between Lexan slides, and irradiated in
the thermal column of the Massachusetts Institute of Technology
(M.I.T.) reactor to obtain neutron-induced autoradiographs (NIAR),
(17,18).

Table 1. Sex, Age, Weight and Dose at Injection, Days Post-
          Injection and Age and Weight at Death

Dog No	Sex	Age at Injection (d)	Weight at Injection (kg)	Injected Dose (µCi/kg)	Days Post-Injection (d)	Age at Death (d)	Weight at death (kg
T31P3	M	520	13.00	0.305	41	561	11.02
T35P3	M	550	11.90	0.303	362	912	11.87
T29P3	M	552	12.10	0.296	561	1113	13.15
T27P3	M	556	11.50	0.332	755	1311	10.71
M11P3	M	600	10.50	0.309	1197	1797	12.39
F5P3	F	651	8.22	0.288	1503	2154	9.35
M4P3	M	608	8.51	0.292	1950	2558	9.94

A low neutron fluence $\phi = 2 \times 10^{15}$ n/cm^2 was used for quantitative analysis, and a higher fluence $\phi = 5 \times 10^{16}$ n/cm^2 was used
for qualitative analysis. The Lexan slides were etched in a solution of 5N KOH for approximately 9 min at 70° C, with continuous
agitation. Microradiographs of each irradiated bone section were
also taken.

The density of induced fission fragment tracks in compact bone
was determined by counting fission fragment tracks at a magnification of 430X (microscopic field of 0.0484 mm^2). Such measurements
were made in alternate microscopic fields within an individual
section disregarding fields partially filled with bone at the

periosteal and endosteal surface regions. The total number of microscopic fields sampled varied from 70 to 140, depending on the size of the bone section examined.

To estimate the ^{239}Pu concentration in cortical bone (C_{Pu}), from the track density T, the following formula was used (20):

$$C_{Pu} = \frac{TF}{\sigma\phi\eta R} \qquad (1)$$

where σ is the thermal neutron cross section for fission of ^{239}Pu (7.42 X 10^{-22} cm^2), ϕ is the thermal neutron fluence, η is the empirically determined fission fragment track detection efficiency (0.488), F is the conversion factor (2.43 X 10^{-11} pCi/^{239}Pu nucleus), and R is the average range of fission fragments in methylmethacrylate (18 μm). Therefore:

$$C_{Pu} = 1.86 \ 10^{-2} \ T$$

where C_{Pu} is in units of pCi/cm^3 and T in units of tracks/cm^2.

Morphometric parameters for cortical bone were determined by examining each microradiograph using a Quantimet 720 Image Analyzer at a magnification of 4X (19). The number of fields examined varied from 10 to 20 depending on the size of the bone section examined. The following parameters were determined:

a) bone porosity, expressed as ratio between the area of all cavities and the area of compact bone surface

b) the surface/volume ratio calculated from the following equation (20):

$$S_{vb} = K(P/A) \qquad (2)$$

where K is a constant equal to $4/\pi$, P is the perimeter of all cavities present in compact bone, including forming and resorbing cavities such as Haversian and Volkmann's canals, and A is the cortical bone area. All results are expressed as mean $\pm$ SEM.

RESULTS AND DISCUSSION

Table 2 shows the ^{239}Pu concentration, the percent porosity and the surface/volume ratio for the mid-ulnar shaft of the experi-

mental animals. Table 3 gives the same data for the dorsal spine
of the thoracic vertebrae of these animals.

Table 2. ^{239}Pu Concentration, Per Cent Porosity, and
Surface/Volume Ratio in Mid-Ulnar Shaft of Dogs at
Various Times Post-Injection

Dog No.	Days Post Injection	^{239}Pu Concentration $\pm$ S.E. (pCi/cm^3)	Porosity %	S/V cm^{-1}
T31P3	41	370 $\pm$ 41	3.6 $\pm$ 0.1	67.4 $\pm$ 4.0
T35P3	362	517 $\pm$ 33	2.7 $\pm$ 0.2	65.7 $\pm$ 12.2
T29P3	561	318 $\pm$ 28	2.1 $\pm$ 0.1	59.3 $\pm$ 4.4
T27P3	755	850 $\pm$ 71	1.7 $\pm$ 0.1	43.6 $\pm$ 0.2
M11P3	1197	394 $\pm$ 20	3.0 $\pm$ 0.6	54.8 $\pm$ 9.4
F5P3	1503	498 $\pm$ 33	3.2 $\pm$ 0.3	47.6 $\pm$ 0.3
M4P3	1950	476 $\pm$ 37	4.1 $\pm$ 1.0	57.3 $\pm$ 2.7

Table 3. ^{239}Pu Concentration, Per Cent Porosity and
Surface/Volume Ratio Dorsal Spine of Thoracic Vertebrae
of Dogs at Various Times Post Injection

Dog No.	Days Post Injection	^{239}Pu Concentration $\pm$ S.E. (pCi/cm^3)	Porosity %	S/V cm^{-1}
T31P3	41	833 $\pm$ 63	6.1 $\pm$ 0.7	68.4 $\pm$ 8.3
T35P3	362	580 $\pm$ 41	2.6 $\pm$ 0.4	49.8 $\pm$ 5.6
T29P3	561	742 $\pm$ 54	2.1 $\pm$ 0.5	42.2 $\pm$ 6.6
T27P3	755	960 $\pm$ 71	2.3 $\pm$ 0.1	44.0 $\pm$ 1.0
M11P3	1197	787 $\pm$ 65	3.5 $\pm$ 0.6	54.3 $\pm$ 9.2
F5P3	1503	843 $\pm$ 56	3.1 $\pm$ 0.5	53.6 $\pm$ 7.6
M1P3	1950	722 $\pm$ 48	3.1 $\pm$ 0.1	47.8 $\pm$ 1.9

Except for dog T27P3, all the animals injected as young adults show similar fission track densities in cortical bone, irrespective of the time from injection to death. The concentration of Pu in the dorsal spine of the thoracic vertebrae is generally a factor 1.5 to 2 higher than in the mid-ulnar shaft, which may be due in part to the different rate of blood flow in the two bones. In the mouse skeleton, the density of endosteal deposition of plutonium is determined by the rate of blood flow in the mouse skeleton (21).

The variation of the percentages of porosity and of surface/volume ratios among the animals is within a factor of 2 in most cases, although different areas of the same bone section can show differences up to a factor of 10. The variation does not seem to be related to increased age of the animals, nor can any correlation be established with fission track density. The neutron-induced autoradiographs obtained using a neutron fluence of 5 X 10^{16} n/cm^2, in conjunction with the microradiographs of the irradiated bone sections, clearly show the microdistribution pattern of plutonium in cortical bone; the bulk of plutonium is deposited on forming, resorbing and resting (Haversian and Volkmann's canals) bone surfaces soon after the time of injection (Figs. 1-4). While the new bone is more uniformly labeled, the very similar distribution pattern observed at different times after injection shows that the remodeling rate in these animals is fairly slow, probably due to radiation injury to the bone which disturbs the remodeling activity (22,15,23). The finding that the fission track density is almost constant at various times post injection is in agreement with the results of other radiochemical studies indicating that Pu retention time in cortical bone is extremely long (24,25).

Our results are particularly relevant to microdosimetric evaluation. During their lifespans, bone cells located within the alpha particle range in the cortical bone surfaces will receive a dose considerably higher than the average dose to the skeleton. Assuming an average plutonium concentration of 400 pCi/cm^3 in the whole skeleton, a skeletal mass of 1000 g and bone density of 2.0

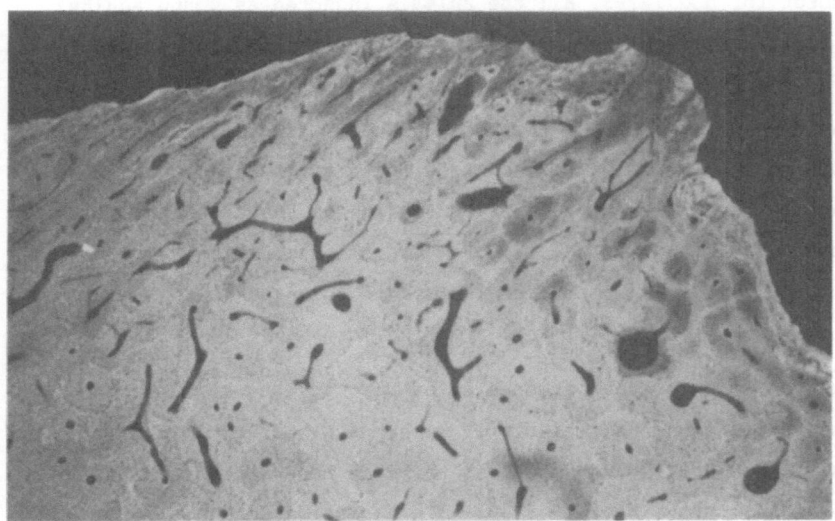

Figure 1.   Microradiograph of a region of tendon insertion of the
mid-ulnar shaft of dog T35P3 killed at 362 days post-
injection.   Note recently formed hypomineralized
osteones (arrows) and forming osteones (arrow heads)
concentrated near the periosteal surfaces, X5.6

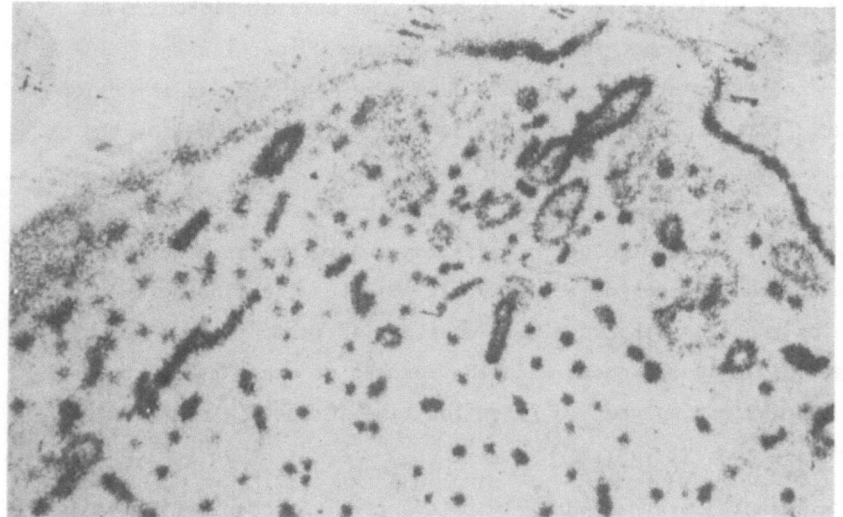

Figure 2.   Corresponding neutron-induced autoradiograph to Figure
1.   Note heavy deposits of fission tracks lining the
bone surfaces.   Even at 362 days post-injection, the
bulk of the tracks are lining resting surfaces
(Haversian and Volkmann canals) labeled at the time of
injection X5.6.

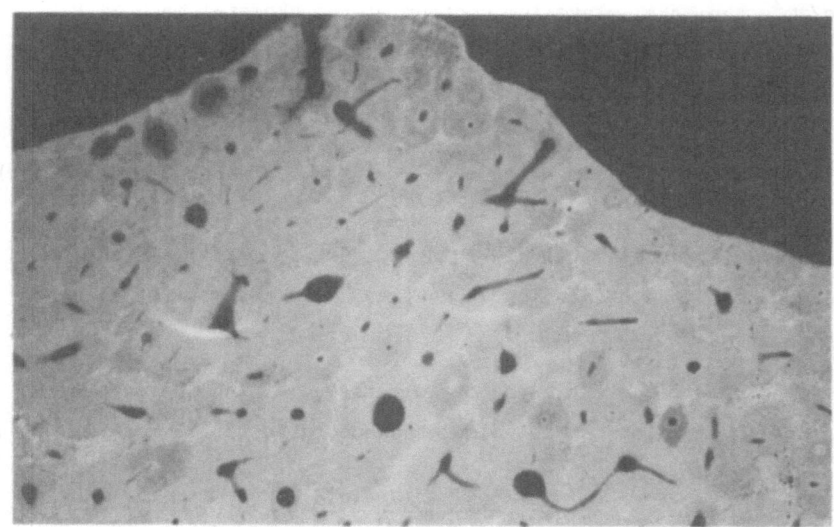

Figure 3. Microradiograph of mid-ulnar shaft from dog M11P3 killed at 1197 days post-injection. Few hypomineralized osteones (arrows) are located near the periosteal surface, X5.6.

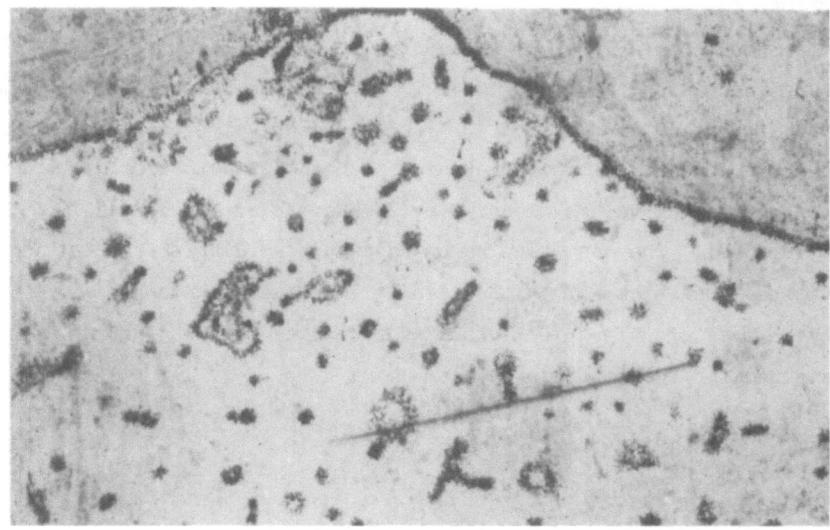

Figure 4. Corresponding neutron-induced autoradiograph to Figure 3. This is a typical example of depressed cortical bone remodeling. The bulk of the heavy deposit of fission tracks are located on resting surfaces (Haversian and Volkmann's canal) labeled 1197 days previously at the time of injection, X5.6.

g/cm^3, the total plutonium content of the skeletal mass is 0.2 µCi. The average dose rate to the skeleton (assuming a uniform distribution of Pu) is calculated according to the formula:

$$D_{bone} = \frac{51.2 \ IE_\alpha}{M} = 0.053 \ \text{Rad} \ d^{-1} \tag{3}$$

where I is the skeletal plutonium content in µCi, E_α is the energy of ^{239}Pu α-emission in MeV, and M is the mass of mineral bone in grams.

The dose rate to a layer of soft tissue lining the Haversian canals q µm thick can be calculated according to the formula (26):

$$D(q,d) = \frac{51.2 \ IE_\alpha K(q,d)}{M} \ \text{Rad} \ d^{-1} \tag{4}$$

where I is the plutonium content in µCi, E_α is the energy of ^{239}Pu α-emission in MeV, M is the mass of soft tissue in grams, and K (q,d) is the average fraction of that energy absorbed in an endosteal tissue layer of q µm thickness, if the decay occurs d µm below the endosteal surface.

Let us consider a typical Haversian canal having a diameter of 50 µm and a length of 2.5 mm (27). Its volume and surface will be 4.91 X 10^{-6} cm^3 and 3.93 X 10^{-3} cm^2, respectively. Assuming an average concentration of plutonium in bone of 400 pCi/cm^3, the Pu content in the volume occupied by the Haversian canal will be 1.96 X 10^{-9} µCi. The dose rate assuming a uniform distribution of Pu to the 10µm thick soft tissue lining the Haversian canal, which has a mass of 3.14 X 10^{-6} grams if a density of 1.0 g/cm^3 is assumed for the soft tissue, is:

$$D(10,0) = 0.042 \ \text{Rad} \ d^{-1} \tag{5}$$

Because in reality the distribution of plutonium is non-uniform, this calculation underestimates the dose rate to the soft tissue lining the Haversian canal. A conservative estimate of the dose rate can be obtained, assuming that plutonium is deposited only on the surfaces of all cavities present in cortical bone proper. In this case, the plutonium activity deposited on the surface of the cortical bone proper, assuming a surface/volume ratio of 54 cm^{-1}, is 2.91 X 10^{-8} µCi. If there is no burial of plutonium and it is deposited on the bone surface, the dose rate to the 10 µm thick soft tissue lining the Haversian canal is:

$$D(10,0) = 0.62 \text{ Rad } d^{-1} \tag{6}$$

The wide range of values observed in the different dose rate calculations outlines the need for detailed Pu microdistribution studies if realistic microdosimetric evaluations are required.

SUMMARY

^{239}Pu microdistribution has been studied in cortical bones (cross sections of mid-ulnar shaft and the dorsal spine of the thoracic vertebrae) of beagle dogs injected with about 0.3 µCi/kg ^{239}Pu monomeric citrate and killed between 41 and 1950 days post injection. The concentration of ^{239}Pu in the dorsal spine of the thoracic vertebrae was generally a factor 1.5 to 2 higher than in the mid-ulnar shaft. Nearly all the dogs exhibited similar track density in the cortical bone proper independent of the time interval from injection to death. The plutonium was deposited on existing bone surfaces at the time of injection and subsequently some of the ^{239}Pu redistributed into a more uniform deposit of lower concentration as the result of bone remodeling. A similar distribution pattern was observed at different times after injection showing that the remodeling rate was slow and/or radiation injury had depressed the bone remodeling rate. The dose rate to the 10 µm thick soft tissue lining the Haversian canal, assuming that Pu was deposited only on the surface, was a factor of 10 higher than the calculated dose rate assuming a uniform distribution of Pu in the bone.

ACKNOWLEDGEMENT

This research was supported by U.S. DOE Contract DE-AC02-76EV-00119.

REFERENCES

1. Arnold J.S. and Jee W.S.S. (1957). Bone growth and osteo-clastic activity as indicated by radioautographic distribution of Pu^{239}. Am. J. Anat., 101, 367-417.

2. Arnold J.S. and Jee W.S.S. (1962). Pattern of long term skeletal remodeling revealed by radioautographic distribution of ^{239}Pu in dogs. Health Phys., 81, 705-707.

3. Twente J.A. and Jee W.S.S. (1961). Determination of Pu^{239} content of bone tissue: A comparison of radiochemical, track counting, and photoelectric density techniques. Health Phys., 59, 142-148.

4. Jee W.S.S., Arnold J.S., Cochran T.H, Twente J.A., and Mical R.S. (1962). Relationship of microdistribution of alpha particles to damage. In: Dougherty, T.F., Jee, W.S.S., Mays, C.W. and Stover, B.J. (eds.). Some Aspects of Internal Irradiation, pp. 27-45, (Pergamon Press, Oxford).

5. Bleaney B. (1967). Radiation dose-rates near bone surfaces in rabbits after an injection of plutonium. Phys. Med. Biol., 12, 145-160.

6. Bleaney B. and Vaughan J. (1971). Distribution of ^{239}Pu in the bone marrow and on the endosteal surface of the femur of adult rabbits following injection of $^{239}Pu(NO_3)_4$. Brit. J. Radiol., 44, 67-73.

7. Vaughan J. (1973). Distribution, excretion and effects of plutonium as a bone seeker. In: Hodge, H.C., Stannard, J.N. and Hursh, J.B. (eds.) Handbook of Experimental Pharmacology, Vol. 36: Uranium, Plutonium, Transplutonic Elements, pp. 349-502 (Springer-Verlag, Berlin).

8. Schlenker R.A., Oltman B.G. and Cummins H.T. (1976). Micro-scopic distribution of ^{239}Pu deposited in bone from a human injection case. In: Jee, W.S.S. (ed.). The Health Effects of Plutonium and Radium. pp. 321-328 (J.W. Press, Salt Lake City).

9. Wronski T.J., Smith J.M., and Jee W.S.S. (1980). The micro-distribution and retention of injected ^{239}Pu on trabecular bone surfaces of the beagle: implications for the induction of osto-sarcomas. Radiat.Res., 83, 74-89,

10. Priest N.D. and Giannola S.J. (1980). ^{241}Pu deposition and redistribution in the rat rib. Int. J. Radiat. Biol., 37, 281-298.

11. Green D., Howells G.R. and Thorne M.C. (1978). Plutonium-239 deposition in the skeleton of the mouse. Int. J. Radiat. Biol., 34, 27-36.

12. Green D, Howells G.R. and Thorne M.C. (1981). A semiauto-mated technique for assessing the microdistribution of ^{239}Pu deposited in bone. Phys. Med. Biol., 26:379-387.

13. Loutit J.F., Brues A.M., Marinelli L., Spiers F.W. and Vaughan J.(1968). A Review of the Radiosensitivity of the Tissues in Bone, ICRP Publication 11 (Pergamon Press, Oxford).

14. Jee W.S.S. (1983). The skeletal tissues. In: Weiss, L. (ed.). Histology, pp. 200-255, (Elsevier Biomedical, New York.

15. Jee W.S.S. (1962). Histopathological endpoints in compact bone receiving alpha emitters. In: Dougherty, T.F., Jee, W.S.S., Mays, C.W. and Stover, B.J. (eds.). Some Aspects of Internal Irradiation, pp. 95-113 (Pergamon Press, Oxford).

16. Pool R.R., Morgan J.P., Parks N.J., Farnham J.E. and Littman M.S. (1983). Comparative pathogenesis of radium-induced intra-cortical bone lesions in human and beagles. Health Phys., 44 155-177, Suppl. No. 1.

17. Jee W.S.S., Dell R.B. and Miller L.G. (1972). High resolu-tion neutron-induced autoradiography of bone containing ^{239}Pu. Health Phys., 22, 761-763.

18. Fellows M.H., Clark L., O'Toole J.J., Kimmel D.B. and Jee W.S.S. (1975). An improved technique for neutron-induced auto-radiography of bone containing plutonium. Health Phys.,29, 97-101.

19. Woodbury L.A., Woodbury N.A., Wronski T. and Jee W.S.S. (1976). In: Jee, W.S.S. (ed.). Preliminary studies on the use of the Quantimet-720 for the measurement of radiographs of bone sections, Research in Radiobiology. pp. 285-304 (COO-119-251, Division of Radiobiology, University of Utah, Salt Lake City.

20. Elias H and Hyde D.M. (1980). An elementary introduction to stereology (Quantitative microscopy). Am. J. Anat., 159,12-446.

21.   Humphreys E.R, Green D, Howells G.R. and Thorne M.C. (1982).   Relationship between blood flow, bone strucure, and ^{239}Pu deposition in the mouse skeleton.   Calcif. Tissue Int., 34, 416-421.

22.   Jee W.S.S. and Arnold J.S. (1960).   Effects of internally deposited radioisotopes upon blood vessels of cortical bone. Proc. Soc. Exptl. Biol. & Med., 105, 351-156.

23.   Jee W.S.S. (1964).   The influence of reduced local vascularity on the rate of internal reconstruction of adult long bone cortex.   In: Frost, H.M. (ed.).   Bone Biodynamics, pp. 259-277, (Little Brown, Boston).

24.   Stover B.J. and Atherton D.R. (1974).   Kinetics of the skeletal retention of ^{239}Pu(IV).   Radiat. Res., 60, 525-535.

25.   Bruenger F. (1983).   Personal communication.   Radiobiology Division, Department of Pharmacology, Univ. of Utah.

26.   Thorne M.C. (1976).   Aspects of the dosimetry of plutonium in bone.   Nature, 259, 539-541.

27.   Beddoe A.H. (1977).   Measurements of the microscopic structure of cortical bone.   Phys. Med. Biol., 22, 298-308.

19

Removal of Plutonium and Americium from Various Parts of Rat Skeleton

V. VOLF

INTRODUCTION

In recent communications on prolonged oral chelation treatment after injection of ^{238}Pu and ^{241}Am in rats (Vo84a,b) even small amounts of Zn-DTPA in drinking water were demonstrated to reduce substantially the organ contents of both actinides. The different effect of treatment on the proximal and distal parts of the femur and humerus was considered to be due to differences in bone growth and remodelling.

In this study a detailed analysis of whole skeletons was performed with the aim of estimating the relative radiation risk for various parts of the skeleton due to deposited ^{238}Pu and ^{241}Am both in untreated animals and after chelation treatment.

EXPERIMENTAL

Young adult female Sprague-Dawley rats were injected i.v. with ^{238}Pu and ^{241}Am citrate (about 19 kBq/kg body weight). For treatment, Zn-DTPA was added to the drinking water in concentrations which resulted in an intake of approximately 30 and 300 μmol/kg body weight/day; the administration started at 4d or 30d after administration of actinides and continued until the end of the experiment at 105 d.

Tab. 1 shows the concentration of ^{238}Pu and ^{241}Am per g fresh bone in selected regions representing about 65% of the skeleton. On average the ^{238}Pu values were 1.6 times higher than those of ^{241}Am and the concentrations of both actinides in the extremities were higher than

211

those in the axial skeleton, especially after treatment. The latter suggests that DTPA preferentially removed activity from the axial skeleton. The ratios between the femur and whole skeleton were always greater than one and increased after treatment. It is evident that the use of the femur as an indicator of actinide concentration in total skeleton would have resulted in an overestimation and with respect to treatment effectiveness in an underestimation.

The relative effects of the three treatment schedules investigated on the actinide concentration in different bones are summarized in Fig. 1. Obviously some regions such as the mandible, distal parts of the extremities and tail were relatively refractory to treatment. On the other hand, in some parts of the long bones, such as the proximal humerus and proximal tibia, the actinide concentrations were reduced to the same extent as in the predominant parts of the axial skeleton. There were some further differences in the effect of treatment on the two actinides, e.g. the relatively less effective treatments with small amounts of DTPA reduced ^{241}Am concentrations in the spine (except of tail) and in the pelvis to a greater extent than those of ^{238}Pu.

With respect to the differences observed between the two halves of the long bones, the following should be noted. In untreated rats, the concentrations of ^{238}Pu in proximal humerus, ulna and tibia as well as in the distal radius and femur were substantially higher than those in the other halves of these bones. The same was true for ^{241}Am, except that the concentration in the ulna was higher in the distal than in the proximal half. Treatment diminished these differences, since actinides were removed preferentially from the sites which showed higher concentrations in untreated animals.

As seen in Fig. 2, there was a good correlation between the changes of ^{238}Pu and ^{241}Am concentrations in the proximal and distal halves of femur and tibia. Both ^{238}Pu and ^{241}Am data from control as well as treated rats could be fitted by single regression curves, which suggests common uptake and removal mechanisms. Corresponding values for humerus, however, could be fitted only by two separate regression curves for ^{238}Pu and ^{241}Am; but their parallel slope suggests that the mechanism of treatment effect was common to both actinides. The values in ulna and radius changed in a more complicated way, perhaps reflecting differences in tissue binding and/or availability of ^{238}Pu and

^{241}Am.

Tab. 2 summarizes radiation dose rates at the end of the present experiment in various parts of the skeleton. In order to estimate the relative radiation doses due to ^{238}Pu and ^{241}Am, the dose rates were normalized to equal injected activities. The skeletal weight fractions indicate that about 30% of the bone mass is found in the extremities and 70% in other bones, the axial skeleton. The average skeletal dose rates with ^{241}Am were only about 60% of those with ^{238}Pu, both in control and treated rats. While dose rates higher than the skeletal average were found in untreated rats in about 30% of axial skeleton and about 15% of the extremities, in treated animals only about 20% of the axial skeleton was irradiated with more than the average skeletal dose rate. With ^{241}Am the fraction of highly irradiated extremities increased to about 30%.

The data suggest that prolonged treatment with DTPA changes the radiation dose distribution within the skeleton, which may be of importance in elucidating the mechanisms responsible for the development of bone tumors. Furthermore, there were some differences between ^{238}Pu and ^{241}Am removal from the axial skeleton and distal extremities which occurred after prolonged treatment with DTPA. The validity of these findings is supported by the fact that in the present experiment both actinides were followed under exactly the same conditions.

The highest dose rates in untreated rats were estimated for highly trabecular bone regions, which were also the sites of the greatest dose rate reduction following treatment. Fig. 3 shows the relative concentrations of ^{238}Pu and ^{241}Am in three selected skeletal segments, taking the average concentration in the whole skeleton as 1. In untreated animals, values greater than 1 were obtained in the spine (except the tail) as well as in proximal humerus and proximal tibia. These differences were less pronounced especially after early administration of larger amounts of DTPA, which decreased the values in the spine (except the tail) to less than 1. On the other hand, the relative concentrations of both actinides in the tail, distal humerus and distal tibia increased after treatment, more with ^{241}Am than with ^{238}Pu.

It is well known that the spine, proximal humerus and proximal tibia are predominant sites for the development of experimentally induced osteosarcomas (Th73). One may speculate that decorporation treatment should therefore be more efficient in reducing the tumor risk than could be expected from the reduction of the average skeletal concentration. However, the few results obtained with ^{239}Pu after relatively short treatment with large amounts of DTPA (Bu68, Ro67) indicate that the reduction of bone tumor incidence was less than would be expected from the fraction of the activity removed. No such data are available for ^{241}Am. Clearly more experimental work is necessary on the quantitative effects of therapeutic removal of actinides from the skeleton on the induction of bone tumors or other serious late effects.

CONCLUSION

1. A wide range of radiation dose rates due to actinides deposited was observed in various parts of the skeleton. In untreated rats, the highest values were found in highly trabecular bone, the lowest in highly cortical bone. Treatment reduced the radiation dose rates preferentially in bones with high trabecularity, which turn over more rapidly than the cortical bones. This suggests that the efficacy of a prolonged treatment depends upon the bone remodelling rate.

2. Simultaneous administration of ^{238}Pu and ^{241}Am enabled a direct comparison of their kinetics under identical conditions. The average normalized skeletal radiation dose rates due to ^{241}Am were only about 60% of those due to ^{238}Pu, both in control and treated rats. The effect of treatment in most of the axial skeleton was somewhat greater with ^{241}Am than with ^{238}Pu, that in the distal extremities was distinctly less pronounced with ^{241}Am than with ^{238}Pu.

3. Prolonged oral chelation treatment (ca. 30 μmol/kg/d) proved effective even if started one month after injection of the actinides. If treatment began earlier, it was more effective, especially when a ten times higher concentration of Zn-DTPA was administered. The radiation dose rates were preferentially reduced in those bone regions which are also principal sites for the development of tumors after incorporation of actinides. More experimental evidence is needed on the late consequences of the changed distribution of radiation doses due to Pu and Am deposits remaining in the bone after a decorporation treatment.

Table 1. EFFECT OF ORAL Zn-DTPA ON THE CONCENTRATION OF ACTINIDES IN DIFFERENT PARTS OF RAT SKELETON

Bone	Actinide concentration (% of injected amount/g fresh bone)							
	Plutonium-238				Americium-241			
	Controls	Late low DTPA	Early low DTPA	Early high DTPA	Controls	Late low DTPA	Early low DTPA	Early high DTPA
Skull	1.7±0.7	1.0±0.1	1.1±0.05	0.7±0.03	1.2±0.1	0.8±0.1	0.7±0.03	0.5±0.01
Spine	2.9±0.1	1.9±0.1	1.6±0.03	1.1±0.06	1.7±0.1	1.0±0.1	0.8±0.03	0.6±0.02
Pelvis	3.2±0.1	2.2±0.1	2.0±0.02	1.4±0.11	1.9±0.1	1.1±0.1	0.9±0.04	0.7±0.02
Humerus	3.7±0.1	2.3±0.1	2.0±0.06	1.6±0.15	2.0±0.1	1.2±0.1	1.0±0.02	1.0±0.04
Femur	2.9±0.1	2.0±0.1	1.7±0.04	1.4±0.11	1.7±0.1	1.2±0.1	1.0±0.04	0.8±0.04
Whole skeleton	2.5±0.1	1.7±0.1	1.5±0.02	1.1±0.06	1.6±0.1	1.0±0.1	0.8±0.03	0.7±0.02
Femur/Skeleton	1.2±0.01	1.2±0.02	1.2±0.04	1.3±0.04	1.1±0.03	1.1±0.02	1.2±0.02	1.2±0.02

Zn-DTPA was added to drinking water (low DTPA: 3×10^{-4} molar; high DTPA: 3×10^{-3} molar) from day 4 (early DTPA) or day 30 (late DTPA) up to day 105 after i.v. injection of about 19 kBq/kg of Pu-238 and Am-241 citrate. Arithmetic means ± S.E., 5 rats per group.

Table 2. EFFECT OF ORAL Zn-DTPA ON NORMALIZED RADIATION DOSE RATES IN RAT SKELETON 15 WEEKS AFTER INJECTION OF 238Pu AND 241Am.

| Bone | Skeletal fraction | Normalized dose rate (mGy/d/37 kBq injected per kg) | | | | | |
| | | Plutonium-238 | | | Americium-241 | | |
		Controls	Late low DTPA	Early high DTPA	Controls	Late low DTPA	Early high DTPA
Skull	0.15	11	7	5	8	5	3
Mandibulae	0.05	9	8	5	7	5	3
Scapulae	0.02	17	12	7	11	6	4
Ribs + Sternum	0.08	12	9	6	8	5	3
Cervical spine	0.03	19	12	6	10	6	3
Thoracic spine	0.07	21	13	7	11	6	3
Lumbar spine	0.08	23	15	6	12	7	4
Sacral spine	0.04	25	15	9	13	7	4
Tail	0.12	14	10	7	10	7	5
Pelvis	0.06	21	14	9	12	7	5
Humeri prox.	0.02	29	15	10	15	8	6
dist.	0.02	17	14	11	10	8	7
Radii + Ulnae	0.03	15	12	9	11	9	7
Femora prox.	0.04	13	9	7	8	6	5
dist.	0.05	24	16	11	13	9	6
Tibiae prox.	0.04	26	15	9	16	9	6
dist.	0.03	9	8	7	8	7	6
Feet + Ankles	0.07	10	8	6	9	8	6
Whole skeleton	1.00	16	11	7	10	7	4

For explanations see Table 1.

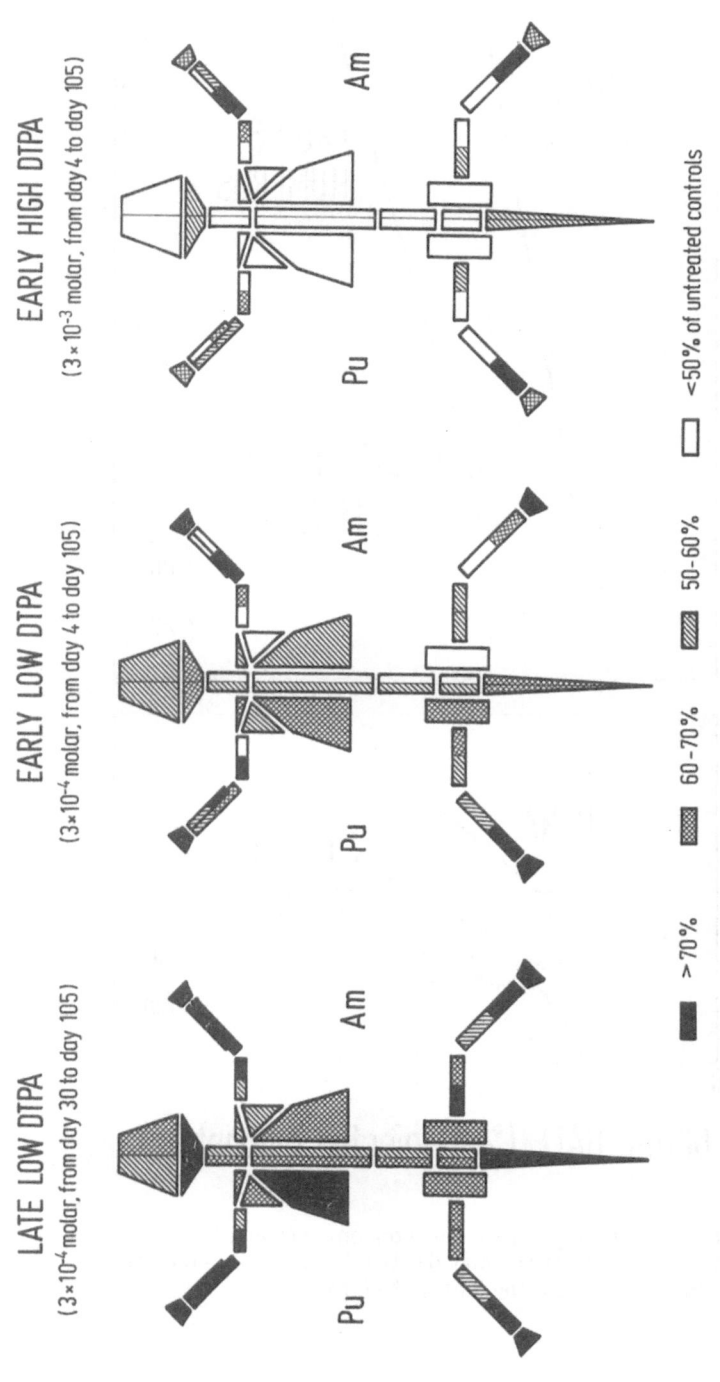

FIGURE 1 Reduced concentrations of Pu-238 and Am-241 in rat bones after prolonged drinking Zn-DTPA. Values are expressed as percentage of those in the respective skeletal parts of untreated animals.

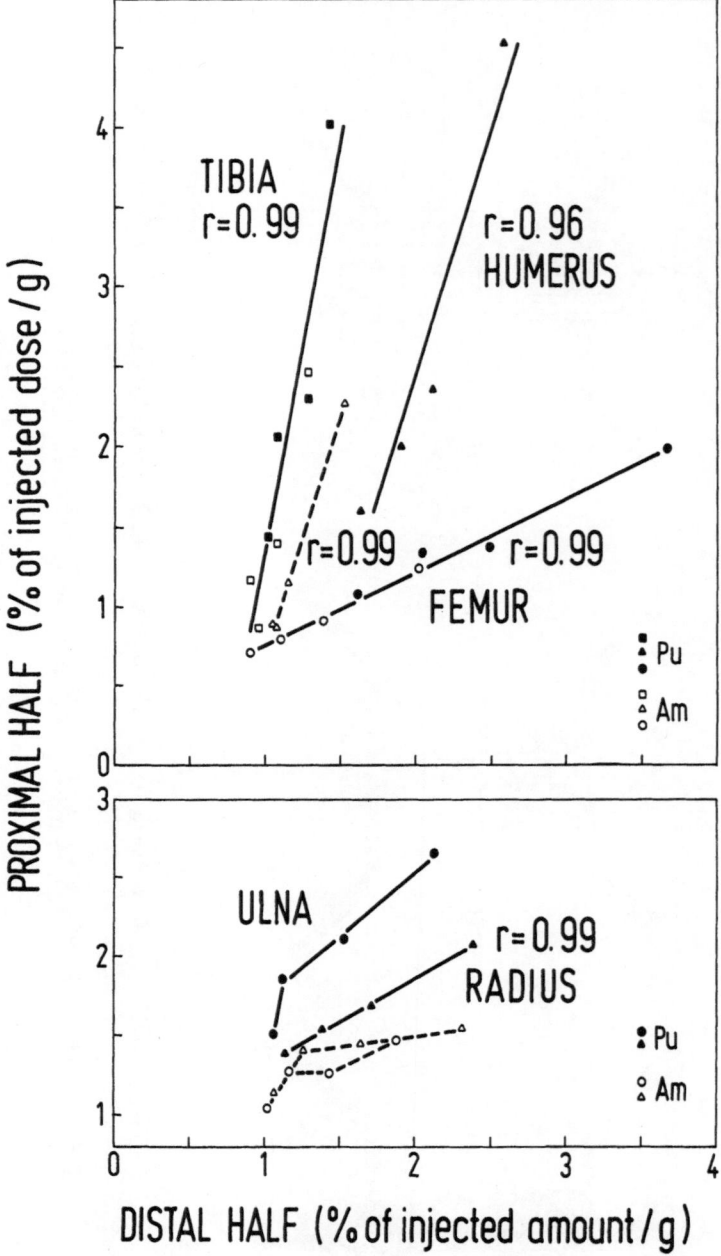

FIGURE 2   Relationship between the concentration of Pu-238 and
Am-241 in proximal and distal halves of long bones,
both in treated and untreated rats.

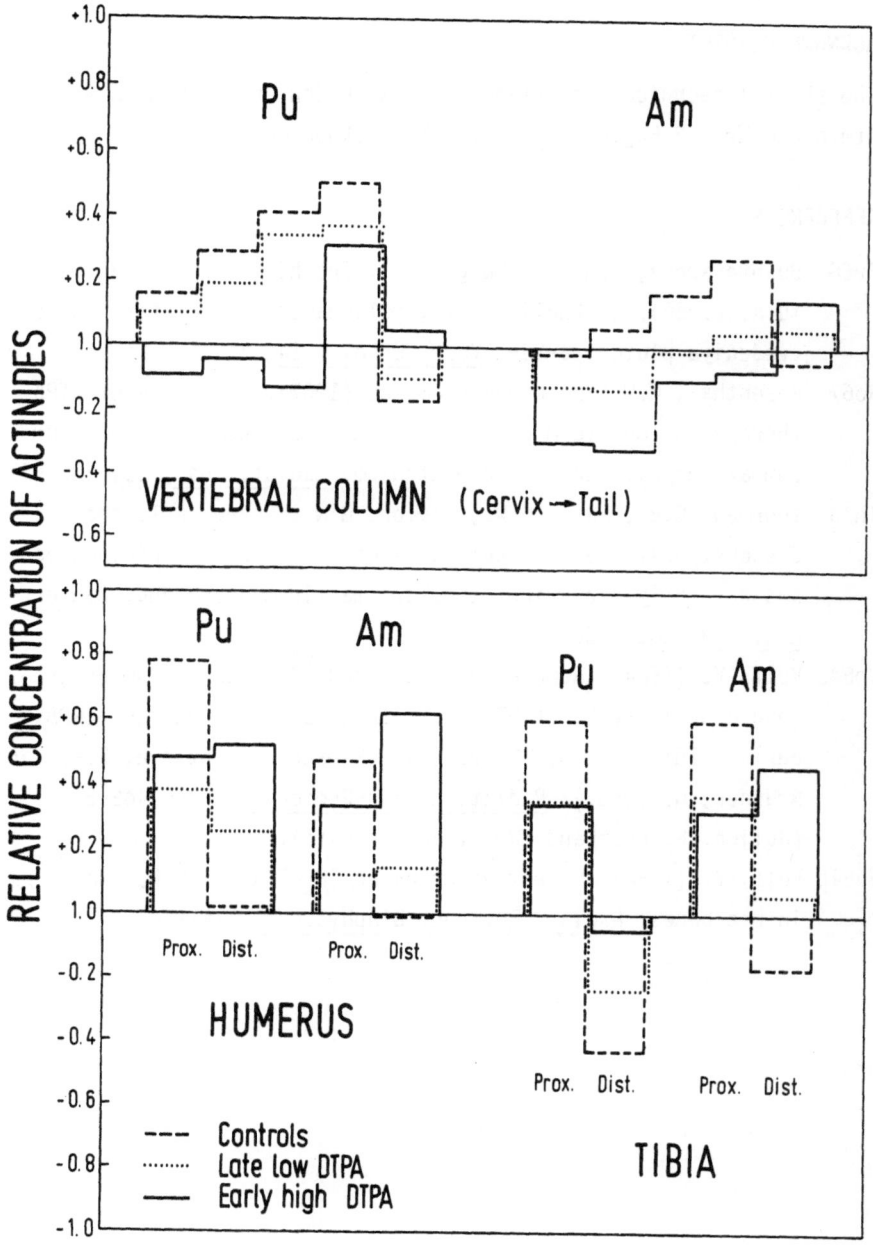

FIGURE 3   Relative concentrations of Pu-238 and Am-241 in rat bones
after oral treatment with Zn-DTPA (average concentration
in whole skeleton = 1).

ACKNOWLEDGEMENT

The skilful technical assistance of Miss P.Schlenker, Mrs. B.Braun-
stein and Mrs. B.Eggmann is gratefully acknowledged.

REFERENCES

Bu68   Bukhtoyarova, E.M., Lemberg, V.K., Erokhin, R.A. and Belyayev,
       Yu.A. (1968). Opukholi u krys, poluchavshikh pentatsin posle
       vvedeniya plutoniya-239. Vopr. Onkol., 14, 71-74.
Ro67   Rosenthal, M.W. and Lindenbaum, A. (1967). Influence of DTPA
       therapy on long-term effects of retained monomeric plutonium:
       Comparison with polymeric plutonium. Radiat. Res., 31, 506-521.
Th73   Thurman, G.B., Mays, C.W., Taylor, G.N., Keane, A.T. and
       Sissons, H.A. (1973). Skeletal location of radiation-induced
       and naturally occurring osteosarcomas in man and dog. Cancer
       Res., 33, 1604-1607.
Vo84a Volf, V. (1984). Removal of deposited ^{238}Pu and ^{241}Am by pro-
       longed oral intake of DTPA. 6th International Congress IRPA,
       Berlin. In: Kaul, A., Neider, R., Pensko, J., Stieve, F.-E. and
       Brunner, H. (eds.). Radiation-Risk-Protection. pp. 442-5.
       (Jülich: Fachverband für Strahlenschutz).
Vo84b Volf, V. (1984). Effect of drinking Zn-DTPA on ^{238}Pu and ^{241}Am
       in rat bones. Radiat. Environ. Biophys., 23, 141-143.

20

The Retention of Plutonium in Human Bone: A Reconnaissance

D. M. TAYLOR

The retention time of a long-lived radionuclide in human bone is an important parameter for the assessment of the maximum quantity of that radionuclide which may be allowed to accumulate in the skeleton without producing an unacceptable risk of inducing bone tumours or other serious injury. Plutonium-239 and other transuranium radionuclides arising in the nuclear fuel cycle are of special interest because they could be released into the human environment as a result of a severe accident in a nuclear installation. The only direct study of plutonium metabolism in man (La50) plus data from experimental studies in dogs, rats and mice suggests that the loss of plutonium from bone could be fitted by monoexponential functions with half-times about equal to,or greater than,the natural life expectation of the species. Based on this data the International Commission on Radiological Protection (ICRP72) suggested that the retention of plutonium in human bone should be assumed to follow a monoexponential function with a half-time of 100 a.

More recent analyses of the retention of plutonium in the bones of dogs, rats, mice and monkeys have indicated that the rate of loss from bone can no longer be best described by a simple monoexponential model. Stover et al. (St72,St74) concluded that in the beagle the retention of plutonium in the humeri and lumbar vertebrae could be fitted best by an exponential term plus a constant fraction model. The calculated equations were:

$$\text{Humerus} = 0.71 \exp -0.0022 \, t + 0.29$$
$$\text{Vertebrae} = 0.69 \exp -0.0018 \, t + 0.31$$

where retention in each bone is 1.0 at t = 0 days. The half-time of the exponential portion is about 1 year, or circa 7 % of the life-expectation of the beagle.

Similar long-term studies in rats (Ho75,Ta83) and mice (An83) have shown that skeletal retention can be described by 2- and 3-component exponential functions, respectively. In both species the longest component has a half-time greater than the natural life expectation. Durbin et al. (Du83) reported a 2-component exponential clearance of plutonium from monkey bones; however, in this species the longest half-time measured in the 1100 day study was only about 3 years or about 10 % of the probable life-span of the monkey.

All these animal studies were carried out using low doses of [239]Pu or [238]Pu and the likelihood of radiation-induced changes in bone retention having occurred appears remote.

Since 1945, and especially in the late 1950 s and early 1960 s the whole human population has been inhaling or ingesting small amounts of plutonium which were released into the atmosphere as a result of nuclear weapon testing. During the past two decades McInroy and his colleagues at the Los Alamos National Laboratory have been measuring the concentrations of this "fall-out" [239,240]Pu in autopsy samples of human tissue, including liver and bone (McI79, McI81). Since about 1970 the levels of "fall-out" plutonium in the atmosphere and human food chain have been very low and it appeared likely that any downward trend in the plutonium concentrations in human bone since about 1970 would give an indication of the rate of metabolic loss of the radioelement from skeletal tissue. Data for human vertebrae collected from persons living in several different states in the United States of America, who had a median age of about 60 a at death (McI81), give an indication that the concentration of plutonium did decrease between 1970 and 1977. In order to attempt to derive a clearer picture of the retention of plutonium in human bone the data of McInroy et al. (McI79) have been re-analysed.

The analysis of the bone data is complicated by the fact that the available samples were often relatively small and the plutonium concentrations were so low that the radioactivity in the measured sample

was often lower than the "minimum reporting level". Out of over 400
vertebral samples measured about 70 % fell into this latter category,
the data for these samples were ignored in the subsequent mathematical
analysis. The initial mathematical analyses were made using the data
published by McInroy et al. in 1979 (McI79) but the main analysis was
made from an updated listing kindly supplied by Dr. McInroy. From this
listing 125 values for the concentration of "fall-out" plutonium in
vertebrae (expressed as dpm/kg fresh bone) were grouped according to
year of death for each year from 1969 to 1978 and the complete data
were tested for their fit to a log-linear concentration vs time relationship using a least squares computational method. This analysis
revealed a significant downward trend in plutonium concentration with
time. Since the data sets for the years 1969-72 contained a few exceptionally high values which could have exaggerated the apparent downward trend, 11 results were eliminated and a new analysis was made
using 114 data sets. This second analysis yielded a regression line
with a significant downward slope (P<0.001 at 112 degrees of freedom)
and a half-time of about 8 a, Figure 1. A similar analysis of the 33
samples of human rib collected between 1972 and 1977 also showed a
downward trend in plutonium concentration with a half-time of about 5a,
which was probably significant at the 5 % level.

Although there appears to be a significant downward trend in the
retention of "fall-out" plutonium in human vertebrae and rib, the
question must be asked 'is this a valid observation?'. There are many
uncertainties inherent in the data, firstly for each year group there
is considerable scatter in the results with a few very high values;
further, as mentioned earlier, about 70 % of the samples analysed were
below the minimum reporting level. An additional complication is that
the yearly data sets do not have a uniform geographical distribution
and in making this analysis it is assumed that all subjects were
exposed to equal amounts of "fall-out": Examination of the data for
each year shows no obvious indication of geographical variation. The
age of the sampled population could also influence the yearly data,but
for the years studied the median age of the subjects at death was about
60 a and the age distribution was similar for each year. No information
on pathological changes in the bone samples is given, and it is assumed
that any age-related changes in bone physiology were similar in each

year group.

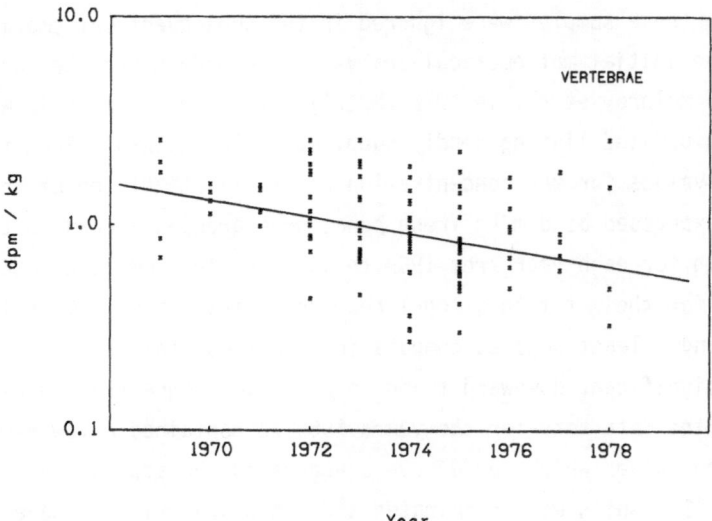

FIGURE 1   The retention of ^{239,240}Pu from "fall-out" in human
            vertebrae (Data from McI79 and McI-Personal communication).
            The calculated half-time of the regression line is 7.6 a
            (95 % confidence limits 6.1 to 9.8 a, n=114 P<0.001).

Recently Broadway and Strong (Br83) commented that in bone samples
from children and young adults analysed by the U.S. Environmental
Protection Agency the ^{239,240}Pu concentrations decreased between 1972
and 1975. These bone samples were composited yearly with respect to
age and geographical location but the type of bone analysed is not
stated. The authors ascribe this decrease to lower plutonium intake
due to decreased atmospheric "fall-out". However, this would not
account for the apparently lower concentration in bone unless there
was also some loss of previously deposited plutonium or, as is possible in the juveniles, an increase in bone mass due to the growth of
"low-plutonium" bone. Analysis of human vertebrae for ^{90}Sr (Pa73) also
revealed a decrease in concentration with time which appears to be
similar to that observed for plutonium. A similar parallel between the
long-term loss of actinide and alkaline earth elements has been observed in animals (Ta83).

The "fall-out" plutonium data suggest the possibility of some,
perhaps quite rapid, loss of plutonium from human vertebrae and rib.

Such a loss would not have been predicted by the human plutonium injection cases (La50) in which the 3 vertebral samples measured gave no indication of radioelement removal between 5 and 546 d post injection. The data used in the present analysis cover a period of only 9 years and in view of the scatter of the reported values the possibility of at least one further component to the bone retention function cannot be excluded. Indeed, by analogy with the beagle and other animal data, such an additional component, or components, would be expected. More recently Singh and Wrenn (Si84) have analysed samples of human rib and vertebrae taken at autopsy from about 40 persons residing in northern Utah and other parts of the U.S.A.. These unpublished data for the years 1979 to 1984 show no evidence of a downward trend with time and the combined values have a median of about 0.6 dpm/kg. The lack of a downward trend in these later analyses may reflect only the short time span of the observations and the scatter of the individual values, or it may be indicative of a long-lived component to the bone retention function. Assuming that there are no systematic analytical differences between the two laboratories, the data of Singh and Wrenn (Si84) may indicate that the "fall-out" plutonium concentration in vertebrae, and probably also in rib, is beginning to level out at a value of about one third to one half that observed in 1969-70 and that, as in the beagle, human bone retention may be described by an exponential plus a constant term relationship, the constant term representing the balance between loss due to bone turnover and re-, or new, deposition in new bone.

It should be emphasised that the results discussed here were obtained from analysis of vertebrae or ribs and both of these bones comprise mainly trabecular bone which is generally considered to have a rate of remodelling which is considerably greater than that of compact bone. Thus the loss of plutonium from human vertebrae may be more rapid than that from mainly compact bones such as femur; the ^{90}Sr studies suggest that this difference could be as large as a factor of four (Pa73). A differential loss of plutonium from vertebrae and other bones has been reported in macaque monkeys (Du83) but not in the dog (St72,St74). Virtually no information is available which would allow us to assess directly the retention time of plutonium in human compact bone. In the absence of such information it would be prudent to assume that plutonium will behave like ^{90}Sr and that the retention time in compact bone may be longer than that in trabecular structures.

If we were to assume that the retention of plutonium in human vertebrae is representative of the whole skeleton, then on the basis of the above analysis of the data of McInroy et al. the half-time of retention in the skeleton would be only 8 a. Such a short half-time is consistent neither with the relatively slow excretion of plutonium observed in the injection cases nor with any of the long-term animal studies. However, if an exponential plus constant term model is assumed for man with about 60 % of bone plutonium being removed with a half-time of about 8 a and the remainder with infinitely long half-time, it can be calculated that the time required to lose the first 50 % of the skeletal plutonium would be about 20 years. This value also appears to be too short to reconcile with the information on excretion and the rate of loss of plutonium from liver previously calculated from the human "fall-out" data (Ta84). The present analysis does not permit the confident prediction of the retention time of plutonium in human bone; however, it does suggest that the analyses of "fall-out" plutonium concentrations in human tissues if continued in adequate numbers, and providing that atmospheric plutonium levels do not increase, can yield useful information on retention patterns in bone and liver. It is highly desirable that such studies, especially with well-defined populations should be continued into the future. In designing such studies it would be appropriate to review the suitability of vertebrae as indicators of the average skeletal plutonium.

Until further human data are available it would appear prudent to retain the present ICRP Model for the retention of plutonium in human bone, with a half-life of 100 a. However, the "fall-out" plutonium studies in human bone do provide a strong indication that plutonium in bone may in fact be rather more mobile than has been assumed in the past.

Acknowledgements

The author wishes to thank Drs. N.Singh, R.C.Thompson and McD.E. Wrenn for helpful discussions and criticisms. Special appreciation is expressed to Dr. J.F.McInroy and to Drs. Singh and Wrenn who very generously made their unpublished data available for study.

An83 Andreozzi,U., Clemente,G.F., Ingrao,G. and Santori,G., 1983, Long term ^{238}Pu and ^{239}Pu retention and organ distribution in mice at low doses. Health Phys. 44 Suppl. 1, 505-511.

Br83 Broadway,J.A. and Strong,A.B., 1983, Radionuclides in Human Bone Samples, Health Phys. 45, 765-768.

Du83 Durbin,P.W., Jeung,N. and Schmidt,C.T., 1983, Distribution and Retention of ^{238}Pu in Macaque Monkeys. In: Proc.Seventh Internat. Congr. Radiat. Res. Amsterdam. July 3-8, 1983, pp E5-03 (Amsterdam, Martinus Nijhoff).

Ho75 Hollins,J.G. and Storr,M.C., 1975, An analysis of the retention of plutonium by the tissues of the rat. Radiat. Res. 61, 468-477.

ICRP 72 International Commission on Radiological Protection, 1972, The Metabolism of Compounds of Plutonium and Other Actinides. ICRP Publication 19 (Oxford, Pergamon Press).

La50 Langham,W.H., Bassett,S.H., Harris,P.S. and Carter,R.E., 1950, Distribution and excretion of plutonium administered to man. Los Alamos Scientific Laboratory Report LA-1151 (Sept.1950) (reprinted Health Phys. 38, 1031-1060).

McI79 McInroy,J.F., Campbell,E.E., Moss,W.D., Tietjen,G.L., Eustler, B.C. and Boyd,H.A., 1979, Plutonium in Autopsy Tissue: A Revision and Updating of data reported in LA-4875. Health Phys. 37, 1-136.

McI81 McInroy,J.F., Boyd,H.A. and Eustler,B.C., 1981, Deposition and retention of plutonium in the United States general population. In: Wrenn,M.E., Actinides in man and animals, pp 161-179 (Salt Lake City, R.D. Press).

Pa73 Papworth,D.G. and Vennart,J., 1973, Retention of ^{90}Sr in human bone at different ages and the resulting radiation doses. Phys. Med. Biol. 18, 169-186.

Si84 Singh,N. and Wrenn,McD.E., 1984, Personal Communication to D.M. Taylor 6 September 1984.

St72 Stover,B.J., Atherton,D.R. and Buster,D.S., 1972, Retention of ^{239}Pu(IV) in the beagle. In: Radiobiology of Plutonium. Stover, B.J. and Jee,W.S.S. (Eds.) p 149-169 (Salt Lake City, J.W.Press).

St74 Stover,B.J. and Atherton,D.R., 1974, Kinetics of Skeletal Retention of ^{239}Pu(IV). Radiat. Res. 60, 525-535.

Ta83 Taylor,D.M., 1983, The comparative retention of bone-seeking
radionuclides in the skeleton of rats. Health Phys. 45, 768-772.

Ta84 Taylor,D.M., 1984, The retention of plutonium and americium in
liver: A interspecies comparison. In: Kaul,A., Neider,R., Pensko,
J., Stieve, F.-E. and Brunner,H. (Eds.). Radiation-Risk-Protec-
tion, pp 431-434 (Berlin, Fachverband f. Strahlenschutz eV).

21

Distribution of Plutonium-239 and Americium-241 in the Human Skeleton

J. F. McINROY and M. J. SWINT

The concentration of ^{239}Pu and ^{241}Am in each bone of two nuclear workers having 25 years exposure was determined. The defleshed bones of the right half of each skeleton were ashed and dissolved in acid. Each radioisotope was isolated, electrodeposited on to planchets, and counted by alpha pulse height spectrometry. The long bones of the arms and legs were separated into the shaft and the proximal and distal ends. Gross distributions in the cancellous and mineral bones were measured.

Percent distribution in major bone sites

Bones	(Am)	(Pu)
Head	14.1	14.3
Spine and pelvis	17.8	28.7
Shoulder and rib cage	9.0	8.3
Arms and hands	13.1	11.2
Legs and feet	46.0	37.5

Excluding the respiratory system, 48% of the plutonium was in the liver and 44% in the skeleton: americium was distributed 6% in the liver and 84% in the skeleton.

The distribution of plutonium and americium in these two skeletons was similar. The teeth were found to have a relatively low, but consistent, concentration of americium and plutonium. The concentration of these nuclides in the bones was best expressed in terms of activity per gram ash. From these data, distribution coefficients can be obtained and used for the extrapolation of measurements from the smaller bone specimens obtained from routine autopsies to the whole skeleton.

Editors note: Manuscript not received for publication by 5 February 1985

22

Uranium, Thorium and Plutonium in Bones from the General Population of the United States

N. P. SINGH, L. L. LEWIS and M. E. WRENN

INTRODUCTION

This paper describes the concentrations of alpha-emitting isotopes of thorium (^{228}Th, ^{230}Th and ^{232}Th), uranium (^{234}U, ^{235}U and ^{238}U) and plutonium (^{238}Pu, ^{239,240}Pu) in vertebrae, ribs and sternum from former residents of two areas in the United States. These radionuclides were measured in the same sets of bone samples. Measurements of α-emitting isotopes of thorium, uranium, and plutonium reported in the open literature have never been made on the same samples as are reported here. A brief review of measurements of uranium, thorium and plutonium in human tissues follows.

The concentrations of ^{228}Th, ^{230}Th and ^{232}Th have formerly been measured and reported in soft tissues and vertebrae of two populations in the United States: Washington, DC, and Grand Junction, CO (Wr81,Si81,Ib83). Among the soft tissues measured, lymph nodes contained the highest concentrations of ^{228}Th, ^{230}Th and ^{232}Th for both populations. For the Washington, DC, population, the concentrations of ^{228}Th averaged 2.6 pCi/kg; concentrations of ^{230}Th and ^{232}Th were 4.6 pCi/kg and 2.8 pCi/kg, respectively. In the Grand Junction population, the concentrations of ^{228}Th averaged 5.1 pCi/kg, while ^{230}Th and ^{232}Th concentrations were 11.1 pCi/kg and 7.8 pCi/kg, respectively. In vertebrae, the mean concentrations of ^{228}Th were 0.77 and 0.70 pCi/kg for Washington, DC, and Grand Junction, respectively; the mean concentrations of ^{230}Th were 0.42 and 1.20 pCi/kg; and the mean concentrations of ^{232}Th were 0.10 and 0.16 pCi/kg.

The concentrations of uranium in human organs have been previously reported. Hamilton (Ha72) analyzed a number of tissue samples from the United Kingdom and from his measurements estimated the total amount of uranium in these organs to be 86.3 µg. Welford et al (We67,We76) reported the concentrations of uranium ^{238}U/gm wet weight of bone.

The concentrations of plutonium isotopes have been determined in soft tissues and bones of the general populations of different countries by several investigators (Mc79; Wr78, Ta73; Os63; Mu80; Si83). Among the tissues sampled the highest concentration of plutonium was found in liver, ranging from a median of 0.32 pCi/kg in southern Finland (Mu80) to 1.3 pCi/kg in Pennsylvania, USA (Mc79).

MATERIALS AND METHODS

Collection of Tissues

Samples of vertebrae, ribs and sternum were collected from eight former residents of Pennsylvania and from five former residents of Colorado. Autopsy samples were generally from accident victims or persons who died suddenly of coronary diseases. None of the subjects had chronic, debilitating disease or metabolic disease known to affect the metabolism of uranium, thorium and plutonium. For each subject, the tissue samples were placed in individual plastic bags and packaged in separate labeled containers. The specimens were frozen after autopsy and transported to our laboratory packed in dry ice. The date of death, age at death, sex, residential history, smoking and drinking history, past medical history and occupational data were obtained for each case.

Radiochemical Procedures

Thorium, uranium, and plutonium were determined using the method of Singh et al (Si84). Solvent extraction and alpha spectrometry were employed in the quantitative determination of these three actinides. The bone specimens, spiked with ^{232}U, ^{229}Th and ^{242}Pu tracers, were wet ashed with HNO_3, followed by alternate additions of a few drops of HNO_3 and H_2O_2. Uranium was reduced to the tetravalent state with 200 mg $SnCl_2$ and 25 ml HI. Uranium, thorium and plutonium were then coprecipitated with calcium as oxalates, heated to 550°C, dissolved in 50 ml HCl, and the acidity adjusted to 10 M.

Uranium and plutonium were extracted into a 20% tri-lauryl amine (TLA) solution in xylene, leaving thorium in the aqueous phase. Plutonium was back-extracted from the TLA phase by shaking with a 1:1.5 volume of 0.05 M NH_4I in 8 M HCl, which reduces Pu(IV) to Pu(III). Uranium was then back-extracted with an equal volume of 0.1 M HCl. Thorium, which remained in the aqueous phase, was evaporated to dryness, dissolved in 4 M HNO_3, and the acidity adjusted to 4 M. It was then extracted into a 20% TLA solution in xylene pre-equilibrated with 4 M HNO_3, and back-extracted with 10 M HCl. Uranium, thorium, and plutonium were then electrodeposited separately onto platinum discs and counted by an alpha spectrometer with a multi-channel analyzer and surface barrier silicon diodes.

RESULTS AND DISCUSSIONS

The concentrations of alpha-emitting isotopes of thorium, uranium and plutonium in vertebrae, ribs and sternum are given in Tables 1-3. The concentrations of ^{232}Th in vertebrae were very low (mean of 0.10 ± 0.02 pCi/kg) compared to ^{230}Th (mean of 0.70 ± 0.26 pCi/kg)

TABLE 1

URANIUM, PLUTONIUM AND THORIUM IN VERTEBRAE OF COLORADO AND PENNSYLVANIA RESIDENTS
(pCi/kg wet weight)

ID #	U-238	U-235	U-234	Pu-239,240	Pu-238	Th-232	Th-230	Th-228
Colorado								
80-C9	4.66±0.43	0.20 ±.10	5.75±0.49	0.30±.12	0.20 ±.10	-0.0004±.16	1.11±0.36	0.85±0.40
80-C10	1.14±0.16	0.04 ±.04	1.67±0.19	0.17±.08	-0.06 ±.09	0.06 ±.08	0.87±0.18	1.03±0.18
80-C11	0.48±0.13	0.05 ±.05	0.79±0.18	0.35±.12	0.03 ±.06	0.07 ±.07	0.38±0.12	0.59±0.12
80-C13	1.51±0.34	-0.005±.11	1.79±0.38	0.28±.16	-0.12 ±.13	-0.05 ±.08	0.83±0.22	0.98±0.24
80-C14	0.56±0.11	-0.01 ±.03	0.63±0.13	0.23±.08	0.01 ±.07	0.11 ±.05	0.36±0.11	0.32±0.13
80-C15	0.37±0.10	0.03 ±.03	1.21±0.15	0.02±.05	-0.07 ±.05	0.30 ±.12	3.66±0.37	0.54±0.16
79-C16	0.68±0.13	0.02 ±.02	0.72±0.14	0.13±.07	-0.03 ±.06	0.20 ±.08	0.28±0.11	1.45±0.22
x̄±S.D.	1.21±1.45	0.04 ±.07	1.63±1.74	0.22±.11	-0.004±.10	0.096 ±.11	0.96±1.14	0.88±0.39
Pennsylvania								
80-P4	0.30±.06	0.03 ±.02	0.34±.07	0.21±.05	0.03 ±.02	0.14 ±.04	0.29±.06	4.82±0.24
80-P6	0.26±.05	0.03 ±.02	0.38±.06	0.34±.04	0.07 ±.03	0.16 ±.04	0.35±.06	0.60±0.08
80-P7	0.25±.07	0.02 ±.03	0.21±.07	0.13±.03	0.03 ±.02	0.03 ±.03	0.31±.07	0.32±0.07
80-P8	0.13±.05	0.02 ±.02	0.25±.06	0.22±.05	0.005±.03	0.07 ±.02	0.11±.03	0.34±0.05
80-P9	0.67±.06	0.03 ±.01	0.68±.06	0.22±.04	0.03 ±.02	0.11 ±.05	0.31±.07	0.47±0.09
80-C17	0.30±.05	-0.004±.02	0.45±.06	0.25±.06	0.01 ±.03	0.08 ±.04	0.19±.06	1.28±0.14
x̄±S.D.	0.32±.23	0.03 ±.006	0.37±.19	0.22±.075	0.033±.023	0.102 ±.053	0.27±.09	1.31±1.96
Difference of Means	0.89	0.01	1.26	0.008	-0.037	0.006	0.69	0.43
t-test	1.34	0.20	1.58	0.142	0.83	0.109	1.32	0.62
Probability	0.10	0.42	0.07	0.44	0.21	0.46	0.11	0.28

TABLE 2

URANIUM, PLUTONIUM AND THORIUM IN RIBS OF COLORADO AND PENNSYLVANIA RESIDENTS

(pCi/kg wet weight)

ID #	U-238	U-235	U-234	Pu-239,240	Pu-238	Th-232	Th-230	Th-228
Colorado								
80-C9	2.81±0.36	0.08 ±.08	4.47±0.45	0.28±.11	-0.05±.17	0.43±.23	1.08±.33	0.49±.28
80-C10	1.93±0.32	-0.005 ±.10	1.62±0.37	0.03±.14	-0.15±.13	0.99±.18	1.48±.21	1.75±.24
80-C15	0.56±0.30	0.0001±.13	1.51±0.44	0.05±.14	0.20±.20	0.09±.25	2.15±.65	0.75±.50
x̄±S.D.	1.77±1.13	0.025±.077	2.53±1.68	0.12±.14	0.00±.18	0.50±.46	1.57±.54	1.0 ±.67
Pennsylvania								
80-P4	0.26±0.09	0.04 ±.04	0.26±.10	0.11±.05	0.01±.05	0.28±.07	0.58±.10	2.84±0.21
80-P5	0.14±0.08	0.02 ±.04	0.31±.11	0.37±.08	-0.03±.04	0.57±.11	0.72±.13	2.38±0.22
80-P6	0.25±0.09	0.04 ±.02	0.53±.12	0.41±.06	0.01±.04	0.11±.06	0.48±.11	0.52±0.12
80-P7	0.36±0.15	0.004 ±.07	0.46±.17	0.23±.04	0.02±.06	0.03±.06	0.56±.13	0.30±0.11
80-P8	0.34±0.09	0.02 ±.03	0.25±.09	0.25±.06	-0.01±.02	0.07±.06	0.59±.11	0.33±0.09
80-P9	0.18±0.04	-0.004 ±.02	0.34±.06	0.19±.06	-0.07±.04	0.11±.06	0.28±.08	0.76±0.13
x̄±S.D.	0.26±0.09	0.020 ±.018	0.36±.11	0.26±.11	0.012±.034	0.20±.20	0.54±.15	1.19±1.12
Difference								
of Means	1.51	0.005	2.17	0.14	0.012	0.30	1.03	0.19
t-test	3.50	0.24	3.41	1.64	0.16	1.47	4.65	0.27
Probability	0.005	0.41	0.006	0.072	0.44	0.09	0.001	0.40

TABLE 3

URANIUM, PLUTONIUM AND THORIUM IN STERNUM OF COLORADO AND PENNSYLVANIA RESIDENTS

(pCi/kg wet weight)

ID #	U-238	U-235	U-234	Pu-239,240	Pu-238	Th-232	Th-230	Th-228
80-C9	3.96±.61	0.31 ±.19	6.54±.79	0.23 ±.17	-0.07±.20	-0.01±.03	-0.002±.04	0.02±0.04
80-P4	1.36±.51	-0.30 ±.22	1.61±.56	0.43 ±.22	0.54±.24	0.77±.41	0.28 ±.50	4.31±0.93
80-P5	0.25±.27	-0.07 ±.07	0.27±.31	-0.002±.07	0.04±.16	0.15±.30	1.12 ±.47	3.83±0.79
80-P6	1.26±.43	-0.004 ±.11	1.46±.45	1.46 ±.39	0.52±.23	0.16±.31	0.17 ±.34	6.72±1.07
80-P7	1.30±.32	-0.0002±.09	1.82±.42	0.17 ±.14	-0.05±.14	0.55±.29	1.22 ±.50	1.46±0.43
80-P8	0.43±.37	0.05 ±.16	1.73±.53	0.53 ±.36	-0.09±.38	0.35±.35	0.11 ±.46	2.07±0.63
80-P9	1.07±.43	0.07 ±.17	1.12±.48	0.26 ±.19	-0.15±.18	0.31±.11	1.50 ±.26	0.70±0.29
x̄±S.E.	1.38±.46	0.01 ±.07	2.08±.77	0.44 ±.18	0.11±.11	0.33±.10	0.63 ±.24	2.73±0.89

and ^{228}Th (mean of 1.05 ± 0.33 pCi/kg). In general, the concentration of ^{228}Th was highest, probably due to the accumulation of ^{228}Ra, which is highly soluble, readily available through the food chain, and which decays to ^{228}Th.

Among uranium isotopes, the concentrations of ^{235}U in vertebrae were lowest with a mean of 0.03 ± 0.01 pCi/kg wet weight. In general, the concentrations of ^{234}U in vertebrae were higher than the concentrations of ^{238}U; the mean concentration of ^{234}U was almost 30% higher than the mean concentration of ^{238}U. The concentrations of ^{238}U and ^{234}U were exceptionally high in one case (80-C9): 4.66 ± 0.43 pCi ^{238}U/kg and 5.75 ± 0.49 pCi ^{234}U/kg. The concentrations of ^{238}Pu in vertebrae were negligible. The concentrations of ^{239,240}Pu ranged from 0.02 ± 0.05 to 0.35 ± 0.12 pCi/kg wet weight, with a mean of 0.22 ± 0.03 pCi/kg wet weight.

The mean concentrations of thorium isotopes in ribs were similar to those in vertebrae. The mean concentration of ^{228}Th was highest (1.12 ± 0.32 pCi/kg) followed by ^{230}Th (0.88 ± 0.20 pCi/kg) and ^{232}Th (0.30 ± 0.11 pCi/kg).

The concentrations of ^{238}U and ^{234}U in ribs were again highest in subject 80-C9, showing an exceptionally high intake of uranium. The mean concentration of ^{234}U was higher than the mean concentration of ^{238}U. The concentrations of ^{235}U were very low. As in vertebrae, the concentrations of ^{238}Pu were negligible. The concentrations of ^{239,240}Pu ranged from 0.03 ± 0.14 to 0.41 ± 0.06 pCi/kg, with a mean of 0.21 ± 0.04 pCi/kg wet weight.

The concentrations of the thorium, uranium and plutonium isotopes in sternum were higher than the concentrations of these isotopes in vertebrae and ribs. However, the analytical errors in the determinations were also higher than the errors in vertebrae and ribs. This is probably due to the small size of the sternum samples available for radiochemical analyses. The mean concentrations of ^{228}Th were highest (2.73 ± 0.89 pCi/kg wet weight), followed by ^{230}Th (0.63 ± 0.24 pCi/kg wet weight) and ^{232}Th (0.33 ± 0.10 pCi/kg wet weight).

The mean concentration of ^{234}U (2.08 ± 0.77 pCi/kg wet weight) was again higher than the mean concentration of ^{238}U (1.38 ± 0.46 pCi/kg wet weight). The concentrations of ^{238}Pu were again negligible. The mean concentration of ^{239,240}Pu was 0.44 ± 0.18 pCi/kg wet weight.

The concentrations of alpha-emitting isotopes of uranium, plutonium and thorium in vertebrae of the Colorado and Pennsylvania populations are not significantly different from each other (cf Table 1). However, the concentrations of ^{234}U, ^{238}U and ^{230}Th in ribs of the Colorado population are significantly higher than those from the Pennsylvania population. No statistical analysis could be performed for the concentrations of uranium, plutonium and thorium isotopes in the sternum of the two populations because only one sample was obtained from Colorado.

A histogram showing the concentrations of ^{232}Th, ^{230}Th and ^{238}U and ^{239,240}Pu is given in Figure 1. The concentrations of ^{228}Th

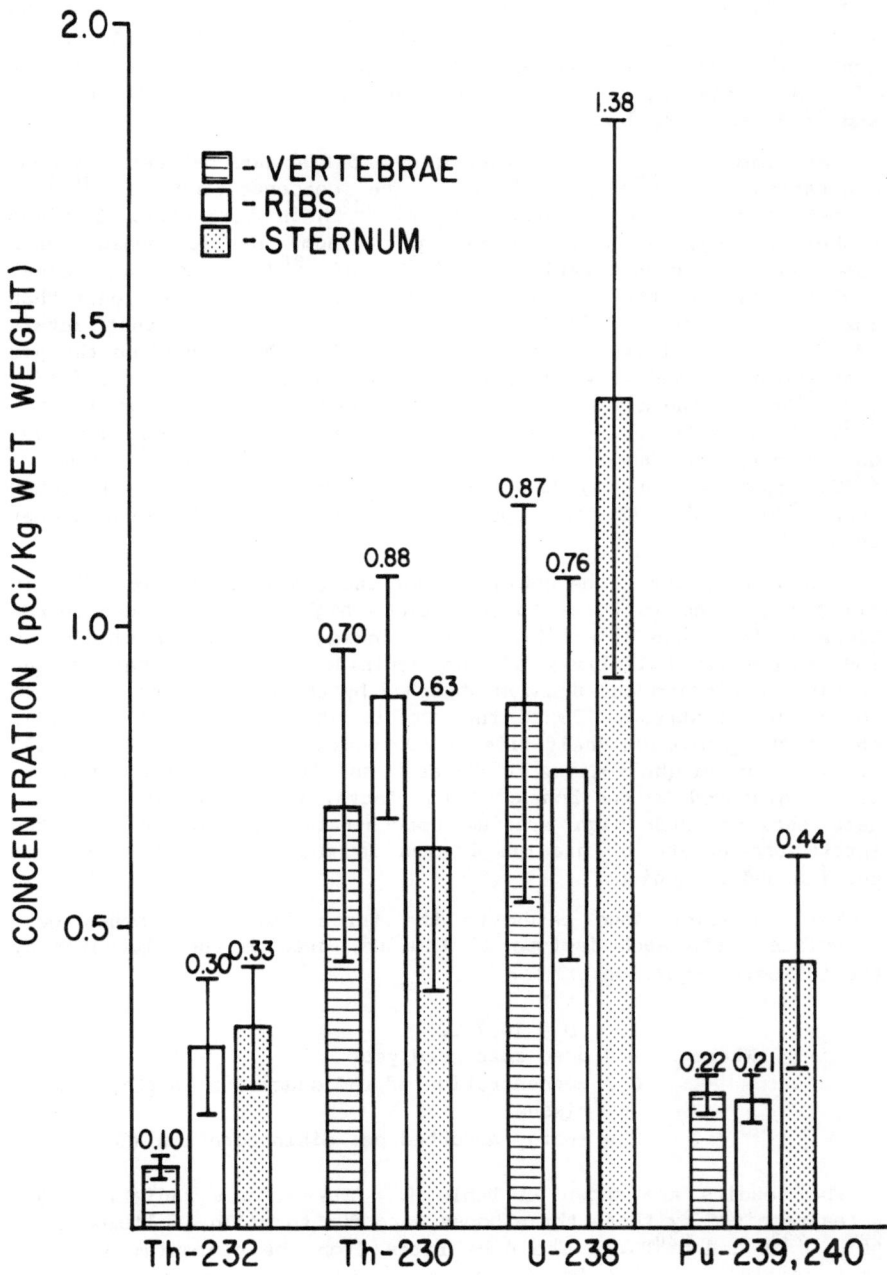

Figure 1
Comparison of mean concentrations of selected isotopes in bones
from the general population.

^{234}U, ^{235}U and ^{238}Pu were not included in this histogram for the following reasons: in bone the concentration of ^{228}Th mostly represents the concentration of its parent ^{228}Ra; the concentration of ^{234}U is similar to its parent ^{238}U, and the concentrations ^{235}U and ^{238}Pu are very low.

The unique point to be noted is the difference between the concentrations of ^{232}Th and ^{230}Th. The concentration of ^{230}Th is almost 7 times higher than that of ^{232}Th in vertebrae, 3 times higher in ribs, and 2 times higher in sternum. Earlier measurements show that the concentrations of ^{232}Th and ^{230}Th in soil are equal (UN77), and that the concentration of ^{230}Th is 1.5 times higher than the concentration of ^{232}Th in air (Se73). Assuming that intake of ^{230}Th is 1.5 times greater than that of ^{232}Th (based on the air measurements), and knowing that the biological half-lives of ^{232}Th and ^{230}Th in bone are equal, we would expect the concentration of ^{230}Th in bone to be 1.5 times higher than ^{232}Th. The fact that our measurements show much higher concentrations of ^{230}Th than ^{232}Th suggests that (1) the intake of ^{230}Th in man is much higher than ^{232}Th and/or (2) the uptake of ^{230}Th in man is much higher than ^{232}Th.

The other point to be noted is that the concentration of ^{238}U in all three bones is three to four times higher than the concentrations of ^{232}Th and ^{239,240}Pu. In reviewing the translocation rates and biological half-lives of the actinides, we find that of the thorium, plutonium and uranium absorbed by the body and translocated to the blood stream, 70% of the thorium (half-life of 8000 days), 45% of the plutonium (half-life of 100 years), and only 20% and 2.3% of the uranium (half-lives of 20 days and 5000 days, respectively) is translocated to the bones. These facts, in conjunction with our data showing such high uranium concentrations, suggest that the intake and uptake of uranium in man is much higher than that of thorium and plutonium.

The radiation dose rates to the three individual bones were calculated from each isotope of thorium, uranium and plutonium by the following equation:

$$D = 18.7 \ C\bar{E}$$

Where   D = dose rate mrad/year
                  C = concentration of radionuclides in pCi/g of tissue
                  $\bar{E}$ = energy absorbed per disintegration (MeV).

The results are shown in Table 4. The maximum radiation dose rates received by these three bones were due to ^{228}Th, followed by ^{234}U, ^{238}U and ^{230}Th. The dose rates from the plutonium isotopes were negligible. The total dose rates to vertebrae and ribs were 0.37 and 0.38 mrad/year, respectively, but the dose rate to sternum was much higher (0.70 mrad/year). However, the total dose rates, including the alpha-emitting daughters of ^{228}Th and ^{230}Th to vertebrae, ribs, and sternum were 0.37, 0.39 and 0.70, respectively. It was assumed that the daughters were in equilibrium with parent ^{228}Th and ^{230}Th, which seems reasonable because Lloyd et al

Table 4

RADIATION DOSE RATES TO VERTEBRAE, RIBS, AND STERNUM

ISOTOPE	VERTEBRAE	RIBS	STERNUM
U-238	0.07	0.06	0.11
U-235	0.003	0.002	0.001
U-234	0.10	0.10	0.18
Pu-239,240	0.02	0.02	0.04
Pu-238	0.001	0.001	0.01
Th-232	0.01	0.02	0.02
Th-230	0.06	0.08	0.06
Th-228	0.11	0.11	0.28
TOTAL	0.37	0.39	0.70
Th-228 daughters*	0.61	0.61	1.55
Th-230 daughters*	0.38	0.50	0.38
TOTAL	1.36	1.50	2.63

* Assuming equilibrium

(L184) reported a maximum disequilibrium of 16% in bones of beagles injected with different levels of ^{228}Th

SUMMARY

Alpha-emitting isotopes of thorium (^{228}Th, ^{230}Th, and ^{232}Th), uranium (^{234}U, ^{235}U and ^{238}U), and plutonium (^{238}Pu, ^{239,240}Pu) were determined in thirteen vertebrae, nine ribs and seven sternum samples obtained from former residents of Colorado and Pennsylvania. In vertebrae, the mean concentration of ^{234}U was highest (1.14 ± 0.41 pCi/kg), followed by ^{228}Th (1.05 ± 0.33 pCi/kg), ^{238}U (0.87 ± 0.33 pCi/kg), ^{230}Th (0.70 ± 0.26 pCi/kg), ^{239,240}Pu (0.22 ± 0.03 pCi/kg), ^{232}Th (0.10 ± 0.02 pCi/kg), ^{235}U (0.03 ± 0.01 pCi/kg), and ^{238}Pu (0.01 ± 0.02 pCi/kg). The mean concentrations of these isotopes in ribs and sternum were similarly ordered. The concentrations of all the isotopes of uranium, thorium, and plutonium were highest in sternum, except ^{230}Th , which was highest in ribs.

The concentration of ^{230}Th was found to be 2 to 7 times higher than the concentration of ^{232}Th, which suggests that the intake and/or the uptake of ^{230}Th in man is much higher than that of ^{232}Th. The concentration of ^{238}U was 3 to 4 times higher than the concentrations of ^{232}Th and ^{239,240}Pu in all bones, which suggests that the intake and uptake of uranium in man is much higher than that of thorium and plutonium.

The radiation dose rates to vertebrae, ribs and sternum due to all these isotopes of uranium, thorium, and plutonium were calculated. The total dose rates to vertebrae and ribs were 0.37 and 0.38 mrad/year, respectively, but the dose rate to sternum was much higher (0.70 mrad/year). The maximum dose contribution came from ^{228}Th, followed by ^{234}U, ^{238}U, and ^{230}Th.

ACKNOWLEDGMENTS

This work was performed under DOE Contract Number DE-AC02-76EV-00119. The authors sincerely thank Diane Fouts for editing and typing the manuscript.

REFERENCES

Ha72   Hamilton EI. 1971. The Concentration of Uranium in Man and His Diet. Health Phys. **22**: 149-153.

Ib83   Ibrahim SA, Wrenn ME, Singh NP, Cohen N and Saccomano G. 1983. Thorium Concentrations in Human Tissues from Two U.S. Populations. Health Phys. **44** Suppl. 1: 213-220.

L184   Lloyd RD, Jones CW, Mays CW, Atherton DR, Bruenger FW, and Taylor GN. 1984. ^{228}Th Retention and Dosimetry in Beagles. Radiat. Res. **98**: 614.

Mc79   McInroy JF, Campbell EE, Moss WD, Tietjen GL, Eustler BC and Boyd HA. 1979. Plutonium in Autopsy Tissue: A Revision and Updating of Data Reported in LA-4875. Health Phys. **37**:1.

Mu80   Mussalo H, Jaakkola T, Miettinen JK and Laiho K.   1980. Distribution of Fallout Plutonium in Southern Finns.   Health Phys. **39**: 245.

Os63   Osborne RV.   1963. ^{239}Pu and Other Nuclides in Ground Level Air and Lungs During Spring 1962.   Nature **199** 143.

Se73   Sedlet J, Golchert NW, and Duffy TL.   1973.   Environmental Monitoring at Argonne National Laboratory - 1973.   U.S. Atomic Energy Commission Report, Argonne National Laboratory, ANL-8007.

Si82   Singh NP, Wrenn ME, Ibrahim SA, Cohen N and Saccomano G. 1982.   Thorium Concentrations in Human Tissues from Two Geographic Locations of the United States.   In: Natural Radiation Environment, Vohra, Mishra, Pillai, Sadasiven, eds., pp. 258, Willey Eastern Ltd.   New Delhi.

Si83   Singh NP, Wrenn ME and Ibrahim SA.   1983.   Plutonium Concentration in Human Tissues: Comparison to Thorium. Health Phys. **44** (Suppl. 1) 469.

Si84   Singh NP, Zimmerman CJ, Lewis LL and Wrenn ME.   1984. Quantitative Determination of Environmental Levels of Uranium, Thorium and Plutonium in Bone.   J. Nucl. Instruments and Methods in Phys. Res. **223** 558.

Ta73   Takizawa Y.   1973.   Studies on Mechanism of Transfer of Radioactive Nuclides from the Environment to the Human Body in the Nigata District, Northern Japan.   Act. Med. et Biol. **20** 147.

Un77   UNSCEAR.   1977.   Sources and Effects of Ionizing Radiation. United Nations Scientific Committee on the Effects of Atomic Radiation.   Report to the General Assembly.

We67   Welford GA and Baird R.   1967.   Uranium Levels in Human Diet and Biological Materials.   Health Phys. **13**: 1321-1324.

We76   Welford GA, Baird R and Fisenne IM.   1976.   Concentration of Natural Uranium in the Human Body.   Health Phys. Soc. Tenth Midyear Symposium, 239-244.

Wr78   Wrenn ME and Cohen N.   1978.   Determination of ^{239,240}Pu Tissue Concentration in Non-Occupationally Exposed Residents of New York City.   New York University Progress Report 1. Rep. COO-2968-2.

Wr81   Wrenn ME, Singh NP, Cohen N, Ibrahim SA, and Saccomano G. 1981.   Thorium in Human Tissues, Nuclear Regulatory Commission Report NUREG/CR-1227.

23

Metabolic Behaviour of Plutonium in Mice

U. ANDREOZZI, L. ADDIS and S. QUAGGIA

INTRODUCTION

Data giving precise informations on long term effects and life-time
retention at low levels of α-emitting radionuclides are still insufficient. Therefore, an experiment has been initiated at the laboratories
of ENEA Casaccia, to verify the retention kinetic in target organs,
such as skeleton and liver,and its individual variability as a function of injected activity. Furthermore,the incidence and latency time
of late biological effects (life expectancy, bone tumours and other
pathological findings at death) are being studied to be correlated to
the actual retention of the α-emitting radionuclide 239-plutonium.

METHODS

Monomeric 239-plutonium was introduced by single i.v. injection through the lateral tail vein as trisodium citrate solution at pH 6.5 in
2-3 month old BC3F1 male mice. About 2500 mice divided in six groups
receiving doses ranging from 1.2 to 120 nCi/Kg body weight, and 700
controls, housed in special facilities, have been followed until
spontaneous death.

At death, mice have been autopsied and selected organs collected

243

for radiometric measurements and istopathological analyses. Activity
in the skeleton was estimated from measurements by liquid scintillation technique in femur.

RESULTS AND DISCUSSION

Comparison of long term survival (life span) between treated and untreated control groups, reported in Fig. 2, strongly indicate that
no appreciable difference can be seen attributable to plutonium
contamination at the initial activity levels up to 300 pCi/mouse.
More refined analyses (mortality intensity rate as a function of time)
are in progress to confirm these preliminary conclusions and to correlate them with pathology at death. However, the results to date
are in line with expectation based on the low levels of life-time
estimated absorbed dose, of the order of 0.1 Gy average to the skeleton at 300 pCi/mouse injected activity.

Radiometric determinations at various times over the entire lifespan of the animals, reported in Fig.1, show that the kinetic of 239-
plutonium retention in the skeleton is essentially the same as previously found in our mouse strain with much higher initial contamination. The level of fractional retention, however, is consistently
higher and possible statistical and radiological significance of this
difference is being investigated. It appears that a factor of 10 in
the initial activity injected per mouse does not greatly affect the
shape of the curve, nor the general level of fractional retention,
at least at these low levels of plutonium contamination.

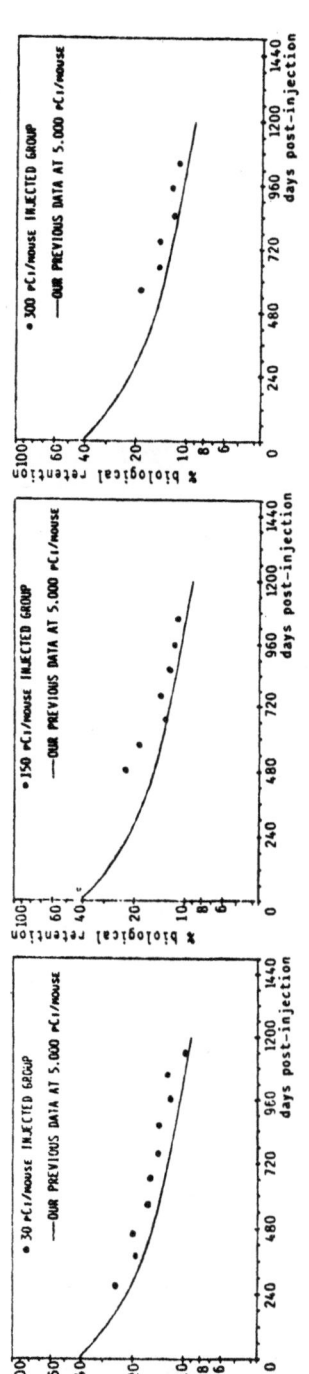

Fig. 1. Biological retention curves in mouse skeleton of the three lowest activity injected groups compared with skeleton retention curve at 5000 pCi/mouse injected group (our published data).

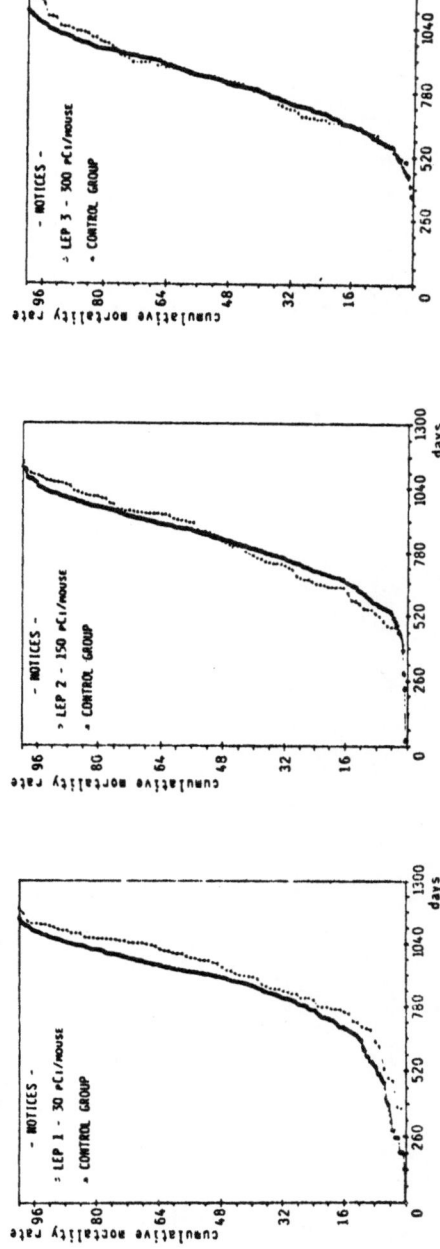

Fig. 2. Cumulative mortality rate of the three lowest activity injected groups compared with the corresponding control groups.

Part 5
Microdosimetry of
Radionuclides in Bone

Part 5
Microdosimetry of
Radionuclides in Bone

24

Microdosimetry of Bone: Implications in Radiological Protection

M. C. THORNE

INTRODUCTION

The generally accepted recommendations for limiting exposures to
ionising radiations are those set out by the International Commission
on Radiological Protection (ICRP). These recommendations concern
limitation of exposure to external irradiation and also limitation of
intakes of radioactive materials into the body by ingestion or inhalation. The basic recommendations of the Commission are set out in
ICRP Publication 26 [ICRP 77] and recommendations concerning limiting
of intakes of radioactive materials are set out in Publication 30
[ICRP 79].

In assessing the carcinogenic and heriditary effects of ionising
radiations on man, the ICRP has opted to use a linear dose-response
relationship without threshold. Thus, the risk of such effects in a
particular individual is taken to be directly proportional to the
radiation dose received, independent of the time, or rate of delivery, of that dose.

Although this proportionality between risk and dose is taken to
apply to all organs and tissues of the body, the constant of proportionality differs between organs and tissues, reflecting observed
differences in radiosensitivity. Allowance for these differences in

249

radiosensitivity is included in the ICRP recomendations by the use of weighting factors for the individual organs and tissues. Named organs and tissues in the ICRP system include 'bone surfaces', which are regarded as the tissues at risk with respect to osteosarcoma induction, and the haemopoietic bone marrow, which is regarded as the tissue at risk with respect to myeloid leukaemia induction.

In this review, a brief description is given of the ICRP system of dose calculation for inhaled or ingested radionuclides. Attention is then concentrated on the techniques used for bone dosimetry and the assumptions implicit in those techniques. Other models and dose-response relationships are commented on and consideration is given to methods by which radionuclide deposition and movement in skeletal tissues can be investigated.

THE ICRP SYSTEM OF DOSE CALCULATION

When a radionuclide is inhaled or ingested, dose rates to individual organs and tissues vary with time after intake because of the redistribution of the radioactive material and its excretion. To take this time dependence into account, the ICRP introduced the concept of committed dose equivalent, $H_{50,T}$, the dose delivered to any organ or tissue T in the 50 years following entry of the radioactive material into the body. Formally, this calculation can be written as:

$$H_{50,T} \text{ per unit intake} = \sum_i \int_M D_{50,i} \, Q_i \, N_i \, dm / \int_M dm$$

where   M   is the mass of the specified organ or tissue;

$D_{50,i}$ is the absorbed dose in tissue element dm, due to radiation type i, in the 50 years following intake;

Q_i is the quality factor for that type for radiation; and

N_i is the product of all other modifying factors, e.g. dose rate.

The quality factor is introduced to take account of the relative biological effectiveness of various radiation types. While relative biological effectiveness differs between endpoints and may be dependant upon total dose and dose rates, administratively it has been convenient to specify single values of Q for particular radiation types. Thus the ICRP has specified the following values for use with radionuclides incorporated into the body:

Q=1 for beta particles, electrons, and electromagnetic radiation, including gamma radiation, X-rays and bremsstrahlung;

Q=10 for neutrons emitted in spontaneous fission and for protons;

Q=20 for alpha particles, heavy recoil particles and fission fragments.

The Commission has also stated that its recommended risk and weighting factors are appropriate for irradiation at low dose rates [ICRP 77]. For this reason, N is taken as unity.

On the basis of the considerations discussed above, it is possible to write:

$$H_{50,T} = \sum_i Q_i \bar{D}_{50,i}$$

where $\bar{D}_{50,i}$ is the average dose to organ or tissue T in the 50 years following the entry of the radioactive material into the body.

The dose to organ or tissue T derives from radioactive emissions originating in that organ or tissue, and also from radioactive emissions originating in any other organ or tissue and entering, or traversing, the target organ. Formally this can be expressed as:

$$H_{50,T} \propto \{\text{Integrated retention in S}\} \times \{\text{Dose equivalent in T from unit retention in S}\}$$

In this expression, S, the source organ, can be identical with T the target organ. In appropriate units:

$$H_{50,T} = 1.6 \times 10^{-10} \sum_s \sum_j [U_S \sum_i SEE(T \leftarrow S)_i] \qquad Sv$$

where U_S is the total number of radionuclide transformations in
                 S over the 50 years following intake;

$SEE(T \leftarrow S)$ is the Specific Effective Energy absorbed in T per
                 transformation in S, and has units of MeV g^{-1} per
                 transformation;

1.6×10^{-10} is the conversion factor from MeV g^{-1} to J kg^{-1};

                 the summation is over all emissions i from all nuc-
                 lides j in source organs S.

Values of $SEE(T \leftarrow S)_i$ are calculated using the expression:

$$SEE(T \leftarrow S)_i = Y_i \ E_i \ AF(T \leftarrow S)_i \ Q_i / M_T$$

where Y_i is the fractional yield of radiation type i per trans-
                 formation;

E_i (MeV)   is the average, or unique, energy of the radiation;

$AF(T \leftarrow S)_i$ is the average fraction of energy absorbed in T from
                 randomly distributed transformations in S;

Q_i is the quality factor; and

M_T (g)   is the mass of organ or tissue T.

By use of these equations, calculations of $H_{50,T}$ are reduced to the
calculation of values of U_S and $AF(T \leftarrow S)_i$. These are discussed below
in the context of skeletal tissues. However, first it is relevant to
note that values of $H_{50,T}$ are combined into a committed effective
dose, H_E, using the formulation:

$$H_E = \sum_T W_T \ H_{50,T}$$

where the summation is over all organs and tissues T which are subjected to significant irradiation. Values of W_T are listed below.

Organ or tissue	W_T	Risk considered
Gonads	0.25	Serious hereditary defects in the first and second generation of offspring
Breast	0.15	Risk of fatal breast cancer averaged over both sexes and all adult life
Red bone marrow	0.12	Risk of fatal leukaemia
Lung	0.12	Risk of fatal lung cancer
Thyroid	0.03	Risk of fatal thyroid cancer
Bone surfaces	0.03	Risk of fatal bone cancer, primarily osteosarcoma
Remainder	0.30	Risk of other fatal cancer

It will be noted that fatal cancers only are considered when deriving these weighting factors. Thus, although the thyroid is known to be highly radiosensitive, it receives a low weighting factor because of the benign or operable nature of the individual tumours. For nuclides which concentrate in the skeleton, the two weighting factors of particular importance are those for red bone marrow and bone surfaces. In this context, bone surfaces are taken to be a 10μm thick layer of tissue adjacent to the endosteal surfaces of bone.

The Commission recommends limits on H_E for individuals and also recommends limits on values of $H_{50,T}$. The former limit is designed to ensure that risks of inducing cancer and hereditary disease are limited to acceptable levels, whereas the latter limit is designed to prevent effects for which there is a minimum, or threshold, dose below which they do not occur. Values of these limits are as follows:

H_E 0.05 Sv for workers, 0.005 Sv for members of the public in any one year, 0.001 Sv for long-term exposure of members of the public;

$H_{50,T}$ 0.5 Sv for all organs and tissues in workers, except for the lens of the eye, for which a value of 0.15 Sv is used. Values for members of the public are 0.1 of those for workers.

RADIONUCLIDE RETENTION AND ENERGY ABSORPTION IN SKELETAL TISSUES

The ICRP adopt the simplistic approach of assuming that skeletal
retention can be considered separately from the calculation of absorbed fractions. Complex patterns of radionuclide retention and redistribution in skeletal tissues are ignored, and only two extreme
patterns of distribution are considered, i.e.

-    radionuclides which are assumed to be deposited and retained as
     an infinitely thin layer on the surfaces of the calcified bone
     (surface seekers);

-    radionuclides which are assumed to be uniformly distributed
     throughout the volume of mineral bone at all times after depos-
     ition in that tissue (volume seekers).

Deposition in bone marrow is not considered, except in respect of
the diffuse soft tissue distribution which occurs with many elements,
e.g. caesium, and in the case of radioisotopes of indium which are
known to accumulate in the bone marrow. It is noted that the ICRP
report does not include consideration of administration of radionuclides in medical practice. If this topic were to be addressed,
the possibility of colloidal material being deposited and retained in
the bone marrow would have to be considered.

The rationale for assigning radionuclides to one or other of these
classes may be summarised as follows:

-    short-lived radionuclides, i.e. those with radioactive half-
     lives of less than 15 days, have little opportunity to penetrate
     deep into the bone matrix and are considered to be surface
     seekers;

-    long-lived isotopes of calcium, strontium, barium and radium are
     assumed to be distributed relatively rapidly throughout the
     calcium of the bone matrix and are taken to be volume seekers;

- most other long-lived radionuclides are assumed to be surface
  seekers, since they are taken to deposit initially upon bone
  surfaces and to redistribute only slowly by the processes of
  bone remodelling.

The degree to which these assumptions are appropriate to particular
radionuclides is discussed below.

In addition to the distinction between surface and volume seeking
radionuclides, the ICRP also distinguish between deposition in cortical and trabecular bone, since trabecular bone is in close proximity
to haemopoetic bone marrow, whereas cortical bone is primarily associated with fatty marrow, a tissue not thought to be at risk with
respect to myeloid leukaemia induction. With these distinctions between surface and volume distributions, different types of radionuclide emission, trabecular and cortical bone as source organs, and
bone surface and red marrow as target organs, the ICRP found it
necessary to give 20 different values of absorbed fraction (Table 1).

Table 1.   Absorbed fractions specified by the ICRP

Source	Target	Volume		Surface		
		Alpha	Beta	Alpha	Beta $(\bar{E}<0.2\text{MeV})$	Beta $(\bar{E}>0.2\text{MeV})$
Cortical bone	Bone surfaces	0.01	0.015	0.25	0.25	0.015
	Red marrow	0.0	0.0	0.0	0.0	0.0
Trabecular bone	Bone surfaces	0.025	0.025	0.25	0.25	0.025
	Red marrow	0.05	0.35	0.5	0.5	0.5

Several points may be made concerning the values given above.

- Because of the limited ranges of α and β particles, absorbed
  fractions for red marrow from radionuclides in cortical bone are
  always taken as zero.

- For all α or β emitters on trabecular surfaces, geometrical considerations imply that approximately half the energy will be deposited in the bone marrow and half in the mineral bone.

- For all α and β emitters uniformly distributed throughout the bone volume, self-absorbtion by the mineral matrix reduces fractional absorption values in the marrow to less than 0.5. The reduction is more marked for α-emitters because of their limited range in mineralised bone (~25μm).

- Absorbed fractions for bone surfaces are similar for both cortical and trabecular bone, but are somewhat lower for cortical bone because the surface to volume ratio is lower in cortical than in trabecular bone.

- β particles with mean energies of less than 0.2 MeV typically have ranges comparable with α particles and are, therefore, associated with similar absorbed fractions.

- β particles with mean energies of more than 0.2 MeV typically have ranges larger than average bone thicknesses (>100μm). Thus, absorbed fractions are similar for both surface and volume distributions.

Examination of the data given in Table 1 indicates that the skeletal distribution of radionuclides emitting α particles and low energy β particles is critical to their dosimetry. In both cases, the average or unique energy of the emissions is also of significance.

In order to illustrate the effects of energy of emission on skeletal dosimetry, Table 2 lists absorbed fractions in red marrow for α-emitters buried to different depths below the bone surface and emitting α particles with energies of between 3 and 7 MeV [Th 77].

Table 2. Absorbed fractions in red marrow for α-emitters buried to
          different depths in trabecular bone

Depth (μm)	3 MeV	5 MeV	7 MeV
0	0.50	0.50	0.50
4	0.16	0.30	0.37
8	0.03	0.20	0.29
12	0.00	0.10	0.21
20	0.00	0.01	0.11
30	0.00	0.00	0.04

Correspondingly, Table 3 lists absorbed fractions in the 10μm
thick layer adjacent to the labelled bone, i.e. bone surfaces in ICRP
nomenclature [Th 77].

Table 3. Absorbed fraction in bone surface tissues for α-emitters
          buried to different depths in mineral bone

Depth (μm)	Absorbed fraction		
	3 MeV	5 MeV	7 MeV
0	0.43	0.29	0.17
4	0.16	0.17	0.13
8	0.04	0.13	0.11
12	0.00	0.08	0.09
20	0.00	0.02	0.07
30	0.00	0.00	0.03

Thus, for α-emitting radionuclides, burial in bone to a depth of
only a few microns substantially diminishes dose rates to sensitive
tissues. For comparison, the turnover of compact bone is estimated to
be 2.5% y^{-1} [Va 75], which, for a mass of 4 kg, a density ~2g cm^{-3}
and a surface area ~5.6 m^2 [ICRP 74], implies an apposition rate of
9μm y^{-1}. Thus, α-emitting radionuclides with radioactive half-lives
of more than a few months cannot reasonably be assumed to reside
indefinately upon bone surfaces, since their irradiation of sensitive

tissues may be substantially reduced by apposition of new bone over such periods.

It should be noted that the above calculation is over-simplistic and that dose rates to sensitive tissues cannot be determined directly from mean rates of apposition. At any time, some areas of bone will be in an appositional phase, some in a resorptive phase and some in a quiescent, or 'resting' phase. To illustrate the significance of this, consider a simplified situation some time after intake. Assume 80% of the material retained in the skeleton is on resting surfaces and 20% has been buried to a depth of 40μm. In this case, the average depth of burial is 8μm. The absorbed fraction in bone surface tissues for a 5 MeV α-emitter calculated for 8μm depth of burial is 0.13, whereas the weighted value for the surface and buried deposits is 0.23. Corresponding average depth and weighted values for red marrow are 0.20 and 0.40 respectively.

Throughout this discussion, attention has been concentrated on a 10μm thick layer adjacent to the mineralised surface, since this is the tissue identified by the ICRP as sensitive with respect to osteosarcoma induction. However, evidence for a 10μm thick layer is very limited, since the cell type which is transformed is not well-defined and the distribution of such cells has not been quantified. However, data on osteosarcoma incidence in workers who ingested Ra-226 [Ev 74] and patients treated with Ra-224 [Sp 73] indicate that a substantial fraction of the sensitive cells must lie within 40μm of the bone surfaces. Because most α-emitting radionuclides emit α particles of similar energies to those emitted by Ra-226 and its daughters, the toxicity of these radionuclides relative to Ra-226 is not strongly influenced by the spatial distribution of the sensitive cells in the bone marrow. However, the relative toxicity of α-emitters relative to β-emitters and radionuclides emitting low energy β particles relative to those emitting high energy β particles could be strongly conditioned by this distribution. In this context, it is relevant to note that the dosimetric calculations set out in ICRP Publication 30 [ICRP 79] imply that ingestion or inhalation of Sr-90 will result in 1.8 myeloid leukaemias for each osteosarcoma. This is contrary to the general experience in animal experiments, but might be explained if Ra-226 irradiated only a small fraction of the cells at risk with respect to osteosarcoma induction. However, other explanations are possible, in terms of different shaped dose-response curves for α- and β-irradiation for both osteosarcoma and myeloid leukaemia induction.

It should also be noted that the osteosarcomas produced in Ra-226 exposed workers were almost invariably associated with high average skeletal radiation doses (>10 Gy). These doses were high enough to induce gross histological changes. Thus, Lloyd and Henning (Ll 79) reported that in one such case a fibrotic layer of up to 50µm thickness was interposed between the marrow cells and the bone mineral. This layer was essentially acellular and the possibility must exist that much of the radiation dose received by this individual may have been wasted in respect of osteosarcoma induction because of the presence of this radiation-induced fibrotic layer.

REALISTIC MODELS FOR SKELETAL RETENTION AND DOSIMETRY

In a brief review, it is not possible to consider realistic models for a wide range of nuclides. For this reason, attention is concentrated on a model for Pu-239. This topic has been considered in most detail by Priest and his co-workers [Pr 84] and the current version of their model is shown in Fig. 1.

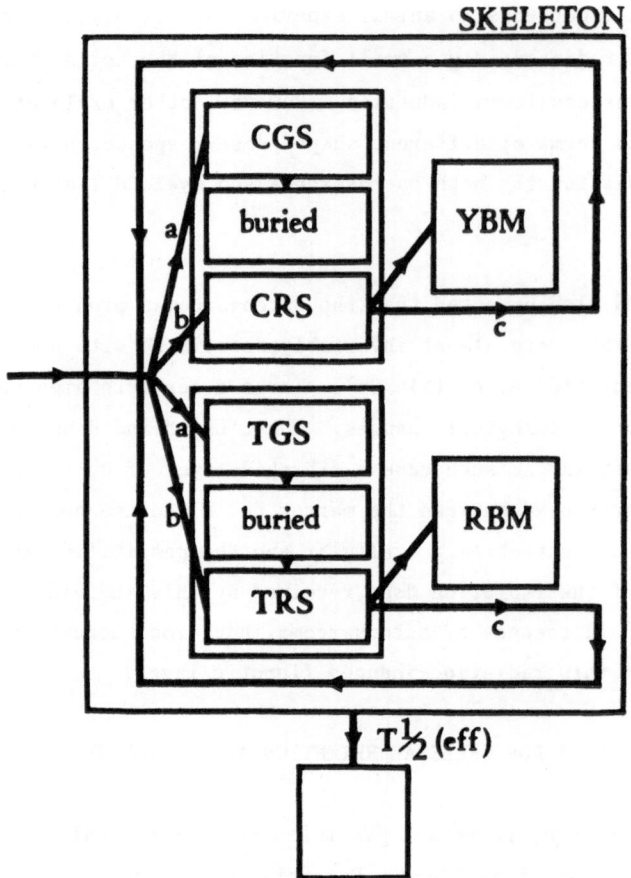

FIGURE 1. The main features of the dosimetric model used to define
         the deposition and translocation of radionuclide within the
         skeleton

Fractions a, b and c represent the radionuclide deposited on
growing bone surfaces, the fraction deposited on resorbing bone
surfaces and the fraction of radionuclide recycled following its loss
from resorbing bone surfaces, respectively. CGS = growing surfaces
of cortical bone. TGS = growing surfaces of trabecular bone. CRS =
resorbing surfaces of cortical bone. TRS = resorbing surfaces of
trabecular bone. YBM = yellow bone marrow. RBM = red bone marrow.
It is assumed that any radionuclide is lost from the skeleton with an
effective half-time that is a combination of the biological retention
half-time of the element in the skeleton and the physical half-life
of the radionuclide [Pr 84].

In this model, activity deposited in the skeleton is partitioned
between growing and resorbing surfaces of cortical and trabecular
bone. Material deposited on resorbing surfaces is assumed to be
removed from those surfaces and either recycled for deposition or
deposited in bone marrow. Cortical bone is assumed to be sufficiently thick that material deposited on the growing surfaces will not
re-emerge over the period of interest. In the case of trabecular
bone, burial is also assumed to proceed at a uniform rate, but the
activity can pass through the bone within the period of simulation
and emerge at a resorbing surface. Removal of activity from the
skeleton as a whole is modelled using a single effective half-life
which is applied to all components of retention.

This model has proved useful in considering the effects of bone
modelling assumptions on annual limits on intake for plutonium.
However, as a physiological representation of the processes involved,
it has a number of limitations.

-    It seems unreasonable to represent clearance from the skeleton
     by a single empirical half-life. More plausibly, some of the
     material which is recycled from bone compartments could be lost
     from the skeleton to be deposited in other tissues, or trans-
     ferred to the excreta. Similarly, material deposited in other
     tissues of the body may be remobilised and transferred to the
     skeleton.

-    Both red and yellow bone marrow are represented as permanent
     stores of resorbed material, except in so far as material is
     taken to be removed uniformly from all skeletal compartments.
     While this concept of permanent retention may be appropriate to
     intravenously injected colloidal material such as thorotrast and
     may also apply to high skeletal burdens of Pu-239, further
     quantitative animal studies are required to identify whether it
     is applicable to low body burdens of Pu-239, or in conditions of
     chronic exposure, where the bone is relatively uniformly labelled.

-     All skeletal surfaces are considered as accreting or resorbing at the time of deposition. In practice, a large fraction of surfaces may be in a resting state. There is a need to determine the extent of deposition on resting and active surfaces and the timescale over which resting surfaces become active and vice versa.

Thus, while it is possible to use this model to give a first estimate of the effects of incorporating microscopic parameters in a model for Pu-239 retention in the skeleton, it is clear that much more work is required before a detailed, physiologically justified, model for Pu-239 dynamics can be constructed. For most other α- and β-emitting radionuclides, the fragmentary data currently available are not sufficient to justify a model as complex as the one discussed above. The scope for research on radionuclide distribution and retention in the skeleton is, therefore, wide. Furthermore, several sensitive techniques are available for this, as is discussed below. However, before discussing techniques, it is appropriate to note that such research is relevant not only to dose estimates used in regulation, but also to the determination of appropriate dose-response curves for radiation-induced osteosarcoma.

DOSE RESPONSE RELATIONSHIPS

In reporting the incidence of osteosarcomas in individuals exposed to irradiation from internally-incorporated α-emitters, it is usual to relate incidence to average skeletal dose. However, a complex relationship may exist between average skeletal dose and the distribution of doses received by sensitive tissues. One factor, that irradiation may induce histological changes in the irradiated tissues, has already been noted. Because such changes may be cumulative dose, or dose rate, related, it is possible that equal average skeletal doses delivered as a result of different patterns of intake of a radionuclide will not correspond to equal doses to sensitive tissues. Even in the absence of gross irradiation-induced changes, effects may be very different for the same average skeletal dose, because the effect may be determined by dose rate, as well as total dose, to the

sensitive tissues.   This will be the case when intra-cellular repair
processes with a characteristic time for repair, or cellular proliferation responses, are involved in induction of the effect.   Thus,
for example, a high dose delivered over a short interval can steri-
lise a large fraction of potentially transformed cells, whereas if
the same dose is delivered over a longer period, cellular proliferation will counter this and give rise to a larger population of viable
transformed cells.   In this context, Mole [Mo 79] has argued that
this protraction effect is seen in both mice and humans injected with
Ra-224, since, for a given injected activity, osteosarcoma incidence
increases as the period over which the injections are given increases.

EXPERIMENTAL TECHNIQUES

Gross retention of radionuclides in the skeleton, or parts of the
skeleton, can be measured using several conventional techniques.
For studies in man external gamma counting is available and in animal, or autopsy, studies this may be supplemented by the α, β or γ
counting of samples.   A more difficult problem is to quantify the
time-dependent behaviour of radioactive materials in the skeleton at
a resolution of a few microns.   This requires the use of histological sections and the extreme variability of bone structure implies
that many sections must be used from several different bones in order
to obtain an adequate measure of the overall pattern of behaviour.

One possibility is to use conventional autoradiographic techniques,
in which α- or β-emissions originating from histological sections
form tracks in a photographic emulsion overlying the section.   These
tracks can be developed and viewed in conjunction with the underlying
section.   This technique is suitable for use with β-emitting radionuclides, or with high levels of α-emitting radionuclides.   However,
it is insufficiently sensitive to be of use at the concentrations of
α-emitters of interest in radiological protection.

In the special case of the fissionable radionuclides U-235 and
Pu-239, an alternative technique is available which is applicable at
very low concentrations of activity.   This is neutron-induced autoradiography (NIAR).   In this technique, histological sections of the

bone, or, more recently, other tissues [Gr 78], are mounted on polycarbonate plastic slides.   These preparations are irradiated with
thermal neutrons in a nuclear reactor, a process with the following
consequences:

-   A fraction of the fissionable atoms present in each section are
    induced to fission.   As a result of each fission, two heavy
    fission fragments are produced and, in most cases, one of these
    enters the polycarbonate plastic leaving a track of damage which
    can be revealed by etching with sodium hydroxide.

-   A reaction occurs between the surface of the section and the
    plastic and this reaction induces a latent image of the struc-
    ture of the section in the plastic which can also be revealed by
    etching with sodium hydroxide.

A typical image produced by this technique is shown in Fig. 2.

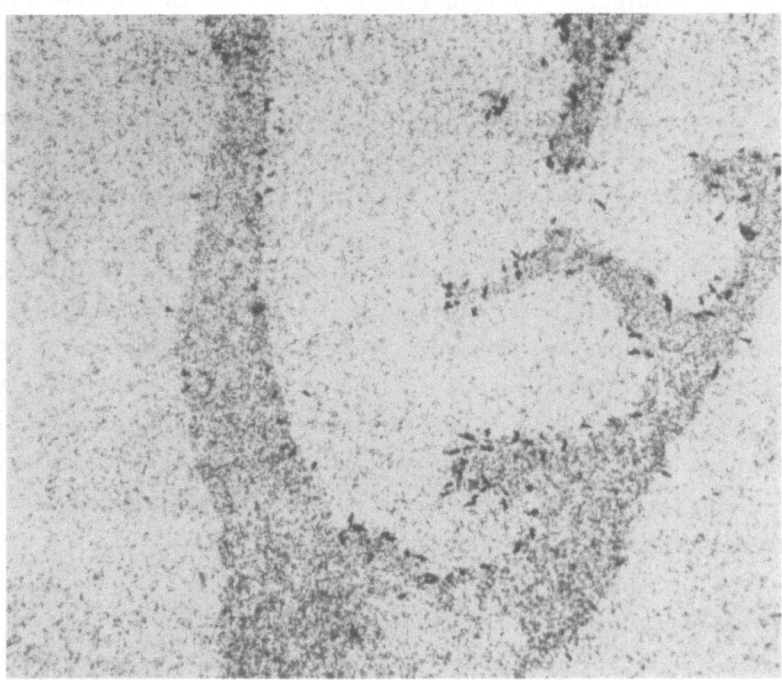

FIGURE 2. NIAR image of mineral bone on Lexan

The technique has been extended to reveal more of the section
structure by a four step technique which involves irradiation with
thermal neutrons; annealing at a temperature high enough to eliminate the latent image, but low enough to preserve the tracks of
damage induced by the fission fragments, irradiation with α-particles
and etching in sodium hydroxide.   In this case, irradiation with
α-particles damages the surface of the plastic, but to a varying
extent depending upon the amount and density of interposing tissue
present in the histological section.   Thus, a negative image of the
section structure is induced on the plastic and can be revealed by
etching.

Given an image of the section structure and superimposed tracks of
fission fragments derived from U-235 or Pu-239, it is possible to
determine the distribution of distances of tracks from particular
structures in the section.   Thus, Green et al. [Gr 79, Gr 81] used
images derived from sections of mouse bone labelled with Pu-239, such
as that shown in Fig. 2, and measured the distribution of perpendicular distances of track-ends from the nearest mineral/marrow interface.   This gave a track-end distribution about the bone surface.
By using a monte-carlo code to simulate the track end distribution
expected from sources of Pu-239 lying at various depths in marrow or
mineral bone, Green et al. were able to interpret the observed track-
end distributions in terms of distributions of Pu-239 relative to the
bone surface.   Some illustrative results from their studies are
shown in Fig. 3.

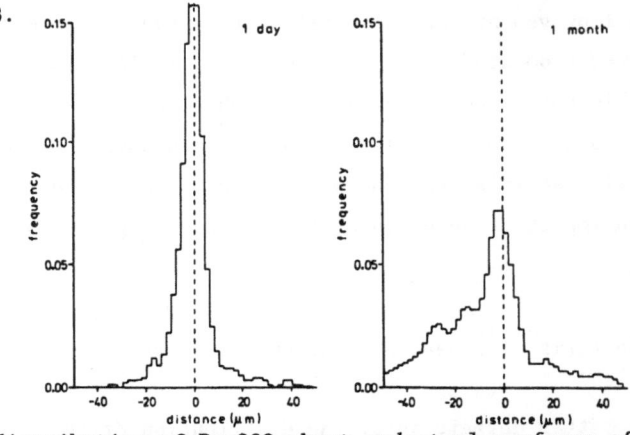

FIGURE 3. The distribution of Pu-239 about endosteal surfaces of the
ilium in the female CBA mouse at 1 day and 1 month after
injection.   Negative distances are into mineral bone.

These various autoradiographic techniques typically have resolutions of better than 3µm and can, therefore, be used to measure radionuclide distributions in the skeletons of experimental animals with an accuracy adequate for dosimetric purposes.   Such measurements are directly useful in the interpretation of animal experiments on radionuclide toxicity, but they are also useful in elucidating mechanisms of radionuclide distribution and retention in the skeleton which may eventually be extrapolated to man.

DISCUSSION

The current system of radiological protection recommended by the ICRP requires the calculation of radiation doses to a wide range of organs and tissues.   In the skeleton, the two tissues identified as being of importance are the red bone marrow, in respect of myeloid leukaemia induction, and a layer 10µm thick over bone surfaces, taken to contain the cells sensitive to osteosarcoma induction.

In the calculation of radiation doses to these tissues, the ICRP separate radionuclide distribution and retention in the skeleton. Consideration of a model for Pu-239 retention illustrates that this distinction is artificial.   Thus, although the ICRP model gives a reasonable basis for defining limits on exposure to radioactive materials, it is clearly susceptible to considerable improvement. Such improvements are also relevant to the interpretation of data derived from studies on experimental animals, since average skeletal dose is not an adequate parameter when relations between this quantity and dose to sensitive tissues can change with the amount of activity administered and where dose rates to sensitive tissues may be an important determinant of the effects produced by a particular dose.

In terms of research requirements there is a need for:

-    better definition of the distribution of the cells at risk,
     particularly with respect to osetosarcoma induction;

- studies of dose-response relationships in which dose and dose-rate to the sensitive tissues are considered as determining variables;

- more quantitative studies on the distribution of radionuclides in skeletal tissues at a resolution of a few microns.

In respect of all these, there is a need for studies in several mammalian species, so that there is some basis for extrapolation of the results to man.

REFERENCES

Ev74.   Evans, R.D., 1974.   Radium in man.   Health Phys., 27, 497-510.

Gr78.   Green, D., Howells, G.R., Thorne, M.C. and Watts, R.H., 1978. Imaging of tissue sections on Lexan by alpha particles and thermal neutrons: an aid in fissionable radionuclide distribution studies. Int. J. Appl. Radiat. Isot., 29, 285-295.

Gr79.   Green, D., Howells, G.R. and Thorne, M.C., 1979.   Quantitative microscopic studies of the distribution and retention of ^{239}Pu in the ilium of the female CBA mouse.   Int. J. Radiat. Biol., 36, 499-511.

Gr81.   Green, D., Howells, G.R. and Thorne, M.C., 1981.   A semi-automated technique for assessing the microdistribution of ^{239}Pu deposited in bone.   Phys. Med. Biol., 26, 379-387.

ICRP74.   ICRP Publication 23, 1974.   Report of the Task Group on Reference Man (Oxford, Pergamon Press).

ICRP77.   ICRP Publication 26, 1977.   Recommendations of the International Commission on Radiological Protection.   Annals of the ICRP, Vol.1, No.3 (Oxford, Pergamon Press).

ICRP79.   ICRP Publication 30, Part 1, 1979.   Limits for Intakes of
Radionuclides by Workers.   Annals of the ICRP, Vol.2, No.3/4
(Oxford, Pergamon Press).

L179.   Lloyd, E.L. and Henning, C.B., 1979.   Cells at risk for the
production of bone tumors in man - an electron microscope study of
the endosteal surface of control bone and bone from a human radium
case.   In: Radiological and Environmental Research Division
Argonne National Laboratory Annual Report, Part 2, pp.39-53,
ANL-79-65 (Pt. 2).

Mo79.   Mole, R.W., 1979.   Carcinogenesis by Thorotrast and other
sources of irradiation, especially other α-emitters.   Environ.
Res., 18, 192-215.

Pr84.   Priest, N.D. and Birchall, A., 1984.   Progress on the dosimetry of bone surface seeking radionuclides.   Radiol. Prot.
Bull., No.59, 20-26.

Sp73.   Spiess, H. and Mays, C.W., 1973.   Protraction effect on bone
sarcoma induction by ^{224}Ra in children and adults.   In: Radiation
Carcinogenesis (Sanders, C.L., Busch, R.H., Ballow, J.E. and Mahlum,
D.D., Eds.), pp.437-450, CONF-720505, USEAC.

Th77.   Thorne, M.C., 1977.   Aspects of the dosimetry of alpha-
emitting radionuclides in bone with particular emphasis on Ra-226
and Pu-239.   Phys. Med. Biol., 22, 36-46.

Va75.   Vaughan, J.M., 1975.   The Physiology of Bone. (London,
Oxford University Press).

25

Localized Alpha-Dosimetry for Cancer Induction Studies

E. POLIG

INTRODUCTION

Radiation causes damage to biological tissue through the absorption of
its energy and the concomitant functional changes caused by lesions on
a molecular level. If frequent enough to overwhelm an organ's capacity
for restoration or repair such lesions may finally become manifest on
the macroscopic level by inhibition or alteration (cancer) of the
organ's function. It has been therefore recognized that the amount or
"concentration" of absorbed energy is the relevant physical parameter
to which the observed effects of radiation have to be linked. This is
in contrast to the concepts of conventional chemical toxicity where
the amount or concentration of the toxic substance itself is related
to its effect. Radiation dosimetry plays a key-role in the toxicology
of radionuclides. If applied to biological tissue or organisms it is a
physico-mathematical theory with intimate connection to the
physiological processes and morphological structure of living matter.

For a sufficiently complete and accurate approach to radiation
dosimetry in biological tissue one has to know
  - the intensity and arrangement of the radiation sources
  - the structure and behaviour of the sensitive targets.
It is an almost trivial suspicion that the strength and spatial
arrangement of the radiation sources, or in other words, the spatial

distribution and concentration of a radionuclide is strongly related
to the structure and function of an organ. The skeleton with its
constituents bone and soft tissue is itself a very "inhomogeneous"
organ and as such stands out from all the remaining organs of the
body. This inhomogeneity of the organ is reflected by a
correspondingly non-uniform distribution of almost all radionuclides
with skeletal affinity. The characterization and quantitation of the
distribution of a radionuclide in the skeleton and its change in time
must therefore be one of the primary goals of radiation dosimetry.

DOSIMETRIC ASPECTS OF THE DEPOSITS

Alpha-emitters depositing in the skeleton may be broadly categorized
into volume-seekers and surface-seekers. Typical representatives of
the former group are the alkaline-earth elements, of the latter group
the transuranic elements. Volume-seekers deposit more or less
uniformly throughout calcified tissue, whereas surface-seekers
deposit, at least initially, on bone surfaces only. It has to be
noted, however, that as a consequence of remodelling processes the
distribution of surface-seekers gradually assumes to a certain extent
the characteristics of a volume-seeker. The differences in deposition
in the skeleton point towards different mechanisms of binding to
skeletal consituents and also have important implications for the
radiation dosimetry of these elements.

The different types of label generated after a single injection of
a surface-seeker depend on the state of the surface element at the
time of injection. At any particular time a surface element in the
skeleton may be either resting, forming or resorbing.

On a resting surface a surface deposition accumulates with a
specific surface activity that increases rapidly shortly after
injection. After the usually rapid decline of the specific blood
activity a secondary surface label will be superimposed on the primary
label due to recirculation of activity that has been resorbed at other
sites in the skeleton. The dose rate calculated for a certain distance
from the bone surface (Fig.1) shows correspondingly first a rapid
increase followed by a slow increase due to the secondary deposits.
The formation of secondary surface labels by redeposition of resorbed

activity can best be seen in slowly turning over parts of the
skeleton, which thus have a high fraction of resting surfaces. Fig. 2
shows the increase of the specific surface activity of 239-Pu in the
epiphysis of rat femurs after the injection of 18.5 kBq/kg. If a
surface element undergoes resorption the dose rate drops quickly to
zero because of the removal of the surface deposit at the beginning of
the remodelling cycle and remains at zero for the rest of the
resorption period. After the onset of bone formation the dose rate
gradually increases because a low level diffuse label will be laid
down along with new bone. During the period of quiescence following
the completion of the formation phase a further secondary surface
deposit slowly accumulates. For the rest of the lifetime such a
surface element then experiences a periodic pattern of build-up of
diffuse deposits and secondary surface labels followed by resorption.
The specific activities of these labels gradually decline
corresponding to the decrease in blood specific activity (Fig.1).

At a bone forming surface the initial rapid increase of dose rates
is followed by a decline due to the burial of the surface deposit.
This decline depends on how much of the formation cycle has been
completed at the time of injection. If injection occurs at an early
time within the formation period the final burial depth may be large
enough to completely shield the bone marrow from further irradiation.
In a late stage of the formation cycle the final burial depth may be
just a few microns with a correspondingly low shielding effect. During
bone formation a diffuse deposit will also be generated with a
concentration related to the blood specific activity. After formation
has ceased a secondary surface deposit slowly builds up. Subsequent
resorption first reduces the dose rate because of resorption of the
secondary deposit and then increases the dose rate again because the
buried surface label is approaching the surface. After complete local
resorption of all radioactivity, this surface element enters the normal
cycle of low level diffuse deposition and formation of secondary
surface deposits, followed by resorption as discussed above for resting
surfaces.

The time dependence of the dose rate at surface elements that are
resorbing at the time of intitial uptake of radioactivity is similar
to the cases of forming and resting surfaces after the first

remodelling cycle has been completed. During resorption a short term
surface deposition may deliver a relatively high dose rate to the
adjacent marrow (Pr80).

The time dependence of dose rates resulting from the deposition of
a volume-seeker like 226-Ra is shown in Fig.3. At a resting surface
the dose rate from the diffuse deposit increases and attains a maximum
within a short time. The slow decrease of the diffuse dose rate due to
the diminishing of the diffuse concentration is interrupted if
remodelling starts and a growing volume deposit at the much higher hot
spot concentration begins to accumulate. After the completion of the
remodelling cycle the hotspot concentration and the resulting dose
rate declines steadily much like the diffuse concentration until a new
remodelling cycle starts by resorbing all or a part of the hotspot and
reducing the dose rates accordingly. We then observe a repeated
pattern of lowering of the hotspot dose rates because of resorption
and a subsequent increase due to the formation of new hotspots at a
lower level of concentration than the previous one. The kinetics of
dose rates for the other two types of surfaces may be visualized by
choosing an appropriate time point at the same curve (Fig.3).

Accumulated radiation doses to a specified location of the marrow
and for a representative part of the skeleton may be calculated by
integration of dose rate curves like those shown in Fig. s 1 and 3
with respect to time, taking into account the relative contribution of
the three types of surfaces and the 'phase shift' between individual
curves of the statistical ensemble of surface elements chosen. By
'phase shift' we mean that for instance for resting surface elements
the time between initial uptake and the occurence of the first
remodelling cycle may vary from one element to the other. This
possibility has been indicated in Fig.1 by a dashed line. This
asynchrony may be accounted for by a shift of the curves using an
appropriate time increment. Summarizing it may be said that the dose
rate behaviour at the different types of surfaces only differs with
respect to the initial phase of uptake until the first remodelling
cycle starts. From then onwards we have a periodic pattern of dose
rate changes with decreasing amplitudes. The period of this pattern is
of course related to the average turnover rate. As a coarse estimate
one may say that this period is the inverse of the turnover rate. For

a turnover rate of 100%/year, as is typical for adult rodents and young adult dogs, this would mean a period of one year, for 10%/year as typical for human trabecular bone a period of about 10 years follows.

What the significance of the initial differences in the dose rate behaviour in causing late effects like cancer is, remains an open question. The dosimetric approach to determining accumulated radiation doses as described above, although superior to determining average skeletal doses, is still formal and unrealistic in the sense that integrating over dose rate curves like those shown in Fig. s 1 and 3 ignores the fact that the widely variable levels of dose rates are delivered to different types of osteogenic cells with different potential for malignant transformation.

Autoradiographic images of the microscopic distribution of radionuclides reveal that the concentrations of deposits are not only changing in time but also that in many cases there is a considerable nonuniformity in space. This holds both for the surface concentration of a surface-seeker as well as for the volume deposition of a volume-seeker. For the initial uptake of surface-seekers the variability of the specific surface activity may be explained at least in part by local differences in the blood supply. Whether the same holds for the observed variation of diffuse concentrations of volume-seekers is unknown. Fig. 4 shows the variation of the specific surface activity of 241-Am after injection of 104.3 kBq/kg in the proximal and distal humerus and of the diffuse concentration of 226-Ra after injection of 322 kBq/kg in the lumbar vertebra of beagle dogs. Such a non-uniformity of local concentrations means that the whole population of a particular type of osteogenic cells is irradiated at different dose rates and thus receives different accumulated doses. This may have important consequences for the overall response of the skeleton (see below).

DOSIMETRIC ASPECTS OF THE TARGETS

The cells at risk for the induction of osteogenic tumours are the osteogenic cells or their precursors mainly located in close proximity to bone surfaces or within bone. Among the different types of cells the osteoblasts as bone forming cells, their precursors, the osteoprogenitors , the lining cells and also fibroblastic cells appearing in association with fibrotic tissue (L183) seem to be the most likely candidates for malignant transformation. To determine average absorbed doses to a population of targets one needs to know the intensity of the radiation field at the location of the targets. For short range alpha-emitters deposited on bone surfaces or in bone and irradiating cells in adjacent marrow this means a precise determination of the distances of the sensitive sites–namely the cell nucleus– from the bone surfaces. Such precision is necessary because of the rapid drop of dose rates with increasing distances from the bone surface. For alpha-particles of range 37 μm originating at a bone surface the dose rate at a distance 3 μm from the surface is about twice as high as at a distance of 10 μm. As cell nuclei of a certain type of cell are not located at a precisely defined distance the relative location of a population of targets may be best described by a probability density. Fig. 5 shows the probability densities of distances for lining cells, osteoblasts and osteoprogenitors as determined in the metaphysis of rats (Po84). The mean distances are increasing in the order of lining cells, osteoblasts and osteoprogenitors. Apart from the local variation of surface or volume concentrations of an alpha-emitter we thus have identified another source of variation, namely the position of the target in the non-isotropic radiation field. From the probability densities of the concentration and the distance, one may calculate a combined probability density of the dose rates for the whole population of cells assuming independence of the two stochastic variables. This has been done in Fig.6 for the dose rates in the dog lumbar vertebra resulting from the diffuse concentration of 226-Ra. It is obvious that because of the wide spread of dose rates the irradiation to the respective cell populations is quite non-uniform.

We thus have the remarkable result that dose rates and absorbed doses are stochastic variables with considerable variation throughout the skeleton and even within a single bone. In fact another stochastic variable comes into play if accumulated doses have to be determined from dose rates, namely the time of irradiation. This is shown for the case of 241-Am contaminated beagle bones in Fig.7. The initial surface deposits on resting surfaces are primarily irradiating lining cells until such surfaces are remodelled and the surface deposits are removed along with old bone. For the population of lining cells as a whole this means that the time of irradiation of individual cells is a random variable equal to the time between injection and resorption of the respective surface element. For exponentially distributed residence times the probability densities of radiation doses as shown in Fig.7 result. Only the specific surface activity was taken into account as the other random variable. The exponential distribution of residence times for surface deposits is a consequence of the assumption that remodelling occurs at random, i.e. is independent of the age of the bone. The mean residence time is then equal to 1/(turnover rate).

Apart from the sources of variability discussed above, namely local intensity of source, position of targets, time of irradiation, there are other stochastic factors related to the target itself or to the physical processes of energy deposition that constitute what is called microdosimetry in a strict sense. Alpha particles traversing the cell nucleus as the sensitive volume deposits energy within this sensitive volume that depends on the track segment length and the LET. Moreover the amount of energy given off is fluctuating because of the random nature of single energy absorption events (straggling). Such fluctuations of local energy deposition take place even if the parameters like distance of targets and local concentrations are assumed to have exactly determined values. The lengths of particle track segments depends among other things on the shape and size of bone cell nuclei. Fig. 8 gives a schematic representation of the nuclei of lining cells, osteoblasts and osteoprogenitors. It has been found that all nuclei can be characterized by oblate spheroids and their dimensions were determined by means of computer simulation from measurements on histological sections (Po 84). Fig.8 shows the variation of shapes by presenting the averages along with shapes having mean dimensions plus or minus one standard deviation. It is common to refer to the energy deposited along a track segment through a sensitive volume divided by the mass of the volume as the specific energy, to distinguish this stochastic quantity from the non-stochastic absorbed dose. Fig.9 shows three single event spectra (for one particle traversal only) of specific energy for

alpha-particles originating on bone surfaces or 10 µm beneath a bone
surface. As sensitive volumes spheres of 2 µm diameter are
considered. In cases where the level of irradiation is so low that
most of the targets are not hit by alpha particles the mean specific
energy of single events is considerably higher than the absorbed dose.
There are also particle traversals with specific energy exceeding the
mean value by far. For high intensity irradiation or irradiation over
prolonged times the spectrum of specific energy may be obtained by
convolution of the single event spectrum and the distribution of hits
(Po83).

DOSIMETRY AND MODELS OF TUMOUR INDUCTION

The primary goal of localized radiation dosimetry in bone is to obtain
risk estimates applicable to humans and derived from experimental data
on animals. As human data on the effects of 226-Ra and 228-Ra are
available we may state the problem more precisely. Can we find a
dosimetric model incorporating all essential physiological and
structural characteristics of the skeleton that describes the tumour
incidences observed in humans and one or more animal species (e.g.
dogs) equally well? If so we may, with some confidence, apply the
machinery of this model to another radionuclide, using the data on
the same animal as input and coming up with the prediction of effects
on humans. This philosophy of modeling is an extension of the simpler
concept of toxicity ratios advanced previously (L172).

Marshall and Groer (Ma77) developed a model of tumour induction by
226-Ra/228-Ra that was fit to observed tumour incidences in humans and
dogs. The model assumed that transformation into malignancy involves
two induction stages and that the rate of promotion is proportional to
bone turnover. It was further postulated that the rate of accumulation
of cells in the two induction stages is proportional to the endosteal
dose rate (0-10 µm from surfaces), the number of cells at risk and a
constant called intiation probability σ . It was possible to fit the
model predictions such as tumour rate and cummulative incidence to
observations in humans and beagle dogs under the condition that the
initiation probability per cell was about ten times greater in the dog
than in man ($5 \cdot 10^{-7}$/rad vs. $4.7 \, 10^{-8}$/rad). If one simplifies the

differential equations of the Marshall and Groer model for the case of
very low dose rates where cell killing and the depletion of cell pools
can be ignored one obtains for the tumour rate P (%/year)

$$P = \frac{\lambda \sigma^2 s}{2} D^2 \qquad (1)$$

with λ = promotion rate, s= total number of endosteal cells, D=
endosteal dose. In view of what has been said above about the spatial
and temporal variation of endosteal dose rates one may introduce two
modifications of the concept characterized by Eq.1. The first is to
allow for the variability of endosteal doses which would change Eq.1
to

$$P = \frac{\lambda \sigma^2 s}{2} D^2 (1 + V_D^2) \qquad (2)$$

with the relative variation V_D of the endosteal dose. As Eq.2 shows
such a variation always tends to increase tumour rates compared to the
case of a uniform dose distribution. For a fit of the model with P
given this would mean that σ is actually lower than was determined by
Marshall and Groer. The second modification would concern the value of
the mean endosteal dose itself. Fig.10 shows how the time dependence of
dose rates for a surface-seeker as depicted in Fig.1 relates to the
presence of different types of bone cells. If only osteoprogenitors or
active osteoblasts can be induced the relevant endosteal dose rate to
these cells for a surface-seeker would be lower than if endosteal
doses are calculated disregarding the presence or absence of sensitive
cells. The reason for this is that usually both osteoprogenitors and
active osteoblasts appear on the scene only during bone formation,
i.e. after the high initial surface concentrations have been removed
already. Curves of cumulative doses for single surface elements
superimpose to yield the endosteal dose and its variance for a
specific type of cell in a bone or the whole skeleton. The random time
shifts between curves of individual surface elements then tend to
produce a smooth resulting curve for the whole population of cells.
Bone turnover determines the mean time interval between remodelling
cycles. For endosteal doses to lining cells this means that increasing
turnover rates tend to reduce the radiation dose because they lower

the mean residence time of the initial surface deposits. For osteoblasts and progenitors increasing turnover rates effect an increase in endosteal doses (Fig.10) simply because these cells appear more frequently on surfaces. Experimentally it has been found in dogs that high turnover bones in the skeleton are also sites of high tumour incidences (Wr80). It is important to note that if osteoblasts or progenitors are assumed to be the cells at risk we do not need to postulate a separate promotion step triggered by a remodelling stimulus to account for the influence of turnover as was necessary in the model of Marshall and Groer. It is likely that future experiments using detailed microautoradiography and localized dosimetry will also shed some light on the number of events necessary for tumor induction.

Because of lack of space only a few particular aspects of the relationship between microdistribution studies, local dosimetry and mechanisms of tumour induction could be discussed. It should be mentioned at this point, however, that there are alternative concepts on which tumour models may be based. One is the hit concept with interaction cross sections and particle fluences as key parameters, the other is microdosimetry with its central parameter specific energy. The results of these differing approaches, however, can always be expressed in terms of endosteal dose.

CONCLUSIONS

From the foregoing the following conclusions may be drawn.

1. If tumour induction is a non-linear process with regard to radiation doses or specific energy the variation of parameters such as local concentrations, distances and dimensions of cell nuclei and time of irradiation has to be taken into account.

2. There is no unique endosteal dose. Instead it has to be specified to which type of bone cells endosteal doses are determined.

3. A model of bone tumour induction based on endosteal doses from alpha-emitters should work for both surface-seekers and volume-seekers.

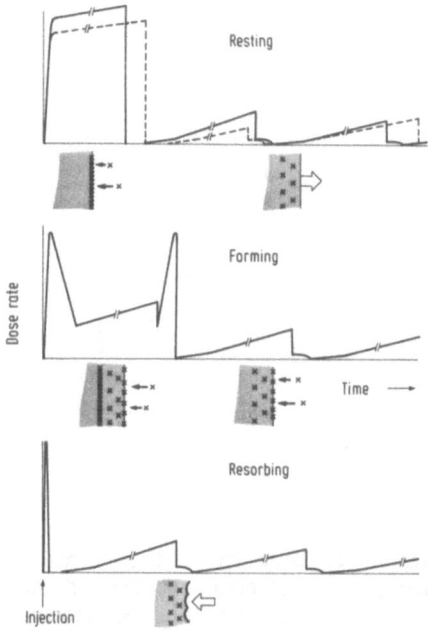

Fig.1 Kinetic behaviour of dose rates from a surface-seeker at surface
elements that are resting, forming or resorbing at the time of
uptake. Crosses represent planar or volume deposits of a
radionuclide. Shaded areas represent bone.
The dashed line represents the dose rate behaviour at another
resting surface element.

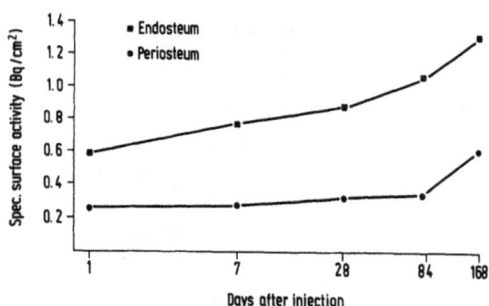

Fig.2 Specific surface activity of 239-Pu in the epiphysis of rat
femurs after injection of 18.5 kBq/kg bodyweight.

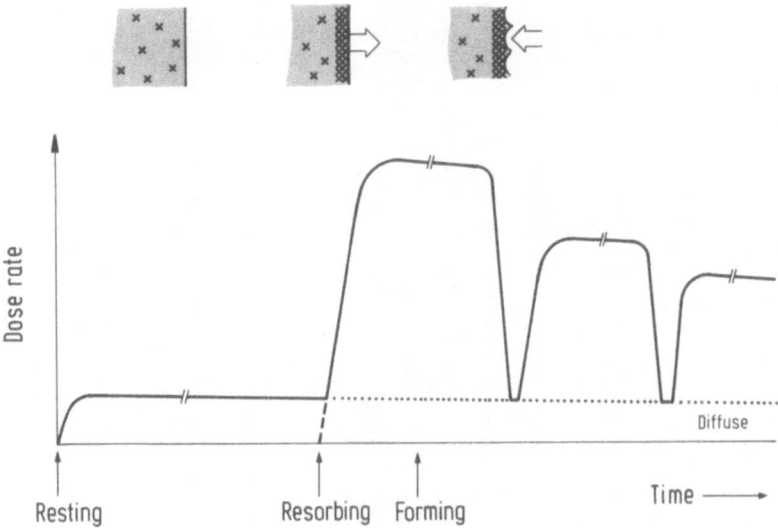

Fig.3 Kinetic behaviour of dose rates from a volume-seeker at a bone
surface element. The different status of surface elements
(resting, forming, resorbing) can be accounted for by choosing
appropriate starting points on the time scale.

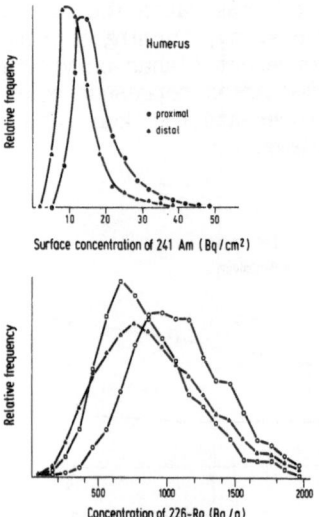

Fig.4 Top: Probability density of surface activity of 241-Am in
beagle humerus 7 days after injection of 104.3 kBq/kg
bodyweight.
Bottom: Probability density of concentration of 226-Ra
in diffuse deposits of beagle lumbar vertebra 5 days after
injection of 322 kBq/kg.

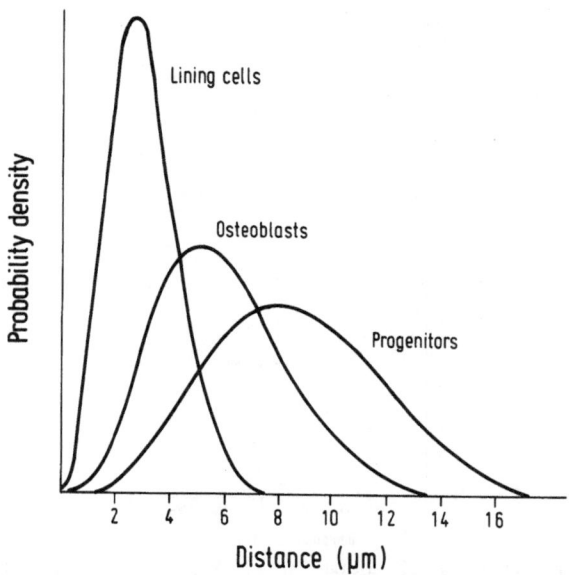

Fig.5 Probability density of distances of lining cells, osteoblasts and osteoprogenitors from bone surfaces in the metaphysis of rats.

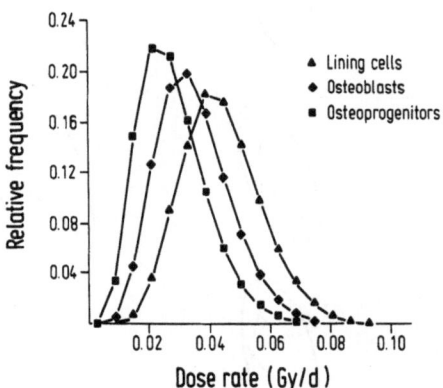

Fig.6 Probability density of dose rates to different types of bone cells in beagle lumbar vertebra 5 days after injection of 322 kBq/kg 226-Ra. Result obtained by taking into account the variations of diffuse concentrations and distances of cell nuclei.

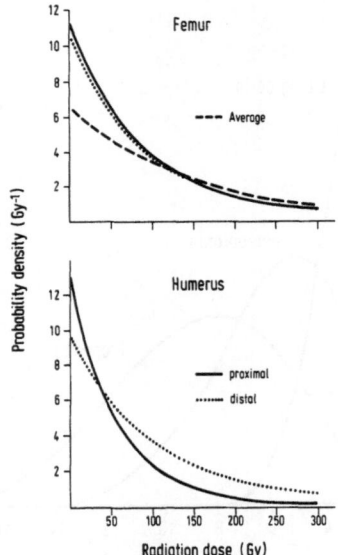

Fig.7 Probability density of accumulated dose to lining cells from
     initial deposits of 241-Am in femur and humerus after injection
     of 133.8 kBq/Kg. Variation of specific surface activity and
     residence time taken into account. For dashed line only
     variation of residence time taken into account.

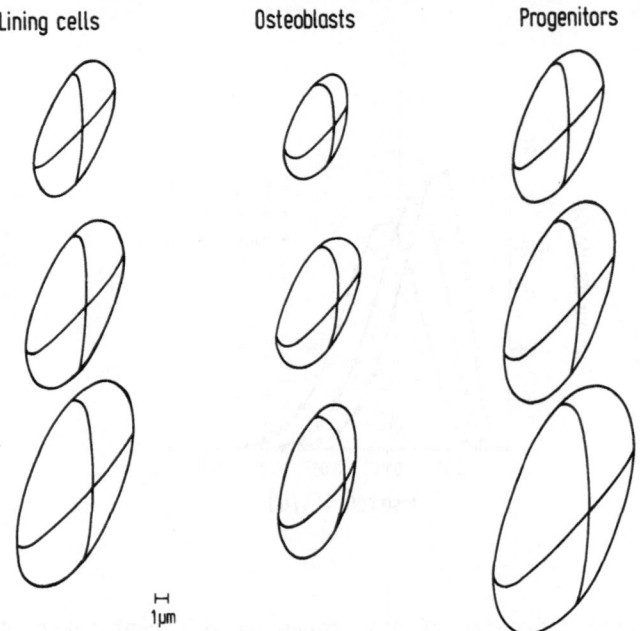

Fig.8 Schematic representation of nuclei of bone cells (oblate
     spheroids). Intermediate shapes represent nuclei with average
     axis dimensions. Shapes on top and bottom represent nuclei
     with axis dimensions mean-/+ standard deviation, respectively.

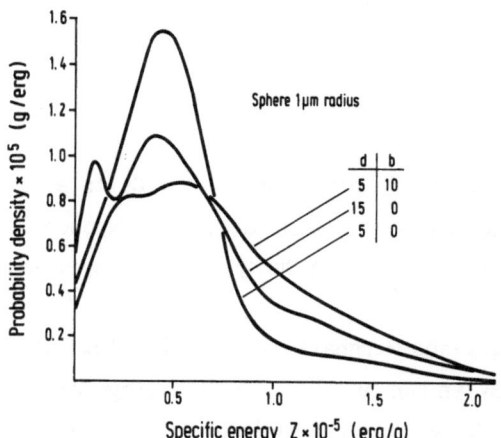

Fig.9 Probability density of specific energy for single traversals
through a spherical target and for 5.14 MeV alpha particles
originating from a planar deposit.

d= distance of the sphere from the bone surface.
b= burial depth of planar deposit in bone.

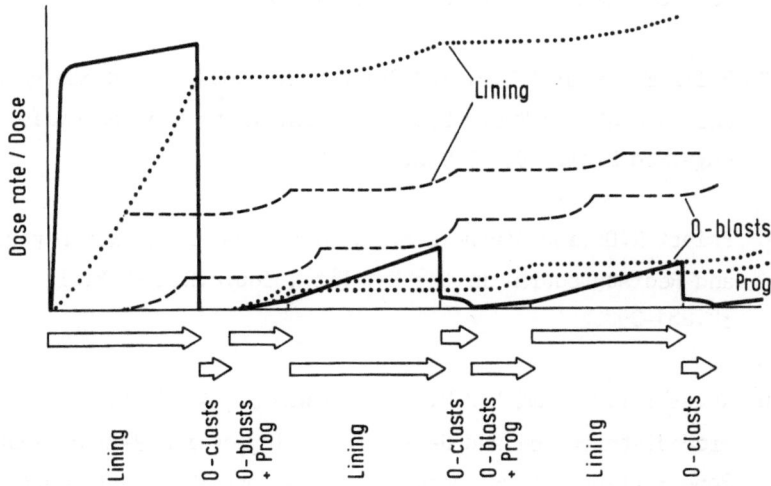

Fig.10 Schematic representation of dose rate and accumulated dose to
different bone cells. The presence of the various types of
cells is indicated by the arrows. The surface is assumed to
be resting at the time of injection.
Dotted line: Accumulated dose to lining cells and osteoblasts.
Dashed line: Accumulated dose if turnover rate is assumed to
be twice the rate for the dotted line.

REFERENCES

L183 Lloyd E.L. and Henning C.B., 1983, Cells at Risk for the
      Production of Bone Tumors in Radium Exposed Individuals
      An Electron Microscope Study , Hlth. Phys. 44, 135-148, Suppl.1.

L172 Lloyd E.L. and Marshall J.H., 1972, Toxicity of 239-Pu relative
      to 226-Ra in Man and Dog , Radiobiology of Plutonium, B.Stover
      and W.S.S. Jee Eds., Salt Lake City, 377-383.

Ma77 Marshall J.H. and Groer P.G., 1977, A Theory of the Induction of
      Bone Cancer by Alpha Radiation , Rad. Res. 71,149-192.

Po83 Polig E.,1983, Specific Energy Spectra at Alpha-Contaminated
      Bone Surfaces ,Rad.Evironm.Biophys. 22,163-175.

Po84 Polig E., Kimmel D.B. and Jee W.S.S., 1984, Morphometry of Bone
      Cell Nuclei and Their Location Relative to Bone Surfaces ,
      Phys.Med.Biol. 29,939-952.

Pr80 Priest N.D. and Giannola S.J., 1980, 241-Plutonium Deposition
      and Redistribution in the Rat Rib , Int.J.Radiat.Biol.
      37,281-298.

Wr80 Wronski T.J., Smith J.M. and Jee W.S.S.,1980, The
      Microdistribution and Retention of Injected 239-Pu on Trabecular
      Bone Surfaces of the Beagle Implications for the Induction of
      Osteosarcoma , Rad.Res. 83,74-89.

26

The Dosimetry of Plutonium-239 in Bones of the Female Mouse and its Relationship to Observed Effects

D. GREEN and G. R. HOWELLS

INTRODUCTION

Studies on the effects of Plutonium-239 in the skeleton have been restricted largely to two species, the Beagle dog and the mouse. In our work, we have studied the distribution and dosimetry of Plutonium-239 in the female CBA mouse in an attempt to assess to what extent the effects observed by other authors can be explained by purely dosimetric considerations.

To help understand the toxicological effects of Plutonium-239 on bone tissue it is necessary to have a quantitative measure of its distribution with a resolution considerably less than the range of the alpha particle, this being some 40 μm in soft tissue and 27 μm in bone. Much of our effort has been addressed to the problem of achieving the required accuracy in localisation of the plutonium atoms.

In any toxicological study it is important that the physiological characteristics of the species used as the test system are well known, and that the major factors influencing the distribution and retention of the toxic agent are characterised.

Animals

Morphometry, 12 week old female CBA mice - no treatment

Radiochemistry, 12 week old female CBA mice intravenously administered Plutonium-239 citrate, 1.8kBq.kg^{-1} body mass and killed at either 1 day, 1 month or 3 months after injection.

Plutonium distribution, 12 week old female CBA mice intravenously

administered Plutonium-239 citrate, $1.8kBq.kg^{-1}$ body mass and killed
at either 1 day, 1 month or 3 months after injection.
Calcein distribution, 12 week old female CBA mice intravenously
administered 20 mg Calcein kg^{-1} body mass and then twice weekly
injections until the animals were killed at either 1 day, 1 month or
3 months after injection.
In all the experiments the ilium, femur and lumbar vertebrae were
taken for analysis.

Morphometric and physiological characteristics of mouse bone

Bone morphometric and metabolic data included measurements of endosteal
surface area; periosteal surface area; bone marrow volume; bone volume;
chord length distribution; blood flow and bone appositional rates.

Details of the methods used for morphometric measurements and bone
metabolic parameters have been published previously (1, 2, 3). The
morphometric measurements were made with a Quantimet 720 image
analyser (Cambridge Instruments) using 5 μm thick sections of plastic
embedded bone. Chord length distributions in longitudinal sections
through the bones were used to evaluate the degree of anisotropy in
the structures, this value being necessary to correct measurements of
endosteal and periosteal surface made on representative transverse
sections (Table 1).

Table 1   Mouse bone morphometry

Bone	L	$\bar{P}_{(E)}$	λ	$\bar{A}_{(m)}$ $\times 10^{-3}$	$M_{(5 \mu m)}$ $\times 10^{-3}$	$M_{(m)}$ $\times 10^{-2}$
	(cm)	(cm)		(cm^2)	(g)	(g)
Femur	1.54	3.02	1.16	7.37	2.69	1.13
Ilium	0.92	1.08	1.18	4.42	0.58	0.41
Lumbar vert.	0.42	2.57	1.19	9.87	0.65	0.41

L = length of bone

$\bar{P}_{(E)}$ = mean cross-sectional endosteal perimeter

λ = degree of anisotropy

$\bar{A}_{(m)}$ = mean cross-sectional marrow area

$M_{(5 \mu m)}$ = mass of a 5 μm thick layer adjacent to endosteal surface

$M_{(m)}$ = mass of marrow

The blood flow measurements were obtained using Fluorine-18 distribution at steady state as a guide in interpretation of Plutonium-239 uptake pattern within the skeleton (4). A good correlation was found between blood flow to unit area of endosteum and plutonium uptake.

Calcein, a vital stain which deposits on accreting bone surfaces was used to qualitatively assess the metabolic activity of the bones (3). It was found that the ilium, femur and lumbar vertebra were all in an active state of growth and turnover at the time of injection. Comparisons were also made between bone accretion as measured by the burial of Calcein lines and plutonium burial rates. Provided allowance was made for resorption of plutonium and its redeposition on bone surfaces then a good correlation existed between the two parameters.

Plutonium-239 distribution studies

The techniques used for the radiochemical determination of Plutonium-239 in bone samples and the microdistribution of plutonium fission fragment tracks in neutron induced autoradiographs (NIARs) have been described previously (5, 6). The radiochemical analysis of Plutonium-239 in the bones for different times after administration of the radionuclide is given in Table 2.

Table 2   Plutonium-239 distribution in bones of the mouse

Bone	Time after injection	Fraction of injected activity $\times 10^{-2}$
Femur	1 day	1.44
	1 mth	1.47
	3 mths	1.30
Ilium	1 day	0.69
	1 mth	0.74
	3 mths	0.48
Lumbar vert. 1 & 2	1 day	1.63
	1 mth	1.44
	3 mths	1.20
Lumbar vert. 4 & 5	1 day	1.95
	1 mth	1.87
	3 mths	1.61

Calcified sections from representative samples of the bones were mounted on Lexan (polycarbonate plastic) slides and irradiated with thermal neutrons in a nuclear reactor. After irradiation the Lexan slides were etched in 28% NaOH for 1 hour to produce a neutron-induced autoradiograph (Fig.1) in which (a), the neutrons interacting with the mineral bone produce an image of it on the surface of the Lexan and (b), Plutonium-239 atoms in the section are fissioned thus producing fission fragments which penetrate the surface of the Lexan and form damage tracks.

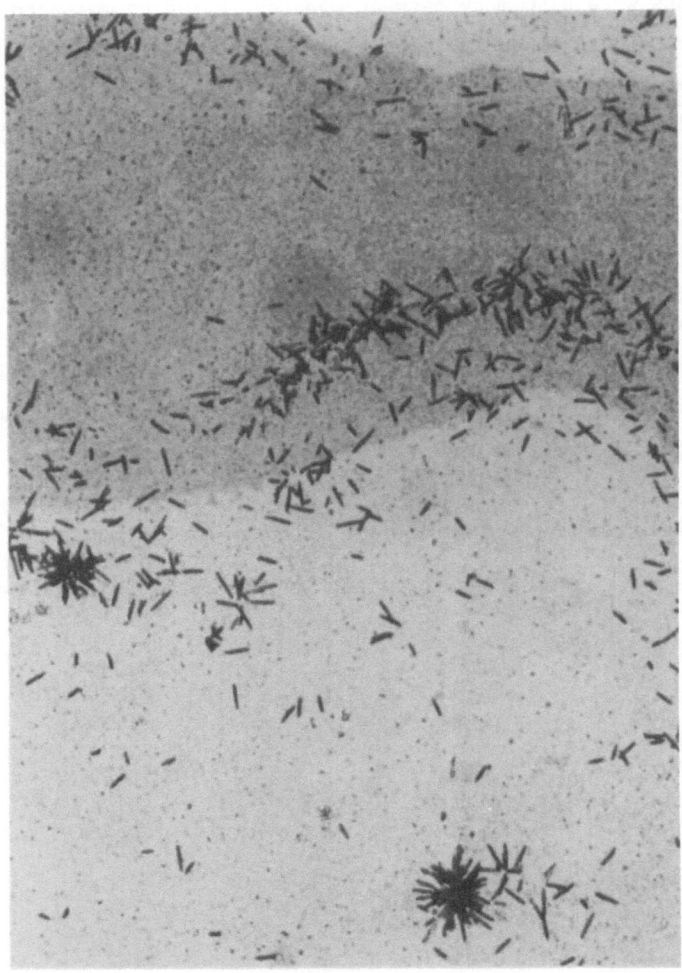

Figure 1   Detail from a neutron induced autoradiograph of mouse bone 3 months after injection of Plutonium-239.

An image analyser was used to record automatically the co-ordinates of each of the edges of the fission fragment tracks and the co-ordinates of the edges of the mineral bone. Thus a map of the tracks relative to the bone edges can be prepared and by suitable mathematical processing, the distribution of the plutonium relative to the bone surfaces can be determined (6, 7).

Resolution of autoradiographic methods

To obtain meaningful dosimetric information from autoradiographs of Plutonium-239 it is necessary to have a quantitative measure of its distribution with a resolution considerably less than the range of the alpha particle, this being some 40 μm in soft tissue and 27 μm in bone. Thorne (8), among others, has shown that the radiation dose received by a 5 μm layer of tissue lining bone surface from a deposit of plutonium at a depth in bone mineral falls almost linearly with the distance the plutonium is buried, and a ± 10% accuracy in the dosimetry of the cells on bone surface requires a resolution of the plutonium deposit of ± 2 to 3 μm. Plutonium fission fragment tracks have a range in Lexan of approximately 19 μm. By calculating the distance from the mid-point of a track to the bone edge it is possible to identify the site of the originating plutonium atom with a resolution of ± 15 μm. Tracks perpendicular to the edge of the bone image do not localize their origin very accurately with respect to it, whereas tracks parallel to it do. By weighting the importance of each track with some function of its inclination (θ) an improvement on the resolution of the plutonium distribution is possible. An effective weighting function was determined by use of a Monte Carlo technique to simulate the distribution of tracks ends arising from a plane source of Plutonium-239. It was found that 80% of the unweighted data lay within ± 11.5 μm of the plane of the plutonium. However, if this data were weighted with $[\cos \theta]^2$, 80% lay within ± 7.0 μm of this plane. A weighting factor of $[\cos \theta]$ was found to be considerably less effective in narrowing the distribution and $[\cos \theta]^3$ and $[\cos \theta]^4$ were found to be only marginally more effective than a weighting factor of $[\cos \theta]^2$. Further improvement in resolution over the ± 7 μm obtained above has been achieved using a simple deconvolution technique in which the plutonium distribution most likely to have produced the observed track distribution is calculated. Details of the calculation have been reported previously (5, 6). Results obtained using a specially prepared plane source of Plutonium-239 indicates that a resolution of ± 2.5 μm may be obtained. It must be emphasised that it is important to use the $[\cos \theta]^2$ factor as well as the deconvolution technique. This is because the weighting factor makes the track distribution used in deconvolution relatively insensitive to track length of the fission fragments in Lexan, to the thickness of the section and to the systematic under-counting of short tracks during digitization.

RESULTS

Figures 2, 3 and 4 show the results of the analysis of the NIARs for each of the three bones at 1 day, 1 month and 3 months after injection respectively. The left hand part of the histogram of each pair shows the distribution of Plutonium-239 with respect to 5 μm layers parallel to endosteal surface. The right hand histogram shows the corresponding calculation of energy deposition rate in successive 5 μm layers of marrow tissue lining endosteal surface. These results, together with the morphometric measurements and radio-chemical results, were used to calculate dose rates to the 5 μm endosteal layer and the whole bone marrow. The results of these calculations are shown in Table 3.

Table 3   Calculated dose-rates in endosteal layer and bone marrow per 37kBq Plutonium-239 kg^{-1} injected ($Gy\ d^{-1} \times 10^{-2}$)

Bone	Endosteal layer			Bone marrow		
	1 day	1 month	3 months	1 day	1 month	3 months
Ilium	10.5	4.5	1.6	4.9	3.9	4.5
Lumbar vert.	10.0	6.6	3.6	4.5	4.4	5.2
Femur	3.3	2.1	1.0	2.7	2.6	2.4

Svoboda et al (9) have measured the effect of Plutonium-239 on the bone marrow in terms of marrow cellularity and ability to form colonies of marrow cells in the spleen (CFU s). Their results for comparable periods to this study are summarised in Table 4.

Figure 2   Plutonium-239 distribution and energy deposition.

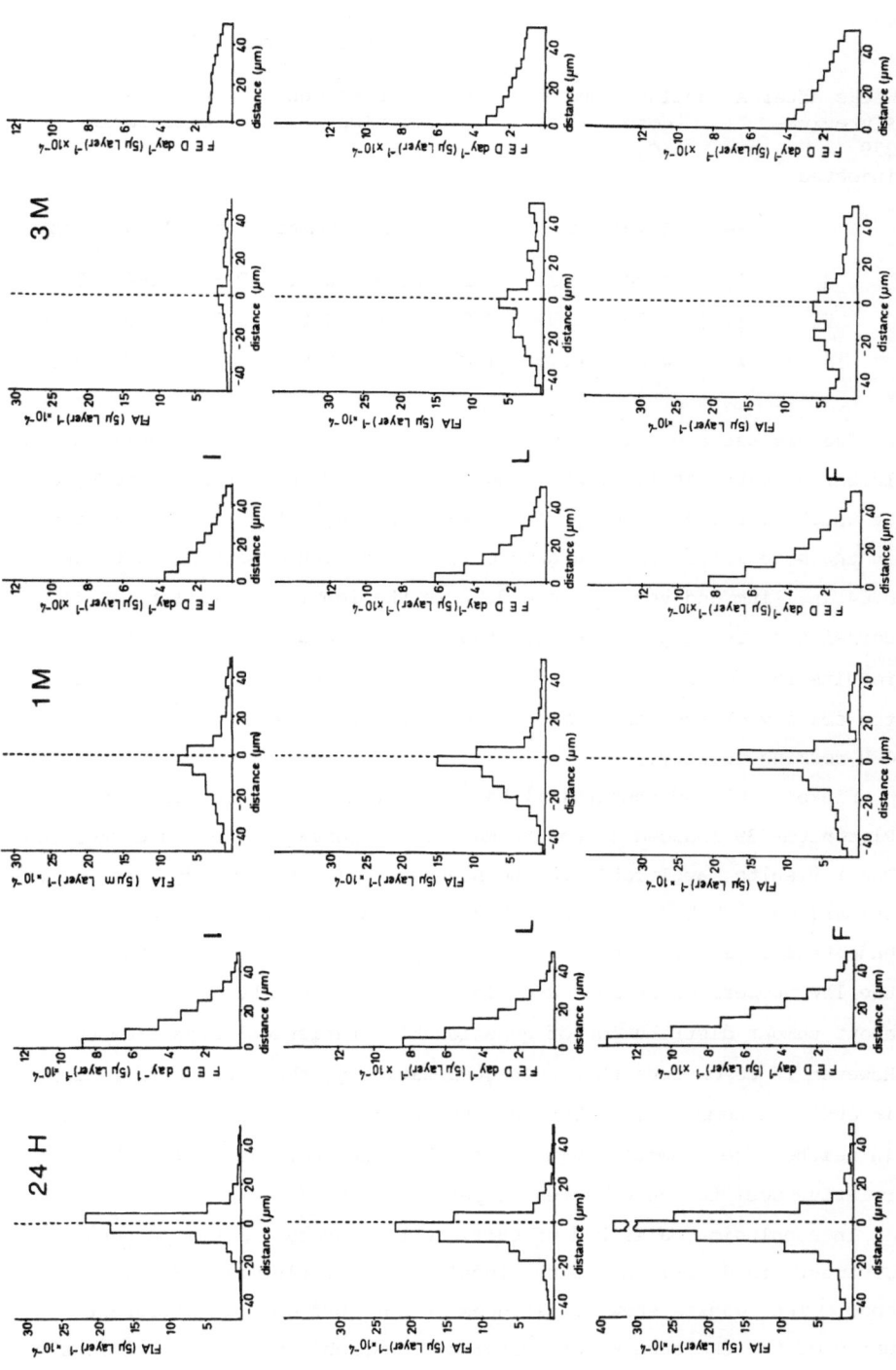

Table 4   Comparison of dose and effect in the bone marrow

Fraction of control values

Weeks after Plutonium-239 injected	Accumulated marrow dose (Gy)			Exogenous spleen colonies			Bone marrow cellularity		
	Femur	Ilium	Lumbar	Femur	Ilium	Lumbar	Femur	Ilium	Lumbar
4	0.72	1.24	1.32	0.55	0.61	0.62	0.80	0.96	0.76
9	1.61	2.79	2.87	0.84	0.68	0.67	0.74	0.86	0.84
15	2.69	4.65	4.79	1.05	0.75	0.64	0.92	0.62	0.64

The highest accumulated marrow doses were measured in the ilium and lumbar vertebra at 15 weeks being 4.65 and 4.79 Gray respectively, and at which time the value for femur was 2.5 Gray. Loss of cellularity in the bone marrow shows a good correlation with dose being 0.62 and 0.64 in ilium and vertebra and 0.92 in the femur. A similar correlation is seen between the radiation dose and effect in the results for colony forming units (CFU s), except that here it is in the ability of the marrow to recover from an initial 40 - 50% loss of CFU forming ability.

Finkel (10) and Loutit (11) have reported on the distribution of Plutonium-239 induced osteosarcoma between bones of the mouse skeleton. Their results, applicable to the bones used for this study, are summarised in Table 5 and compared to the dose received by the endosteal layer over the three months post injection. Unfortunately the low numbers of animals used in their studies makes any conclusions about tumour distribution of questionable statistical significance. However, it is obvious that even qualitatively, there are differences in observed tumour distribution between the two experiments and that in neither does tumour frequency in the bones correlate with the relative dose to the endosteal layer.

In conclusion, a method of sufficient accuracy for the purposes of dosimetry is described for the localisation of Plutonium-239 in mouse bone. The results show differences in absorbed dose in different parts of the skeleton which correlate reasonably well with previously published observations of effects that are the results of cell killing,

i.e. marrow depletion and loss of colony forming potential.
Correlation of osteosarcoma incidence with dose distribution is poor
and this may be due to the low numbers of osteosarcoma results
available.   There is certainly a need for larger toxicity experiments
coupled closely with studies of the relevant dosimetry.   Other
requirements will be to identify the sensitive sites of induction and
other biological factors leading to a tumour.

Table 5   Osteosarcoma induction in mice following administration of
           Plutonium-239

	Osteosarcomas		
Author	Finkel et al	Loutit et al	Dose to endosteal layer
Mouse strain	CFI female	CBA male & female	(Gray)
Injected Plutonium μCi/kg^{-1}	0.16 - 15.6	0.4 - 4.0	
Number of animals	435	60	
Osteosarcomas	136	33	
Lumbar vert. (fraction in single bone)	39 (0.057)	5 (0.030)	5.6
Ilium (fraction in single bone)	6 (0.022)	6 (0.091)	4.1
Femur (fraction in single bone)	11 (0.040)	3 (0.045)	1.7

REFERENCES

1. Green, D., Howells, G.R. and Thorne, M.C. (1981). Morphometric
studies on mouse bone using a computer-based image analysis system.
J. Microsc., 22, 49-58.

2. Green, D. (1981). Some morphological parameters of importance in
the determination of depth of burial measurements of materials in
bone. EULEP Newsletter 26, Ed. J.R. Maisin.

3. Howells, G.R., Green, D., and Sontag, W. (1984). A comparison of
the distribution of 239 Pu and Calcein of the ilium of the female CBA
mouse. Radiat. Environ. Biophys., 23, 127-131.

4. Humphreys, E.R., Green, D., Howells, G.R. and Thorne, M.C. (1982).

Relationship between blood flow, bone structure and [239]Pu deposition in the mouse skeleton. Calcif. Tissue Int., 34, 416-421.

5. Green, D., Howells, G.R. and Thorne, M.C. (1977). A new method for the accurate localisation of [239]Pu in bone. Phys. Med. Biol., 22, 248-297.

6. Green, D., Howells, G.R., and Thorne, M.C. (1981). A semi-automated technique for assessing the microdistribution of [239]Pu deposited in bone. Phys. Med. Biol., 26, 379-387.

7. Howells, G.R. and Green, D. (1981). The temporal and spatial distribution of [239]Pu within bone. In "Bone and Bone seeking Radionuclides". Physiology, Dosimetry and Effects, EUR 7168 EN.

8. Thorne, M.C. (1976). Aspects of the dosimetry of plutonium in bone. Nature, 259, 539-541.

9. Svoboda, V., Kotaskova, R., Lenger, V., and Thomas, J. Effects of [239]Pu on mouse haemopoietic stem cells in different types of bone marrow cavaties. Rad. and Environ. Biophys., 16, 339-345.

10. Finkel, M.P. and Biskis, B.O. (1962). Toxicity of plutonium in mice. Hlth. Phys., 8, 565-579.

11. Loutit, J.F., Sansom, J. and Carr, T.E.F. (1976). The pathology of tumours induced in Harwell mice by [239]Pu and [226]Ra. In "The Health Effects of Plutonium and Radium" ed W.S.S. Jee, Salt Lake City. The J.W. Press.

27

A New Dosimetric Model for Bone Surface Seeking Radionuclides in the Skeleton

N. D. PRIEST and A. BIRCHALL

Values for the fraction of skeletal alpha and beta activity deposited in the bone surfaces and in the red bone marrow following intakes of bone surface seeking radionuclides by adults have been calculated using a multicompartment bone model. This model (Pr84 Th85), unlike the existing ICRP model, incorporates features which allow for the relocation of radionuclide in the skeleton that results from bone remodelling. In one compartment of this model, namely the growing surfaces of cortical bone, radionuclide is taken to be retained and not subject to resorption or recycling. In the corresponding trabecular compartment the radionuclide is taken to be subject to both burial and resorption. Resorbed radionuclide is assumed either to be redeposited onto bone surfaces or to be retained in the bone marrow. The calculations were made assuming that radionuclide is deposited in the skeleton during a fifty year period. The calculations made with this model (see Table) suggest the ICRP recommended values for the fraction of skeletal radionuclide energy deposited in the bone surfaces and red bone marrow following intakes of the more important bone surface seeking radionuclides are about 6 times and 2 times too large, respectively.

Table: Re-calculated and ICRP recommended absorbed fractions

Isotope	Alpha or beta	AF(E)	ICRP	AF(RBM)	ICRP
Short-lived isotopes					
Uranium-230	alpha	0.25	0.25	0.17	0.25
Americium-244	beta	0.12	0.25	0.27	0.25
Plutonium-243	beta	0.05	0.02	0.36	0.25
Intermediate-lived isotopes					
Plutonium-236	alpha	0.06	0.25	0.08	0.25
Promethium-147	beta	0.07	0.25	0.20	0.25
Plutonium-241	beta	0.01	0.25	0.07	0.25
Long-lived isotopes					
Lutetium-176	beta	0.03	0.02	0.30	0.25
Plutonium-239	alpha	0.03	0.25	0.09	0.25
Americium-241	alpha	0.03	0.25	0.13	0.25

The fraction of the total particle energy released in the skeleton that is absorbed in the bone surfaces (AF(E)) and in the red bone marrow (AF(RBM)) calculated for various alpha and beta-emitting actinide and lanthanide isotopes. The equivalent values derived from ICRP data are shown for comparison.

REFERENCES

Pr84 Priest, N D and Birchall, A , 1984, Progress on the dosimetry of bone surface seeking radionuclides. Rad. Prot. Bull. <u>59</u> 20-26.

Th85 Thorne, M C , 1985, Microdosimetry of bone: implications for radiological protection. Paper 24. This publication.

28

Variation of Radiation Exposure due to the Administration of Iron-59 in Patients with Different Diseases

E. WERNER, P. ROTH, U. BÖHNERT, U. ELSASSER, K. HENRICHS, J. DIETRICH and A. KAUL

INTRODUCTION.

The biokinetics of radioisotopes administered in vivo may vary considerably with changes in organ functions. This study was aimed to evaluate the variation in radiation dose in 189 patients with different diseases in whom ferrokinetic investigations were performed for diagnostic purposes.

PATIENTS AND METHODS

The distribution of patients according to diagnosis is shown in Table 1. Ferrokinetic investigations with ^{59}Fe were performed as usual. Additionally, external monitoring of organ activity over sacrum, liver, and spleen and measurements of whole body retention of ^{59}Fe were performed for 3 months.

DATA ANALYSIS AND CALCULATION OF RADIATION DOSE

The tracer data were analyzed using a linear compartmental model for iron metabolism in man. The transfer rates between the compartments were determined iteratively by a non-linear least square fitting procedure. The mean radiation dose D_T in organ T is then given by

$$D_T = \sum_{j \in \varphi} D(T \leftarrow S_j) = \sum_{j \in \varphi} A_j \, S(T \leftarrow S_j)$$

This work was supported by BMI, St. Sch. 757.

where A_j: cumulative activity in source organ j; $S(T \leftarrow S_j)$: mean dose
in target organ T per decay in source organ S_j;
$\wp$: number of source organs. The A_j values are derived from the
matrix of transfer rates. The fractions of blood volume in the
various organs were estimated according to ICRP Publication 23
(ICRP 75).

Table 1: Organ doses and effective dose equivalent (EDE) in ferrokinetic
investigations with ^{59}Fe (mrem/μCi). Mean values $\pm$ 1 SD

Diagnosis (n)	Bone	Bone surface	Bone marrow	Gonads	Liver	Spleen	EDE
Hypoplastic Anaemia (20)	17±5	10±7	34±14	19±5	253±134	247±117	54±13
Haemolytic Anaemia (11)	22±3	13±4	40±8	24±3	101±77	118±106	39±10
Dyserythropoet. Anaemia (11)	23±4	15±10	45±18	25±4	105±73	106±60	39±7
Renal failure No dialysis(30)	23±4	17±4	48±9	25±4	56±35	89±51	37±6
Renal failure Haemodial. (6)	21±2	16±4	45±9	23±3	58±36	108±45	36±6
Renal failure Perit.dial.(10)	24±4	15±3	44±9	26±4	51±16	93±57	37±6
Iron deficiency BL[+)] 0 - 5 (16)	23±3	17±3	48±4	25±3	47±4	72±3	36±2
BL[+)] 5 - 25 (42)	20±3	15±1	42±3	22±3	39±2	62±4	31±3
BL[+)] 25 -105 (29)	15±3	13±2	33±5	16±3	26±6	42±9	22±4
BL[+)] 105 (14)	9±2	11±2	26±4	10±2	15±5	23±8	14±3

+) Mean daily blood loss (ml/day)

RESULTS AND DISCUSSION

The calculated organ doses and effective dose equivalents (EDE) are
given in Table 1. The radiation dose to bone and bone surface shows
a rather small variation within the different groups and with regard
to diagnosis. The radiation dose to the red bone marrow is highest
for the patients with dyserythropoietic anaemias and renal failure.
The largest variations in radiation dose with regard to diagnosis and
also within each group of patients are found for the liver and
spleen. This reflects the varying iron accumulation in these organs
in different diseases. The decrease in radiation dose with
increasing blood losses is to be expected since in iron deficiency
most of the ^{59}Fe is in the circulating blood. The calculation of EDE
is not markedly affected by the variations in organ doses but is

fairly constant for the different diseases. For patients with normal internal iron turnover the data obtained in this study are in accordance with the values published in ICRP Publication 17 (ICRP71).

REFERENCES

ICRP71 International Commission on Radiological Protection (1971). Protection of the patient in radionuclide investigations. Oxford, Pergamon Press, ICRP Publication 17.

ICRP75 International Commission on Radiological Protection (1975). Report of the Task Group on Reference Man. Oxford, Pergamon Press, ICRP Publication 23.

Part 6
Pathology of Metals in Bone

29

Pathogenesis of Radionuclide-Induced Bone Tumors

W. GÖSSNER

The most critical factor in the toxicity of bone-seeking radionuclides is the induction of bone tumors. Therefore this paper will be restricted to problems of osteosarcoma risk after incorporation of bone-seeking radionuclides with special emphasis on the effects of short-lived bone-seekers.

Bone tumor induction by bone-seeking radionuclides provides an excellent experimental model for studies of carcinogenesis by ionizing radiation. Such studies have yielded important information on the mechanism of tumor induction. The experimental findings can also be compared with well established evidence on bone tumor induction in man by alpha-emitters.

OSTEOSARCOMAS IN PATIENTS GIVEN RADIUM-224

In addition to the well-known induction of osteosarcomas following the intake of the long-lived Radium-226 in painters of luminous dials, human cases of bone tumors after medical application of the short-lived Radium-224 have been reported (Ma73; Sp56).

Most of these patients were treated with intravenous injections of "Peteosthor", a preparation containing Radium-224 (Thorium X), which is a short-lived

alpha-emitting isotope of radium with a half-life of
3.66 days. It was hoped that the radiation from
Radium-224 localizing initially on bone surfaces would
have a therapeutic effect in ankylosing spondylitis and
in tuberculosis of bone. Out of 899 patients in the
higher dose group (Study I) given multiple injections of
Radium-224, bone sarcomas developed in 55 cases whose
ages at Radium-224 injection ranged from 2 - 56 years.
All, or virtually all, of the bone sarcomas are ascribed
to radiation since only 0.3 cases would have been expected naturally, based on the general population rate
of 2 bone sarcomas per year/10^5 persons. The distribution of tumor appearance times ranged from 3.5 - 25
years, averaging about 10 - 12 years. The last bone
sarcoma appeared in 1974. Based on present trends few,
if any, additional bone sarcomas are expected among the
remaining Radium-224 patients in this group (Sp70; Ma84).

It is interesting to compare the distribution of
appearance times for bone sarcomas induced by short-
lived Radium-224 vs. long-lived Radium-226 and
Radium-228. Whereas the risk from short-lived Radium-224
seems mainly exhausted after 25 years, the tumors induced by long-lived radium continue to appear throughout
the remaining lifespan. This effect can be attributed to
the continued production of new tumors by radiation received at long times after the initial deposition of the
long-lived radium.

Repeated injections of the short-lived Radium-224 in
humans are still used as a treatment for ankylosing
spondylitis in Germany and other European countries.
This provides a chance to investigate dose-response
relationships in the low dose region for bone-seeking
alpha-emitters (Sc83; Wi83).

At present the treatment generally consists of
10 weekly intravenous injections, each of 28 μCi,
giving a cumulative alpha-dose of about 0.65 Gy to the
marrow-free skeleton of a reference 70-kg-man. This low

dose group (Study II) at present consists of about
1501 patients from 14 hospitals together with about
1557 control patients. Table 1 shows the most important
data from the Radium-224 studies.

Table 1.   Exposure and follow-up parameters for Radium-224 treated
           patients

	STUDY I Juveniles	STUDY I Adults	STUDY II Adults
Total patients	218	681	1501
Deceased patients	81	358	433
Mean injected amount of Radium-224 per kg [/µCi]	29	15	4.8
Mean alpha-skeletal dose [rad]	1100	200	65
Mean injection span [week]	48	26	12
Mean follow-up time [year]	25	22	16

Since 1970 three cases of malignant tumors in the
skeleton have been observed in the low dose group
(Study II) at a skeletal burden of less than 0.9 Gy.

Table 2 shows the frequency of bone tumor cases in
both Radium-224 studies in comparison with that in
radium dial painters.

Table 2.   Bone tumors in the Radium studies

	Radium-224 STUDY I		Radium-224 STUDY II	Radium-226 Dial Painters
Osteosarcoma	41	74.5 %	0	
Chondrosarcoma	3	5.5 %	0	60
Fibrosarcoma	1	1.8 %	1	
Reticulumcellsarcoma	1	1.8 %	1	0
Plasmocytoma (multiple myeloma)	0	-	1	0
Others	4	7.3 %	0	31*
Unspecified	5	9.1 %	0	0
	55	100.0 %	3	

*Sinus or mastoid carcinomas (among 2223 persons total)

In the low dose group 2 of the 3 skeletal tumors were bone-marrow tumors: one reticulum cell sarcoma of bone, and one plasmocytoma. The observation of two bone marrow tumors may indicate an effect on the bone marrow.

Injections of Peteosthor or pure Radium-224 were made at weekly or half-weekly intervals with the injection span ranging from a few weeks to a few years. Therefore questions concerning the relationship between bone dose, dose rate and duration of irradiation periods and osteosarcoma risk have to be answered.

ANIMAL EXPERIMENTS

Application of short-lived radionuclides in animal experiments provides an opportunity to study the effects of both short-term and long-term irradiation, the latter achieved by means of repeated incorporation over longer periods.

Such studies have been carried out in our institute since 1966, and some examples from the large series of experiments have been selected for this paper. These examples are mainly concerned with the dependence of osteosarcoma incidence on the pattern of dose time distribution and radiation quality (Gö76; Mü77; Mü78b; Mü81).

INFLUENCE OF DOSE AND TIME FACTORS FOLLOWING INCORPORATION OF RADIUM-224 IN MICE

Radium-224, an alpha-emitter with a half-life of 3.66 days, occurs in the natural thorium series. In experiments in 4 week old mice a mean skeletal dose of 0.3 Gy is achieved after injection of 1 μCi/kg Radium-224. In older animals the skeletal dose decreased by as much as 30 %. The actual doses in different parts of bone tissue may vary to a high degree. The bone surface dose within a distance of 10 microns may reach a value fourfold higher than the average dose.

The incidence of osteosarcomas after a single injection of Radium-224 has been studied in 4 week old female
NMRI mice. The mean skeletal doses ranged from 0.3 to
15.0 Gy. There was no clear mathematical function between dose and bone tumor incidence. The latter ranged
for all dose groups between 8 and 22 %. The mean latency
periods (i.e. time between injection and first detection
of tumor) lay between 17 and 30 months.

After single injections of Radium-224 more than 90 %
of radioactivity decays within two weeks. Therefore the
question arose whether protracted administration with a
longer irradiation period would be more effective.

The basic scheme of the protraction experiments with
Radium-224 consisted of twice weekly i.p. injections
over periods of 4 to 36 weeks keeping the individual injection amount constant. The total activities injected
lay between 4 and 36 μCi/kg. The total mean skeletal
doses were between 0.9 and 10.8 Gy.

The most important result was that a Radium-224 dose
given protracted over a longer period can produce a multiple of the osteosarcoma incidence produced by a single
injection of the same dose. The longest protraction time
was the most effective; this is shown clearly in the
dose group with 36 μCi/kg over a period of 36 weeks
(Table 3). Compared with the effect of a single injection the bone tumor incidence was increased by a factor
of nearly ten. The highest percentage of bone tumors
achieved was 98 %, but only with a rather high mean
skeletal dose of 8 Gy. The highest tumor incidence was
associated with the shortest mean latency period.

In contrast practically no protraction effect was observed in the lowest investigated dose group of 4 μCi/kg
over a period of 36 weeks, which resulted in a low mean
skeletal dose of 0.9 Gy. Here a bone tumor incidence of
14 % was found, compared with 13 % after single injection of the same amount of Radium-224.

Table 3. The role of time factor: Radium-224

	Protraction 36 weeks	Single Injection		Protraction 36 weeks
Total activity / kg	36 μCi	36 μCi	4 μCi	4 μCi
Osteosarcoma incidence	98 %	11 %	13 %	14 %
Mean latency period	12 months	19 months	21 months	20 months
Mean skeletal dose	8 Gy	10.8 Gy	1.2 Gy	0.9 Gy
Osteosarcoma cases per cent per 1 Gy	12.25 %	1.02 %	10.83 %	15.56 %
Maximal skeletal dose rate	0.08 Gy/d	4.32 Gy/d	0.48 Gy/d	0.009 Gy/d

The situation appears quite different if the results are expressed in per cent of tumor incidence per Gy. Here the highest effectiveness occurred at the lowest dose.

The influence of radiation-free intervals during protracted internal irradiation periods (Figure 1) was studied in another experiment.

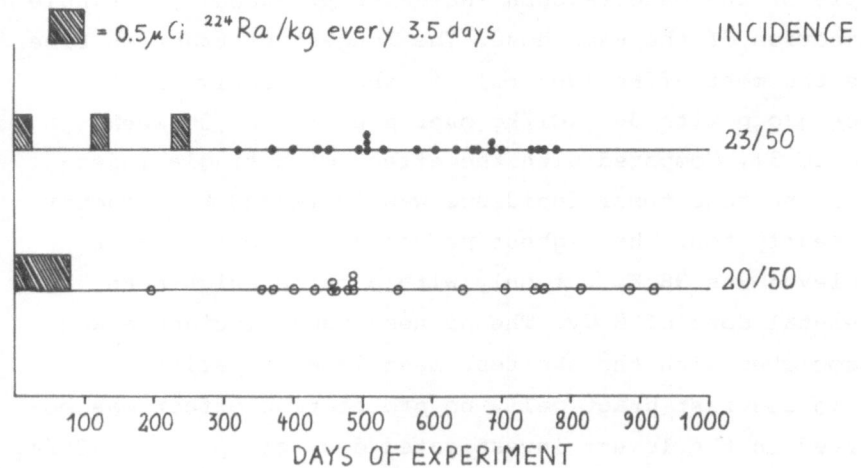

FIGURE 1   Distribution of osteosarcoma cases throughout time after start of internal irradiation period in case of short-term continuous (open circles) and long-term discontinuous (closed circles) alpha irradiation. Incorporated total activity 12 μCi/kg Radium-224.

Female NMRI mice received a total activity of
12 μCi/kg Radium-224 intraperitoneally as fractions of
0.5 μCi/kg every 3.5 days. When treatment was continuous during the 2nd to 4th month the osteosarcoma incidence was 40 % with a mean latency period of 18 months.
Splitting of this continuous treatment period into three
treatment periods of 4 weeks during the 2nd, 5th and 9th
month resulted in an osteosarcoma incidence of 46 % with
a latency period of 19 months. Thus radiation-free intervals do not influence the osteosarcoma risk after internal alpha-irradiation.

BONE TUMOR RISK AFTER INCORPORATION OF THORIUM ISOTOPES

The thorium isotopes for which information about the
biological effects is available include Thorium-232,
Thorium-228 and Thorium-227. An analysis of the behaviour and late effects of these three thorium isotopes,
which have the same biological characteristics but
different physical properties, is therefore of particular interest (Gö82).

Thorium-232 has come to be of considerable importance
since colloidal thorium dioxide was introduced as a contrast medium in diagnostic radiology in 1928. Thorium
dioxide has been widely used since then under the trade
name Thorotrast.

The characteristic lesions produced by Thorotrast in
the human are liver tumors and myeloproliferative diseases. After intravenous injection Thorotrast is taken
up by the reticulo-endothelial cells and becomes encap-
sulated in fibrotic lesions of the liver, spleen and
soft tissues, from which some decay products such as
Radium-228, Thorium-228 and Radium-224 escape and deposit in the bone tissue. It is clear that these bone-
seeking decay-products must contribute to the dangers
involved and induction of osteosarcomas was expected. Up
until now 12 Thorotrast-associated bone neoplasms have
been reported (Ma79).

There are no human data on the behaviour of
Thorium-228 except those which can be derived from the
study of Thorotrast patients.

The animal experiments on short-lived alpha-emitting
bone-seeking radionuclides include, in addition to
Radium-224, the short-lived Thorium-227 (Mü78b).

Thorium-227 has a half-life of 18.7 days, is deposited on the bone surface and decays to Radium-223 which
has a half-life of 11.3 days. Radium-223 can enter
mineral bone.

It is valuable to be able to compare the biological
effects of a short-lived radioisotope with the effects
of a long-lived radioisotope with the same chemical
properties. Studies on the effects of the short-lived
thorium isotope Thorium-227 can be compared with those
of the longer lived Thorium-228 which was investigated
in the radiotoxicity studies in Utah. Thorium-228 is the
most toxic agent of all the internal emitters studied by
the Utah group (see Va73). This high toxic effects, especially the induction of osteosarcomas, is partly due
to the fact that Radium-224 is constantly generated and
a considerable fraction of this nuclide is re-deposited
in the active sites of new bone formation. The high
osteosarcoma risk observed in the protraction experiments with incorporation of low amounts of Radium-224
would explain the high toxicity of this continuous internal production of Radium-224.

Similar conditions are found for Thorium-227 where
Radium-223 is generated, moves into the skeleton and
finally reaches a higher concentration in the bone than
the parent nuclide.

In Figure 2 the cumulative incidence of osteosarcoma
after incorporation of Thorium-227 is plotted versus the
time from the start of the experiment. The number of
animals with newly observed osteosarcomas was determined
each month after the start of the experiment. These
values, expressed as percentage of the initial number of

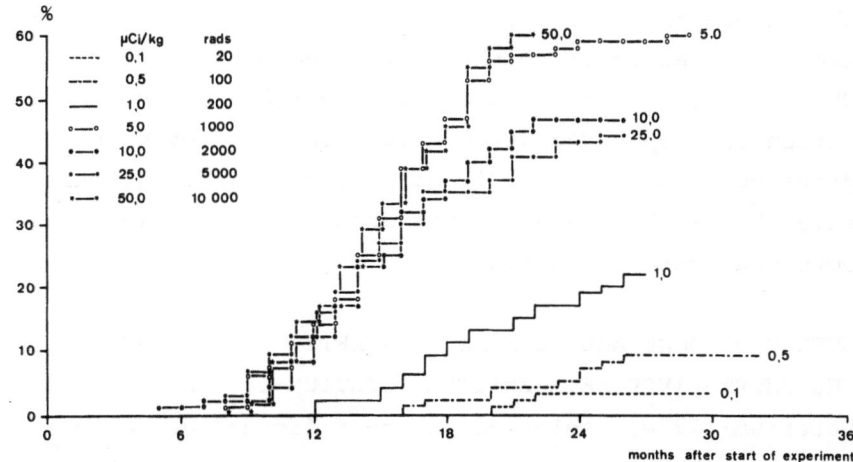

FIGURE 2   Progressive incidence of osteosarcoma after
single injection of Thorium-227 in female NMRI
mice.

animals, were added month by month. After single injections of Thorium-227 the tumor incidence versus time depended strongly on the activity applied. From 0.1 to
5.0 μCi/kg, corresponding to a mean accumulated skeletal dose of 0.2 - 100 Gy, the mean tumor latency time
decreased with increasing activity. It remained constant, however, in the higher dose ranges. After
50 μCi/kg of Thorium-227, with a mean skeletal dose
of 100 Gy, bone necrosis preceded the appearance of bone
tumors. In this Thorium-227 experiment one has to take
into account the fact that the virtual osteosarcoma risk
might also increase beyond 100 Gy if the results were
corrected for mortality by leukemia in groups receiving
between 20 and 50 Gy, since leukemia occurred earlier
than osteosarcoma. Protracted irradiation with
Thorium-227 (5 μCi/kg) over 9 months with injections
every two weeks resulted in an osteosarcoma incidence of
up to 80 %.

The examples described above were obtained from experiments with alpha-emitters, that is to say with
densely ionizing particles. The question arose as to

whether there are analogies or contrasts with beta-emitters, in particular with short-lived beta-emitters.

The differences in the biological effects of beta-radiation and alpha-radiation have been documented in numerous publications (Mü83). As a rough summary it can be said that alpha-radiation has about 10 times higher effects than beta-radiation.

INFLUENCE OF DOSE AND TIME FACTORS AFTER INCORPORATION OF THE SHORT-LIVED BETA-EMITTER LUTETIUM-177 IN MICE

Lutetium-177 was selected as the radionuclide for experiments with beta-emitters. It is a rare earth with a half-life of 6.7 days and a bone-seeker with up to 70 % retention in the skeleton depending on the concomitant carrier amount of the stable element lutetium. The lower the amount of this carrier the higher is the skeletal retention (Mü78a; Mü80).

In general an important aspect of such studies is the assessment of local deposition. This is particularly true for alpha particles with a range in tissue of the order of 20 - 70 μm. However beta particles of 500 keV and more may have ranges of the order of milli-meters. Thus the differences between bone "surface" and "volume" seekers, which are extensively discussed in the case of alpha-emitters, do not play such a role for beta-emitters - at least in the case of small animals such as mice.

The osteosarcomogenic effect of the long-lived beta-emitting alkaline earth Strontium-90 is well estab-lished. Thus for Lutetium-177 skeletal doses were chosen which were known to be effective in the case of Strontium-90.

Most long-term experiments for osteosarcoma induction were performed with Lutetium-177 with a concomitant carrier giving an applied amount of 0.025 mg/kg. The mean skeletal dose was 5.6 Gy per 1 mCi/kg Lutetium-177. Single i.p. injections of 2.8 to 11.1 mCi/kg with a bone tumor incidence between 12 % and 37 % were applied as well as repeated injections of small fractions of activity over 12 weeks with a once weekly injection. Figure 3 shows the cumulative incidence of osteosarcomas in female NMRI mice with three different doses (1, 2, 3 single injections, 4, 5, 6 repeated injections of small fractions). It shows the increased incidence after protraction and the shortening of the latency time. Table 4 shows that with 5.6 mCi/kg the final incidence of osteosarcomas was doubled by protraction increasing from 35 % to 80 %. With 2.8 mCi/kg this protraction effect was lower with an increase of incidence from 12 % to 22 % which, however, was not significant with this number of animals. The latency times were shortened both by the increase of dose and by protraction of the irradiation period. This table also shows the tumor incidence per Gy. Here the highest value was found for a mean skeletal dose of 31.1 Gy protracted over 12 weeks.

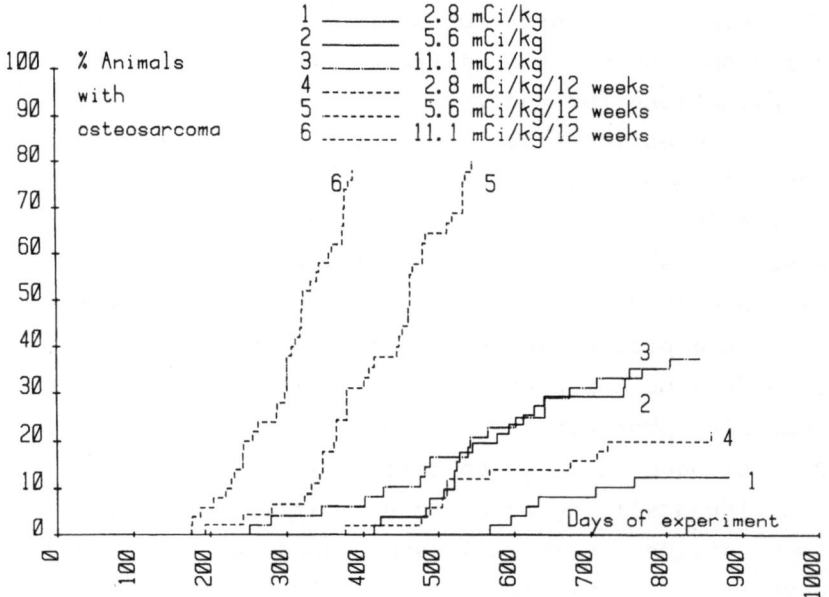

FIGURE 3   Cumulative incidence of osteosarcomas for three Lutetium-177 doses given by one single injection and by 12 weekly injections.

Table 4. The role of time factor: Lutetium-177

	Protraction 36 weeks	Single Injection		Protraction 36 weeks
Total activity / kg	5.6 mCi	5.6 mCi	2.8 mCi	2.8 mCi
Osteosarcoma incidence	80 %	35 %	12 %	22 %
Mean latency period	15 months	19 months	22 months	19 months
Mean skeletal dose	31.1 Gy	31.1 Gy	15.5 Gy	15.5 Gy
Osteosarcoma cases per cent per 1 Gy	2.57 %	1.14 %	0.81 %	1.28 %
Maximal skeletal dose rate	0.4 Gy/d	3.6 Gy/d	1.8 Gy/d	0.2 Gy/d

Compared to the results with alpha-doses these values
are about one tenth, thus suggesting an RBE value of 10
for alpha-emitting bone-seekers in agreement with published data.

ROLE OF DOSE PROTRACTION

The role of dose protraction in the pathogenesis of
osteosarcoma induction is difficult to interpret. Possible explanations for the increase in tumor incidence
with protracted internal irradiation might be provided
by the following two factors:

1. The increased number of irradiated cells.
Bone-seeking short-lived radionuclides deposit preferentially on bone surfaces and in sites of new bone formation. With a protracted injection period additional
sites of new bone formation are irradiated. The result
is that with protraction more cells become irradiated.

2. Prolonged stimulus to cell division.
The continued killing of cells stimulates the surviving
cells to divide. It is well established that continued
pressure for cell division can promote the appearance of
a neoplasm that might otherwise have remained latent.

Protracted irradiation can act both as an initiating and as a promoting agent in the development of cancer. Presumably in this case the initiating event could be non-lethal damage to cells, the promoting effects could be a stimulus to cell division as a compensation for cell death.

As a practical consequence for radiation protection it should be stressed that short-lived radionuclides - in particular with multiple incorporations - may be equally or even more hazardous than a single incorporation of a long-lived radionuclide. This is true in certain dose ranges for both alpha- and beta-emitters.

ROLE OF ENDOGENOUS FACTORS

The protraction experiments with Radium-224 and Thorium-227, which result in a very high osteosarcoma incidence with a rather well synchronized latency time, provide a reproducible animal model of osteosarcoma. This model will be useful in further understanding the pathogenesis of this neoplasm including the influence of various endogenous and exogenous factors on latency time, tumor development and final tumor incidence. The most common biological variables known to alter the neo-plastic response of irradiated animals include sex, age and genetic constitution. The endogenous disposition may or may not play a role as a modifying factor (Gö81).

AGE DISPOSITION

On the basis of the age distribution of osteosarcoma in humans it is generally accepted that skeletal growth may be an important factor in the development of spon-taneous osteosarcoma. Therefore the question arose as to whether skeletal growth may also be of importance in the development of radiation-induced osteosarcoma. In the study of Radium-224 patients Mays and Spiess came to the very cautious conclusion that the skeleton of juveniles might not be unusually susceptible to bone tumor induc-

tion (Ma84). In the dial painters no significant difference in osteosarcoma risk was found in persons first exposed to Radium-226 at less than 18 years of age as compared to another group first exposed when 18 or more
years old.

In order to investigate the role of age further,
1 month and 6 month old female NMRI mice were compared
after incorporation of Thorium-227. Previous experiments
showed that the latency period after incorporation of
5 μCi/kg Thorium-227 is significantly shorter in
6 month old mice than in rapidly growing 1 month old
animals (Gö81; Lu79).

In a recent experiment the osteosarcoma induction in
1 month and 12 month old mice was compared after injection of two different activities of Thorium-227. The
cumulative osteosarcoma incidence was corrected for com-
peting risk and calculated as long as 10 mice per group
survived.

After 5 μCi/kg the corrected cumulative osteosarcoma incidence was 10 % in the 12 month old group and
61 % in the 1 month-old group.

After 1 μCi/kg the corrected cumulative osteosarcoma incidence was 43 % in the 12 month old group and
32 % in the 1 month old group.

500 days after 1 μCi/kg the cumulative osteosarcoma
incidence in the 12 month old group was already 42 %,
whereas in the 1 month old group it was only 6 %.

Thus in the lower irradiation dose range the sensitivity for osteosarcoma induction does not decline
during adult life, but the osteosarcoma appearance time
at this dose level again was shorter in the older
animals (Lu84).

STRAIN DISPOSITION

The comparison of osteosarcoma incidence in different
strains of mice can help to elucidate the still unknown
influence of genetic factors on the susceptibility for
radiation-induced tumor development.

In order to evaluate the role of strain disposition the osteosarcoma induction in female BALB/c and CBA mice was compared. 800 days after incorporation of 5 μCi/kg Thorium-227 the following osteosarcoma incidence was observed:

		Mean tumor appearance time
BALB/c:	53% (26/49)	483 $\pm$ 155 days
CBA:	24% (14/58)	535 $\pm$ 210 days

A major difference between these two strains is their spontaneous and inducible expression of endogenous C-type retroviruses. It is possible that this may contribute to the higher sensitivity of the BALB/c strain to radiation-induced osteosarcoma development (Lu82).

These examples of age and strain disposition clearly demonstrate that these two endogenous factors play an important role with regard to the sensitivity for osteosarcoma induction.

It is clear that many more experiments must be carried out to elucidate the influence of various endogenous, and also exogenous, factors on the induction of radiation-induced tumors. Such experiments more nearly approximate the real situation in humans and should prove valuable when extrapolating results to the human situation.

SUMMARY

The occurrence of osteosarcomas in humans after incorporation of Radium-224 and animal studies with the short-lived bone-seeking radionuclides Radium-224, Thorium-227, and Lutetium-177 have shown that short-lived alpha- and beta-emitting radionuclides, in particular after multiple incorporations, may be equally or even more hazardous than a single incorporation of a long-lived radionuclide.

In addition, in animal experiments it has been shown that age and strain disposition play an important role with regard to the sensitivity for osteosarcoma induction.

REFERENCES

Gö76 Gössner W., Hug O., Luz A. and Müller W. A., 1976,
Experimental induction of bone tumors by short-lived
bone-seeking radionuclides , in: Recent Results in
Cancer Research 54 (Edited by Grundmann E.),
pp. 36-49 (Berlin: Springer Verlag).

Gö81 Gössner W. and Luz A., 1981, Biological factors
as illustrated in work with short-lived alpha-emitters , in: Radiation Protection. Bone and Bone Seeking Radionuclides: Physiology, Dosimetry and Effects
(Edited by Commission of the European Communities,
EUR 7168 EN), pp. 137-153 (Harwood: Academic Publishers).

Gö82 Gössner W., 1982, Biological effects of Thorium ,
in: Radionuclide Metabolism and Toxicity (Edited by
Galle P. and Masse R.), pp. 273-280 (Paris: Masson).

Lu79 Luz A., Müller W. A., Gössner W. and Hug O., 1979,
"Osteosarcoma induced by short-lived bone-seeking
alpha-emitters in mice: The role of age", Envr. Res.
18, 115-119.

Lu82 Luz A., Erfle V., Rohmer H., Schetters H.,
Schäffer E., Linzner U., Müller W. A. and Gössner W.,
1982, CBA- und BALB/c-Mäuse; 2 Inzuchtstämme mit un-
terschiedlicher Empfindlichkeit für die Osteosarkom-
induktion durch Thorium-227 , Verh. Dtsch. Ges. Path.
66, 516.

Lu84 Luz A., Müller W. A., Schäffer E., Murray A. B.,
Linzner U. and Gössner W., 1984, The sensitivity of
female NMRI mice of different ages for osteosarcoma
induction with ^{227}Thorium , Radiat. Environ.
Biophys. (in press).

Ma73 Mays C. W., 1973, Cancer induction in man from
internal radioactivity , Health Phys. 25, 585-592.

Ma79 Mays C. W. and Spiess H., 1979, Bone tumors in
Thorotrast patients , Envr. Res. 18, 88-93.

Ma84   Mays C. W. and Spiess H., 1984, Bone sarcomas in
       patients given Radium-224 , in: Radiation Carcinoge-
       nesis: Epidemiology and Biological Significance
       (Edited by Boice J. D. and Fraumeni J. F.),
       pp. 241-252 (New York: Raven Press).

Mü77   Müller W. A. and Luz A., 1977, The osteosarcomo-
       genic effectiveness of the short-lived ^{224}Ra com-
       pared with that of the long-lived ^{226}Ra in mice ,
       Rad. Res. 70, 444-448.

Mü78a Müller W. A., Linzner U. and Schäffer E. H., 1978,
       Organ distribution studies of Lutetium-177 in
       mouse , Int. J. Nucl. Med. Biol. 5, 29-31.

Mü78b Müller W. A., Gössner W., Hug O. and Luz A., 1978,
       Late effects after incorporation of the short-lived
       alpha-emitters ^{224}Ra and ^{227}Th in mice , Health
       Phys. 35, 33-55.

Mü80   Müller W. A., Schäffer E. and Linzner U., 1980,
       Studies on incorporated short-lived beta-emitters
       with regard to the induction of late effects ,
       Radiat. Environ. Biophys. 18, 1-11.

Mü81   Müller W. A., 1981, Bone dose and tumour induc-
       tion , in: Radiation Protection. Bone and Bone Seek-
       ing Radionuclides: Physiology, Dosimetry and Effects
       (Edited by Commission of the European Communities,
       EUR 7168 EN), pp. 93-110 (Harwood: Academic Pub-
       lishers).

Mü83   Müller W. A., Luz A., Schäffer E. H. and Gössner
       W., 1983, The role of time-factor and RBE for the
       induction of osteosarcomas by incorporated short-
       lived bone-seekers. Health Phys. 44 (Suppl. 1),
       203-212.

Sc83   Schmitt E., Rückbeil C. and Wick R. R., 1983,
       Long-term clinical investigation of patients with
       ankylosing spondylitis treated with ^{224}Ra , Health
       Phys. 44 (Suppl. 1), 197-202.

Sp56 Spiess H., 1956, Schwere Strahlenschäden nach der Peteosthorbehandlung von Kindern , Dtsch. med. Wschr. 81, 1053-1054.

Sp70 Spiess H. and Mays C. W., 1970, Bone cancers induced by Ra-224 (ThX) in children and adults , Health Phys. 19, 713-729.

Va73 Vaughan J. M., 1973, The effects of irradiation on the skeleton , (Oxford: Clarendon Press).

Wi83 Wick R. R. and Gössner W., 1983, Incidence of tumours of the skeleton in [224]Ra treated ankylosing spondylitis patients , in: Biological Effects of Low-Level Radiation, pp. 281-288 (Vienna: International Atomic Energy Agency).

30

Effects of Iron Overload on Bone Remodelling in Pigs

M. C. de VERNEJOUL, A. POINTILLART, C. CYWINER GOLENZER, C. MORIEUX, J. BIELAKOFF, D. MODROWSKI and L. MIRAVET

INTRODUCTION

Although an iron overload in human pathology may be associated with osteoporosis, it cannot be inferred that iron plays a role in bone changes. Osteoporosis in primary hemochromatosis may be related to multi-endocrine deficiency (De60, Ro79) and in Bantu hemochromatosis to vitamin C deficiency (Wa71). Furthermore, in both cases, hepatic failure frequently associated with bone loss, may also induce osteoporosis (Lo78). In *thalassemia major* with secondary hemochromatosis, impaired bone mineralization and apposition associated with iron bone overload have been observed (Ve82). The role of iron in such disorders, however, has not been demonstrated. At the present time, an iron overload is also frequently observed in hemodialized patients (Go79) and it is relevant to know whether an iron overload may play a role in renal osteodystrophy. We have therefore induced an iron overload in pigs of the same magnitude as that observed during human hemochromatosis. Bone remodelling after a 36-day iron overload was studied in growing pigs after a double tetracycline labelling (Fr69) in order to determine whether this treatment leads to bone changes.

MATERIALS AND METHODS

a) Experimental procedure

Ten female L.W. pigs (12-week old) weighing 34±1kg fed a classical diet (0.8% Ca, 0.6% P and 2000 IU of vitamin D3 per kg diet) were divided into 2 groups. Five pigs were used as control and five pigs received 300 mg IM of dextran iron per day during 36 days (i.e. a total of 10.8 g per pig).

All the animals were slaughtered at the end of the experiment (day 36).

b) Biochemical methods

Blood samples were collected 3 times i.e., at the beginning of the experiment (day O), 3 weeks later (day 21) and at slaughter (day 36) to study plasma kinetics of iron, calcium, phosphate, magnesium and alkaline phosphatase . Serum bilirubin, glutamate oxalo acetate transaminase (SGOT), glutamate pyruvate transaminase (SGPT), γ glutamyl transferase (γ GT), siderophilin saturation and plasma 25 hydroxyvitamin D (25-OH D) levels were determined in slaughter samples with methods described elsewhere (Ve82, Pr75). At slaughter plasma 1,25 dihydroxyvitamin D (1,25(OH)$_2$D) level was determined according to Sheppard and De Luca (Sh80),serum vitamin C according to Roe and Kuether (Ro43) and plasma parathyroid hormone (PTH) by radioimmunoassay (Po84).   Liver iron was determined by Pr. Brissot (Hôpital Ponchaillou, Rennes, France) (Br81). Two epiphyses of main metatarsal bones were used to evaluate bone mineral content (ash, calcium, phosphorus and iron). Two-day urine samples were collected during the last week experiment for calcium, phosphorus, and hydroxyproline determination (Po84).

c) Histological methods

The two parathyroid glands were weighed ; one was frozen for lipid staining and the other was routinely fixed and embedded. The liver was weighed, a fragment was preserved for iron determinations and the remainder was routinely fixed and embedded

The pigs were subjected to double tetracycline labelling at 7-day interval with oxytetracycline IM (2O mg/kg body weight for each labelling, two days on for the 1st injection and one day for the 2nd). The pigs were slaughtered 2 days after the last labelling procedure. A fragment of trabecular bone from the iliac crest was removed, kept undecalcified, embedded in methyl methacrylate and sectioned with a Jung K microtome. Five-µm thick sections were cut and stained with toluidine blue and 15-µm thick sections were kept unstained for tetracycline fluorescence evaluation. We measured the trabecular bone volume in an area of 15 mm^2 on three sections, 2 mm below the cortex, at a site located just anterior to the anterosuperior iliac crest. The percentage of trabecular surfaces covered with osteoid seam was measured at a magnification 350. Osteoblast surfaces were measured taking into account plump osteoblast and expressed in percentage of total trabecular surfaces. Osteoclast resorption surfaces were measured taking into account the trabecular surfaces covered by osteoclasts and expressed in percentage of total trabecular surfaces. Howship lacunae devoided of osteoclast were expressed in percentage of total trabecular bone surfaces and denominated reversal surfaces (Ba81). The depth of the lacunae resulting from osteoclast resorption was measured with an image analyzer. The line of an integrating eye piece was positioned parallel to the two edges of the resorption lacunae and the distance from the deeper point of the resorption cavity to the line of the eye gird was measured. Mean osteoid thickness was measured at a magnification 5OO with an image analyzer at equidistant points, which were selected by the intersection of the parallel lines of an integrating eye piece with the trabecular surfaces. Mean wall thickness (MWT) is the thickness of a complete packet (Da81) and was measured in the same way as mean osteoid thickness at equidistant points. Single and double labelled trabecular surfaces were measured on 15 µm undecalcified sections and expressed in percent of total trabecular surfaces. Total labelled surfaces were calculated according to the formula : double labelled + single labelled surfaces/2. Appositional rate (AR) was also measured at equidistant points. Bone forma-

tion rate was calculated from these parameters using the formula : total labelled surfaces x appositional rate and the duration of the formation period (sigma F), using the formula MWT/AR (Fr69).

The parathyroid, hepatic and bone sections were colored with Perls'stain for iron detection (Co77).

d) Statistical methods

The Studentized Range Q test (Newman-Keuls) was used for multiple mean comparisons (MMC) and the variance analysis for paired means (Sn71). All results are expressed as mean ± SEM.

RESULTS

There was no treatment effect on the growth rates (slaughter weight : 58 ±2 control vs 57±1 kg treated, P > 0.05). Plasma iron levels in treated pigs increased linearly and dramatically (table 1). Serum siderophilin saturation, weight and iron content of the liver also increased markedly in treated pigs. Only the SGOT level was elevated by iron overload whereas the SGPT, bilirubin and γ GT serum levels remained unchanged (table 1).

Table 1. Biochemical parameters of iron overload and liver function

		Control pigs	Treated pigs
Plasma iron $\mu g/l$	day 0	17.1 ± 3.2^a	13.3 ± 0.9^a
	day 21	13.6 ± 0.7^a	27 ± 3.5^b
	day 36	14.9 ± 0.9^a	36.9 ± 4.7^c
Siderophilin saturation, %		2.4 ± 2	$3.8 \pm 2^{**}$
Liver weight, kg		1.1 ± 0.04	$1.3 \pm 0.04^{**}$
Iron $\mu g/100$ mg dry liver		24 ± 6	$586 \pm 91^{***}$
SGOT, IU/l		34 ± 3	$54 \pm 6^{*}$
SGPT, IU/l		37 ± 6	42 ± 8
Serum bilirubin, $\mu g/l$		16.4 ± 3	11.7 ± 2
Serum γGT, IU/dl		3.7 ± 0.6	4.2 ± 0.8

a,b,c, values with common superscript are not different($p < 0.05$), MMC. *** $p < 0.01$, ** $p < 0.02$,variance analysis.

Hepatic sections did not show any fibrosis or inflammatory processes. Perls'stain showed iron deposits occurring primarily in the centrolobular region. Large irregular iron deposits were observed in the Kuppfer cells and small regular blue granules in the hepatocytes which at times exhibited a diffuse pale blue coloration. In the control pigs none of the liver sections were Perls' stain positive.

Plasma calcium and phosphate levels decreased in the control while not significantly in treated pigs (table 2). However, with the excep-

Table 2. Plasma calcium, phosphate, magnesium and alkaline phosphatase
(AP) levels

	Day 0	Day 21	Day 36
calcium,mg/dl			
- treated	10.7 ± 0.2^{ab}	10.2 ± 0.3^{b}	9.8 ± 0.1^{b}
- control	11.4 ± 0.1^{a}	11.2 ± 0.4^{a}	10.2 ± 0.2^{b}
Phosphate,mg/dl			
- treated	8.5 ± 0.2^{ab}	7.8 ± 0.4^{b}	7.6 ± 0.4^{b}
- control	9.1 ± 0.5^{a}	8.1 ± 0.2^{ab}	7.0 ± 0.3^{b}
Magnesium,mg/dl			
- treated	1.8 ± 0.03	1.6 ± 0.13	1.7 ± 0.05
- control	1.7 ± 0.04	1.6 ± 0.03	1.7 ± 0.02
AP, BL.u*			
- treated	1.2 ± 0.1	1.1 ± 0.1	1.5 ± 0.2
- control	1.4 ± 0.1	1.6 ± 0.2	1.3 ± 0.1

a,b,   values with no or common superscripts are not different
($P < 0.05$), MMC test. * Bessey-Lowry units (1 u=1 mMol. p.
nitrophenol/h/l at 38°C).

tion of plasma calcium on day 21, higher in the control than in treated pigs, there was no significant difference between the two groups
for plasma calcium, phosphate, magnesium and alkaline phosphatases values, whatever the period. Table 3 shows that 24-hour urine calcium,
phosphate and hydroxyproline were not affected by the iron treatment.

Table 3. Urinary excretions of calcium, phosphate and hydroxyproline
at the end of the study (g/day)

	Control	Treated
Calcium	0.15 ± 0.02	0.17 ± 0.02
Phosphate	0.31 ± 0.08	0.25 ± 0.05
Hydroxyproline	0.20 ± 0.02	0.17 ± 0.02

No significant difference

Table 4. Bone mineral content of epiphysal metatarsal bones.

	Control	Treated
Ash, % D.M.	48.3 ± 0.9	47.9 ± 0.5
Calcium, % D.M.	17.2 ± 0.3	17.0 ± 0.5
Phosphorus, % D.M.	8.6 ± 0.1	8.3 ± 0.2
Magnesium, % D.M.	0.3 ± 0.01	0.3 ± 0.01
Iron , ppm DM	34 ± 1	$360 \pm 43***$

*** $P < 0.01$,   DM : bone dry matter

The plasma levels of 25(OH)D (6.8 ± 2.5 control vs 6.8 ± 1.5 ng/ml
treated), 1.25(OH)$_2$D (68.7± 7.4 control vs 61.5 ± 2.8 pg/ml treated)
and iPTH (1.7 ± 0.1 control vs 2.0 ± 0.1 ng/ml treated) were not modified by the iron treatment as well as serum vitamin C (0.7 ± 0.2
mg/1 , for both groups).

The average parathyroid weights were not significantly different
between the two groups (62 ± 9 control vs 64 ± 14 mg treated). Staining
of frozen sections with oil red revealed the absence of hyperplasia
in both groups. No iron deposit was detectable in treated pigs with
Perls' stain. Bone calcium, phosphate, magnesium and ash contents were
unchanged . Bone iron content was markedly increased in treated pigs
and there was a significant correlation between liver and bone iron
(r = 0.89 p < 0.05).

Table 4. Iliac bone histomorphometry

	Control	Treated
Trabecular bone volume, %	18.1 ± 1.7	17.4 ± 2.0
Osteoid surfaces, %	31.1 ± 3.7	19.7 ± 3.2**
Osteoblast surfaces, %	19.0 ± 1.8	8.5 ± 2.3*
Mean osteoid thickness, μm	4.8 ± 0.4	4.8 ± 0.2
Double labelled surfaces, %	37.9 ± 1.2	30.9 ± 3.1**
Single labelled surfaces, %	11.4 ± 1.1	13.9 ± 1.7
Total labelled surfaces, %	42.8 ± 1.9	36.4 ± 2.0*
Appositional rate, μm/day	2.6 ± 0.14	2.1 ± 0.10*
Bone formation rate, μ^3/μ^2/day	1.12± 0.09	0.81± 0.07**
Mean wall thickness, μm	40.9 ± 2.1	33.2 ± 2.4*
Sigma F, day	15.7 ± 0.3	15.4 ± 0.2
Reversal surfaces, %	2.8 ± 0.5	4.7 ± 0.7**
Osteoclast resorption surfaces, %	5.5 ± 0.9	4.6 ± 0.7
Depth of resorption lacunae, μm	8.0 ± 0.4	8.3 ± 0.3

* p < 0.05,   ** p < 0.01 treated vs control

Bone histomorphometry after double tetracycline labelling (table
4) indicated that trabecular bone volume was unchanged in treated
pigs. Osteoid surfaces were decreased in treated pigs. The osteoid
thickness remained the same in both groups. The osteoblast, double
and total labelled surfaces dwindled in treated pigs. The appositional rate was slightly reduced in treated animals. As a result of the
lower appositional rate of each osteoblast and the decrease in active
forming surfaces, the bone formation rate was markedly reduced in
treated pigs. The mean wall thickness reflecting the quantity of bone

deposited during one remodelling period was decreased in treated pigs. The duration of the formation period was the same(15.7 ± 0.3 days)in control than in treated pigs (15.4 ± 0.2 days). Reversal surfaces were significantly increased by iron overload. Unlike the results concerning bone formation, no substantial difference was noticeable for bone resorption in the treated pigs, the osteoclast surfaces and the depth of lacunae resulting from resorption were unchanged.

Sections from the five control pigs stained with Perls' stain did not show any sign of blue deposit, whereas those from the five treated pigs exhibited a linear iron deposit inside the bone, at the edge of the trabecular surfaces and at the osteoid-mineralized bone interface. Moreover, an iron blue deposit could seldom be detected at the cement line. Iron was present as a large irregular deposit in marrow macrophages. Histochemically stained iron could also be detected in bone cells. In the osteoclasts, there were infrequently large irregular deposits, similar to those seen in marrow macrophages, but mostly, the osteoclasts presented a diffuse pale blue color. The osteoblast cells contained small blue granules.

DISCUSSION

The drastic iron overload presented here avoided rough liver damage, which could have influenced the bone metabolism. In a previous experiment, Lisboa (Li71) induced cirrhosis in dogs by parenteral injections of iron, using the same total dose range as in our experiment but for a longer period (12 months instead of 36 days). Similarly, in HLA-related hemochromatosis (Po70) and transfusional iron overloading (Ca74), many years elapse before hepatic lesions develop. In fact, in our experimental study, we did obtain a massive iron overload since liver iron concentrations reached the same values as those found in adult men with primary hemochromatosis (Br81). Only slight liver parenchymal damage was observed considering the very slight elevated SGOT, the unchanged SGPT and γGT serum levels and the absence of histological alteration. No modification of bone metabolism has been reported in such cases. We observed iron concentrations of the same magnitude both in macrophage and parenchymal cells of the marrow and liver. The same iron distribution was described in massive secondary hemochromatosis (Br77, Va75). The parenchymal iron overload was also similar to that observed during HLA-related hemochromatosis (Br81).

In controls, plasma calcium and phosphate decreased significantly during the study as usually observed in growing pigs (Ul67). There is no clear explanation for the lack of significant decrease between day 21 and 36 in treated contrary to control pigs. From the beginning of the study calcemia was higher in control than in treated pigs despite the random distribution of the ten pigs into two groups. This difference was significant on day 21 but no explanation can be given for this transient result.

Iron overload did not induce any change either in 25(OH)D or in $1,25(OH)_2D$ plasma levels. The parathyroid hormone secretion estimated by anatomical and biochemical methods was unchanged in the treated pigs, while it has been reported in human hemochromatosis to be increased secondary to low vitamin D levels (Pa75) or decreased because of iron deposits in the parathyroid tissue (Br80). Thus the histological changes observed in bone remodelling cannot be interpreted as resulting from modification of the two major regulators of calcium-phosphorus metabolism, i.e., vitamin D and parathyroid hormone. Furthermore the vitamin C serum levels were unchanged by treatment.

Based either on biochemical(plasma alkaline phosphatase and hydroxyprolinuria) or on morphometric parameters, bone remodelling was about four time higher in our animals than in adult man. There was no evidence for mineralization impairment in the treated pigs. Although appositional rate, also called mineralization rate (Me77), was decreased, osteoid thickness remained unchanged. In such cases a mineralization impairment cannot be demonstrated, since it is difficult to consider that the osteoid lamellae deposited slowly by the osteoblast at one edge of the osteoid seam can be mineralized at a higher rate at the interface osteoid-mineralized bone. Both a decrease in a dynamic parameter taking appositional rate into account and an increase in osteoid thickness are required to demonstrate a mineralization impairment (Me77). This did not occur in the iron treated pigs.

The most impressive changes in bone remodelling concerned formation. In treated pigs, the osteoblast and double labelled surfaces were markedly smaller. This decrease in osteoblast number might be

related to a decrease either in osteoblast recruitment or in osteoblast lifespan. The length of the formation period (sigma F) reflects
the lifespan of a group of osteoblasts at one remodelling cycle (Pa
81). Thus, because sigma F was unchanged in treated pigs, the lifespan of osteoblasts was unchanged by treatment. On the other hand,
reversal surface which are candidate to be of primary importance in
the local coupling between resorption and formation (Ba81) grew
substantially.This growth in reversal surfaces already observed
during osteoporosis may be interpreted as a delay in the osteoblast
onset (Bv81). Thus,reduction of active formation surfaces depended
on decreased osteoblast recruitment.

The second point about formation results was the lowered mean wall
thickness which reflects a decreased amount of bone deposited during
one remodelling cycle. This was related to a decrease in both the
extent of active formation surfaces and the appositional rate. No
significant decrease could be observed either in osteoclastic resorption surfaces or in osteoclast activity according to osteoclastic
resorption depth. This unbalance between maintained resorption and
decreased quantity of deposited bone should have induced a decreased
bone mass (Pa82) ; however we did not observe any modification of
trabecular bone volume and of bone ash content. This discrepancy can
be interpreted in two ways. The first hypothesis is that we were not
able to detect an effective decrease in resorption. The second,
which seems more likely, is that the length of the experience was
too short to give the opportunity to detect a decrease in trabecular
bone volume or bone ash content, which are not very sensible methods
for measuring trabecular mass.

The histochemical demonstration of iron by Perls' stain is a
reliable method (Co77). The iron deposit observed in treated pigs
inside the trabecular bone and cement line have already been reported
in children with thalassemia (Ve82). This experimental study demonstrated that the iron deposit at the mineralized bone-osteoid interface did not inhibit mineralization since there was no mineralization
impairment in the treated pigs. In human hemochromatosis iron deposit
have only been demonstrated in osteoclasts (Ve82). The massive acute
overload achieved in this experimental study led to a stainable iron
deposit in both kinds (osteoblast and osteoclast) of bone cells. Some

iron deposit in osteoclasts similar to those observed in marrow macrophage were large and irregular. They are usually considered to be hemosiderine (Co77). This bears out the hypothesis that marrow macrophages might be local osteoclast precursors (Je63). Usually, however, the osteoclasts had a diffuse pale blue color and osteoblasts contained small regular granules. Both kinds of histochemical deposits are typical of primary hemochromatosis (Co77) and, according to Richter and Bessis (Ri65), indicate a ferritin deposit. The presence of iron in the osteoclasts did not seem to modify osteoclast activity. On the other hand iron inside the osteoblast might play a role in the lowered osteoblast activity observed. Local mechanism for osteoblast recruitment is at the present time poorly understood. However, iron might also play a role in decreased osteoblast recruitment, either by accumulation in bone matrix at cement line or by iron accumulation in the macrophage lineage cells, which exists at the reversal surfaces(Ba81).

Finally, a massive iron overload leads to decreased osteoblast numbers and activity. This could be related to the presence of iron inside the bone cells and along the trabecular bone surfaces. It is not known whether the role of iron in remodelling is of primary importance in human pathology when overload occurs more slowly.

Ba81 Baron R., Vignery A., Tran V.P., 1981, "The significance of lacunar erosion without osteoclasts : studies on the reversal phase of the remodeling sequence", Bone Histomorphometry : Jef, W.S. and Parfitt A.M. (Armour Montagu. Paris),35-41.
Bv81 Baron R., Vignery A., Lang R., 1981, "Reversal phase and osteopenia:Defective coupling of resorption to formation in the pathogenesis of osteoporosis", Osteoporosis : De Luca H.F. et al. (University Park Baltimore) 311-320.
Br80 Brezis M., Shalev O., Leibel B., Bernheim J., Ben Isahy D.,1980, "Phosphorus retention and hypoparathyroidism associated with transfusional iron overload in thalassemia", Mineral Electrolyte Metab. 4, 57-62.
Br77 Brink B., Disler P., Lynch S., 1977, "Patterns of iron storage in dietary iron overload and idiopathic hemochromatosis", J. Lab. Clin. Med. 88, 725-731.
Br81 Brissot P., Bourel M., Herry D., Verger J.P., Messner M., Beaumont C., Regnouard F., Ferrand B., Simon M., 1981, "Assessment of liver iron content in 271 patients, reevaluation of direct and indirect methods", Gastroenterology, 80, 557-565.
Ca74 Canale V.C., 1974, "Betha thalassemia, a clinical review", Pediatr. Ann., 3, 6.
Co77 Cooperberg A.A., Rosenberg A., Schwartz J.P., 1977, "Diagnosis value of bone marrow iron deposits in idiopathic hemochromatosis", Arch. Int. Med., 137, 748-751.

Da81 Darby A.J. and Meunier P.J., 1981, "Mean wall thickness and formation periods of trabecular bone packets in osteoporosis", Calcif. Tissue Int., **33**, 199-204.

De60 Delbarre F., 1960, "L'ostéoporose de l'hémochromatose",Sem. hop. Paris, **36**, 3279-3284.

Fr69 Frost H.M., 1969, "Tetracycline-based histological analysis of bone remodeling", Calc. Tiss. Res., **3**, 211-227.

Go79 Gokal R., Millard P.R., Weatherhall D.J., Callender S.T., Leoingham J.G., Oliver D.A., 1979, "Iron metabolism in hemodialysis patients", Q.J. Med., **191**, 369.

Je63 Jee W.S. and Nolan P.D., 1963, "Origin of osteoclasts from the fusion of phagocytes", Nature, **200**, 225-226.

Li71 Lisboa P.E., "Experimental hepatic cirrhosis in dogs caused by chronic massive iron overload", Gut., **12**, 363-368.

Lo78 Long R.G., Meinhard E., Skinner R.K., Varghese Z., Wills M.R., Sherlock S., 1978, "Clinical biochemical and histological studies of osteomalacia osteoporosis and parathyroid function in chronic liver disease", Gut., **19**, 85-90.

Me77 Meunier P.J., Edouard C., Richard D.D., Laurent J., 1977, "Histomorphometry of osteoid tissue. The hyperosteoidoses", Bone histomorphometry : P.J. Meunier (Armour Montagu. Paris), 249-263.

Pa82 Parfitt A.M., 1982, "The coupling of bone formation to bone resorption a critical analysis of the concept and of its relevance to the pathogenesis of osteoporosis", Metab. Bone Dis.Rel.Res.,**4**,1-6.

Pa81 Parfitt A.M., Villanueva A.K., Mathews C.H., Aswani J.A.,1981, "Kinetics of matrix and mineral apposition in osteoporosis and renal osteodystrophy, relationship to rate of turnover and to cell morphology", Bone Histomorphometry : Jee W.S., Parfitt A.M. (Armour Montagu. Paris), 213-219.

Pa75 Pawlotsky Y., Simon M., Hany Y., Brissot P., Bourel M., 1975, "High plasma parathyroid hormone levels and osteoarticular changes in primary hemochromatosis", Scand. J. Rhum. supp. **4**, 15-19.

Po84 Pointillart A., Fontaine N., Thomasset M., 1984, "Phytate phosphorus utilization and intestinal phosphatases in pigs fed low phosphorus : wheat or corn diets", Nut. Rep. Int., **29**, 473-483.

Po70 Powell L.W., 1970, "Changing concepts in hemochromatosis", Post grad. Med. J., **47**, 200-209.

Pr75 Preece M.A., Tomlison S., Ribot C.A., Pietrek J., Korn H.T., Davies D.M., Ford J.A., Dunningham M.G., O'Riordan J.L., 1975, "Studies of vitamin D deficiency in man", Q.J. Med., **176**, 575.

Ri65 Richter G.W. and Bejsis M.C., 1965, "Commentary on hemosiderin" Blood, **25**, 370-373.

Ro43 Roe J.H. and Kuether C.A., 1943, "The determination of ascorbic acid in whole blood an urine through the 2-4 dinitrophenylhydralarzine", J. Biol. Chem., 339-407.

Ro79 Roudier G., Hany Y., Louboutin J.Y., Ferrand B., Bourel M., 1979, "Histomorphometrie et manifestations articulaires de l'hémochromatose idiopathique", Rev. Rhum., **46**, 91-99.

Sh80 Shepard R.M. and De Luca H.F., 1980, "Determination of vitamine D and its metabolites in plasma", Methods in enzymology (New York, Academic Press), 393-414.

Sn71 Snedecor G.W. and Cochran W.G., 1971, "Méthodes statistiques" (Acta, Paris), 302-315.

Ul67 Ullrey D.R., Miller E.R., Brent B.E., Bradley B.L., Hoeffer J.A., 1967, "Swine hematology from birth to maturity", J. Anim. Sci., **26**, 1024-1029.

Va75 Valberg L.S., Simon J.B., Manley P.N., 1975, "Distribution of storage iron as body iron stores expand in patients with hemochromatosis", J. Lab. Clin. Med., **86**, 479-489.

Ve82 Vernejoul M.C. de, Girot R., Gueris J., Cancela L., Bang S., Bielakoff J., Mautalen C., Goldberg D., Miravet L., 1982, "Calcium phosphate metabolism and bone disease in patients with homozygous thalassemia", J. Clin. Endocrinol. metab., **54**, 276-281.

Wa71 Wapnick A.A., Lynch S.R., Seftel H.C., Charlton R.W., Bothwel T.H., Jowsey J., 1971, "The effect of siderosis and ascorbic acid depletion on bone metabolism with special reference to osteoporosis in Bantu", Br. J. Nutr., **25**, 367-370.

31

Skeletal Lesions from Inhaled Plutonium in Beagles

G. E. DAGLE, J. F. PARK, R. E. WELLER, H. A. RAGAN, B. J. McCLANAHAN and D. R. FISHER

INTRODUCTION

Inhalation studies in beagles were initiated in our laboratory to evaluate the dose-effect relationships of inhaled plutonium since inhalation is one of the major routes of accidental exposure.

Early studies showed that inhaled ^{239}Pu oxide induced lung tumors in beagle dogs, but the plutonium translocated to the skeleton was insufficient to produce bone tumors (Pa72). However, in later studies with ^{238}Pu oxide, a soluble fraction of plutonium translocated to the skeleton and induced bone tumors (Pa76).

This report will briefly review the skeletal effects observed in ongoing lifespan studies in beagle dogs at 13, 10, and 7 years, respectively, after inhalation exposure to ^{239}Pu oxide and nitrate or ^{238}Pu oxide. The latter has a specific activity of 15 Ci/g, a half-life of 86 years and decays with alpha emissions of 5.49 MeV. The ^{239}Pu has a specific activity of 0.054 Ci/g; a half-life of 24,000 years and decays with alpha emissions of 5.14 MeV. Plutonium nitrate was chosen to represent soluble material more readily translocated to bone and other tissues than the oxide.

Work supported by the U.S. Department of Energy under Contract DE-AC06-76RLO-1830

METHODS

Beagle dogs were exposed to aerosols of ^{239}Pu oxide or nitrate or to ^{238}Pu oxide, at six dose levels, resulting in average initial pulmonary depositions ranging from approximately 2 to 5800 nCi (Table 1). The dogs, equally divided by sex, were exposed at 18 months of age to ^{239}Pu oxide (1970 and 1971); to ^{238}Pu oxide (1973 and 1974); or to ^{239}Pu nitrate (1976 and 1977). In addition to 20 sham-exposed controls for each isotope, 20 dogs (vehicle controls) were exposed to aerosols of nitric acid.

Table 1. Lifespan dose-effect studies with inhaled plutonium in beagles

Actinide	Number of Dogs	Initial Alveolar Deposition ± SD* (nCi)	(nCi/g Lung)**
^{239}PuO$_2$	8	5800 ± 3300	50 ± 22
	20	1100 ± 170	9.3 ± 1.4
	20	300 ± 62	2.4 ± 0.4
	20	79 ± 14	0.66 ± 0.13
	20	22 ± 4	0.18 ± 0.04
	20	3 ± 1	0.03 ± 0.11
	20	---	---
^{238}PuO$_2$	13	5200 ± 1400	43 ± 12
	20	1300 ± 270	10 ± 1.9
	20	350 ± 81	2.6 ± 0.5
	20	77 ± 11	0.56 ± 0.07
	20	18 ± 3	0.15 ± 0.03
	20	2 ± 1	0.02 ± 0.01
	20	---	---
^{239}Pu(NO$_3$)$_4$	5	5445 ± 1841	47 ± 17
	20	1709 ± 639	13.7 ± 6.2
	20	295 ± 67	2.34 ± 0.77
	20	56 ± 17	0.50 ± 0.25
	20	8 ± 4	0.06 ± 0.04
	20	2 ± 2	0.02 ± 0.02
	20	---	---
	20	---	---

*Estimated from thoracic count at 2 or 4 wk after exposure
**Lung weights estimated at 0.011 x body weight

The dogs were given single 5- to 30-min, nose-only exposures of aerosolized water suspensions of the oxide or of the nitrate solution. The ^{239}Pu oxide was prepared by calcining the oxalate at 750°C for 2 hr (mean AMAD 2.3 µm; mean GSD 1.9). The ^{238}Pu oxide was prepared by calcining the oxalate at 700°C and subjecting the product to steam in argon exchange at 800°C for 96 hr (mean AMAD 1.8 µm; mean GSD 1.9). The ^{239}Pu(NO$_3$)$_4$ was aerosolized from a 0.27 N solution of nitric acid (mean AMAD 0.63 µm; mean GSD 2.0). Ultrafiltration and valence determinations for the ^{239}Pu(NO$_3$)$_4$ solutions showed no appreciable polymerization or disproportionation at the concentration used. The required dose levels were obtained by varying the aerosol concentration and exposure duration.

The dogs were housed, in pairs, in indoor-outdoor runs and provided with routine veterinary care. The animals were observed daily, with hematologic examinations at 3 to 4-mo intervals and annual physical examinations. Bone tumors were detected by clinical examination, annual radiographic examinations, gross and microscopic examination at necropsy, and radiography of disarticulated bones. Radioanalysis of tissues for total alpha activity was performed by liquid scintillation and alpha energy analysis after digestion with HNO$_3$ and ashing in a muffle furnace. Bone-to-bone-marrow ratios were determined by ultrasonic cell disruption of selected bones and separate analysis of bone and marrow.

RESULTS

Bone lesions related to plutonium exposure were observed only in dogs exposed to ^{238}Pu oxide and ^{239}Pu nitrate.

The skeleton accumulated approximately 2% (^{239}Pu oxide), 45% (^{238}Pu oxide) or 50% (^{239}Pu nitrate) of the final body burdens at 13, 10, and 7 years, respectively, after exposure (Figure 1). Skeletal uptake data from the ^{238}PuO$_2$ and ^{239}Pu(NO$_3$)$_4$-exposed dogs were fitted to logarithmic curves, and doses to skeleton were calculated with the following function:

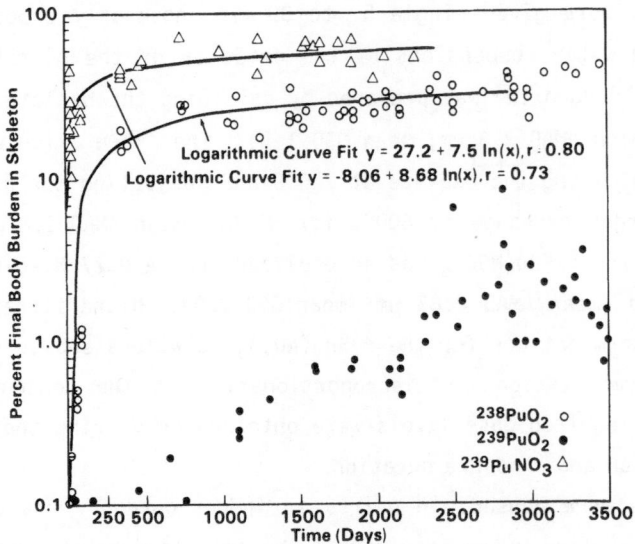

FIGURE 1   Percent of plutonium in skeleton at death of dogs exposed
by inhalation.

$$D_{rad} = \frac{51.23EA}{m} {}_0\!\int^t R(t) \, dt,$$

where

E = alpha particle energy of 5.49 MeV,

A = final tissue body burden in μCi,

m = skeletal mass in grams based on 10% body weight,

R(t) = retention/uptake function for plutonium in bone as determined
from the logarithmic function model and individualized for
each dog, and

t = time at necropsy (minus 60 days for a latency period for dogs
with tumors).

The plutonium concentration in the bones of dogs exposed to plutonium nitrate varied according to location (Figure 2). The sacrum
and lumbar vertebrae nearly always had the highest concentration;
coccygeal vertebrae, radius, tibia-fibula, maxilla, and ulna nearly
always had the lowest concentration; and a large group of bones (center) had concentrations overlapping those of the high and low groups.

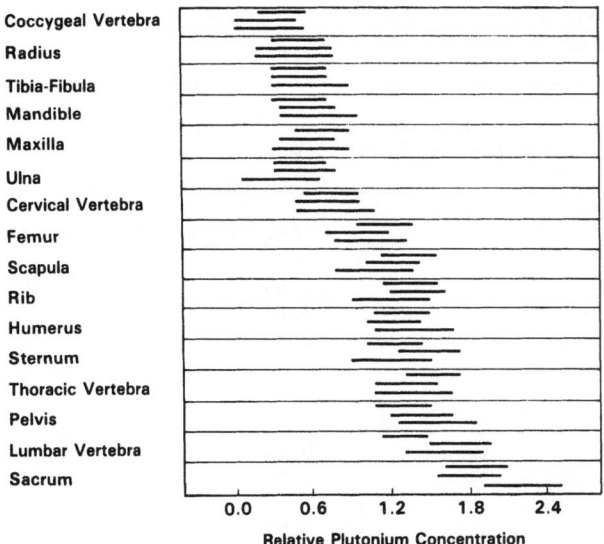

Coccygeal Vertebra
Radius
Tibia-Fibula
Mandible
Maxilla
Ulna
Cervical Vertebra
Femur
Scapula
Rib
Humerus
Sternum
Thoracic Vertebra
Pelvis
Lumbar Vertebra
Sacrum

0.0   0.6   1.2   1.8   2.4
Relative Plutonium Concentration

FIGURE 2   Plutonium concentration in individual bones relative to total skeletal concentration. Each line represents 95% confidence intervals for groups of three to six dogs exposed to different exposure levels of plutonium nitrate.

Studies on the partition of plutonium between bones and bone marrow (Table 2) indicated that 1.6 to 7.4% of the plutonium found in the proximal humeri was actually present in the marrow rather than in the osseous tissue. Since more marrow is present in the diaphyses, proportionally larger amounts of plutonium were deposited in that area. The distal humeri and all areas of the radii, having less marrow, generally had proportionally smaller amounts of plutonium. The lumbar vertebrae had amounts similar to those in the proximal humeri.

We have now observed a total of 48 bone tumors in 41 beagles (Table 3). The tumors were generally well advanced before sufficient lameness or discomfort was detected to warrant a radiographic diagnosis of neoplasia.

Although the majority of tumors were well-differentiated, osteoblastic osteosarcomas, other forms were also observed: complex osteosarcomas (with chondroid differentiation) in two vertebral tumors; fibrosarcomas in one pelvic and one vertebral tumor without clear-cut osteoid differentiation; and a pleomorphic osteosarcoma, with multi-

Table 2. Partition of inhaled ^{239}Pu nitrate between bone and bone marrow in beagles

	Months After Exposure:	43	71	81	93
		Percent of Plutonium in Marrow*			
Humerus					
Proximal		1.55	7.07	3.56	7.40
Diaphyseal		6.26	11.39	6.17	14.79
Distal		0.41	2.31	0.32	2.85
Radius					
Proximal		---	---	0.31	0.79
Diaphyseal		0.79	---	1.42	---
Distal		---	---	0.93	---
Lumbar Vertebra		0.87	5.77	2.85	5.69

*Ratio calculated from: $\dfrac{^{239}\text{Pu in Marrow}}{^{239}\text{Pu in Intact Bone}} \times 100$

Table 3. Bone tumors associated with inhaled plutonium in beagles

	\ Number of Tumors			
	^{238}Pu Oxide	^{239}Pu Nitrate	Total	Dose* (Rad ± SE)
Vertebra	14 (4)	8 (1)	22	146 ± 88
Pelvis	5 (3)	1 (1)	6	131 ± 107
Humerus	1	4 (4)	5	166 ± 78
Scapula	4 (1)	0	4	148 ± 60
Rib	3 (2)	2	5	164 ± 88
Femur	2 (1)	0	2	112 ± 3
Tibia	1 (1)	0	1	135
Sternum	1 (1)	0	1	---
Maxilla	0	1	1	526
Hyoid	1	0	1	101
TOTAL	32	16	48	

*Cumulative absorbed skeletal dose

nucleated giant cells, in one pelvic tumor. Metastases occurred in 40% of the tumors. There was no detectable relationship between total skeletal dose and location of tumors. Serum alkaline phosphatase levels were elevated in dogs with tumors.

Non-neoplastic bone lesions included pronounced radiation osteodystrophy in dogs exposed to high-dose levels. This was characterized by peritrabecular fibrosis, composed of relatively hypocellular connective tissue that tended to surround trabeculae. Although the relationship to plutonium exposure is unclear, there has been a trend toward higher than usual incidence of spondylosis deformans in dogs exposed to $^{238}PuO_2$. In six dogs, hypertrophic osteoarthropathy has been observed secondary to plutonium-induced lung tumors.

DISCUSSION

The results of our studies clearly confirm and extend previous reports on the induction of bone tumors in beagles following inhalation of physicochemical or isotopic forms of plutonium that are translocated to the skeleton (Ha81; Pa76). All of the plutonium-induced tumors observed in the various studies were similar in biological activity and histologic appearance. The principal difference between plutonium-induced bone tumors and those of spontaneous origin may be the appendicular location of the latter in contrast with the axial location of the plutonium-induced tumors. The role of extraskeletal events, such as concurrent lymphopenia, neutropenia, radiation pneumonitis, lung tumors, and hepatopathy, in the induction of bone tumors, remains unclear (Da79; Pa85).

The kinetics of plutonium migration to and from bone should aid in understanding the dosimetry. Stevens (St85) considered the kinetics of bone deposition of plutonium in the $^{239}Pu(NO_3)_4$-exposed dogs on this study and has estimated the half-time in bone to be between 2100 and 2300 days. Based on ratio of life spans, a half-time of 25 to 30 years could therefore be extrapolated for man, in contrast to the 100 years estimated for man by ICRP (IC72). Preliminary microdistribution studies with autoradiography suggest that endosteal deposition of inhaled plutonium is similar to that of intravenously injected plutonium (Smith et al., unpublished data).

The principal biological events associated with plutonium deposition in bone include cell death or sublethal injury due to ionizing radiation, and inflammation and repair mechanisms related to cell death or sublethal injury. These epigenetic or nonstochastic factors are generally included in models (Br80; Ma77; Pe82; Wh82) of alpha-radiation-induced bone cancer. The dogs at the lower dose levels in our study will need to live out their life spans to develop dose-effect relationships for predicting the health consequences of accidental human contamination.

REFERENCES

Br80 Bruenger F. W., Stevens W., Stover B. J., Taylor G. N., Smith J. M., Buster D. S. and Atherton D. R., 1980, The Distribution and Pathological Effects of Pu in Juvenile Beagles , Radiat. Res. 84, 325-342.

Da79 Dagle G. E., Park J. F., Ragan H. A. and Morris J. E., 1979, Toxicology of Inhaled Plutonium in Dogs, in: Biological Implications of Radionuclides Released from Nuclear Industries, pp. 105-119 (Vienna: International Atomic Energy Agency).

Ha81 Hahn F. F., Mewhinney J. A., Merickel B. S., Guilmette R. A., Boeker B. B. and McClellan R. O., 1981, Primary Bone Neoplasms in Beagle Dogs Exposed by Inhalation to Aerosols of Plutonium-238 Dioxide , J. Natl. Cancer Inst. 67, 917-927.

IC72 International Commission on Radiological Protection, 1972, The Metabolism of Compounds of Plutonium and Other Actinides , ICRP Publication 19 (Oxford: Pergamon Press).

Ma77 Marshal J. H., Groer P. G., 1977, A Theory of the Induction of Bone Cancer by Alpha Radiation , Radiat. Res. 71, 149-192.

Pa72 Park J. F., Bair W. J. and Busch R. H., 1972, Progress in Beagle Dog Studies with Transuranium Elements at Battelle-Northwest , Health Phys. 22, 803-810.

Pa85 Park J. F., Dagle G. E., Ragan H. A., Weller R. E. and Stevens D. L., Current Status of Life-Span Studies with Inhaled Plutonium in Beagles at Pacific Northwest Laboratory , in: R. C. Thompson and J. A. Mahaffey, Eds., Life-Span Radiation Studies in Animals: What Can They Tell Us?, 22nd Hanford Life Science Symposium, October 2-4, 1983, Richland, WA (in press).

Pa76 Park J. F., Lund J. E., Ragan H. A., Hackett P. L. and Frazier M. E., 1976, Bone Tumors Induced by Inhalation of ^{238}PuO$_2$ in Dogs , Rec. Results Cancer Res. 54, 17-35.

Pe82 Peterson A. V., Prentice R. L. and Marek P., 1982, Relationship between Dose of Injected ^{239}Pu and Bone Sarcoma Mortality in Young Adult Beagles , Radiat. Res. 90, 77-89.

St85 Stevens D. L. and Dagle G. E., Dose Estimation for Beagles Exposed to Inhaled Plutonium Nitrate Using Nonparametric Statistical Techniques , in: R. C. Thompson and J. A. Mahaffey, Eds., Life-Span Radiation Studies in Animals: What Can They Tell Us?, 22nd Hanford Life Science Symposium, October 2-4, 1983, Richland, WA (in press).

Wh82 Whittemore A. S., 1982, Osteosarcomas Among Beagles Exposed to ^{239}Pu , Radiat. Res. 96, 41-56.

32

The Induction, by ^{239}Pu, of Myeloid Leukaemia and Osteosarcoma in Female CBA Mice (Interim Results)

E. R. HUMPHREYS, J. F. LOUTIT and V. A. STONES

The potential threat to the environment of the by-products of the nuclear power industry is very well recognised and has prompted much research into the effects of α-emitting radionuclides. Most important among these is plutonium first investigated soon after the discovery of the element (Br46, Li47) and continuing today in many animal species (Va73, Ne79). The major late effect from systemic contamination seen in these studies is osteosarcoma and, since this tumour is also seen in humans given isotopes of radium (Ro83), the relationship of its incidence to the amount of α-emitter given has provided the framework upon which the relevant radiological protection standards are based.

In contrast, late effects of α-emitting radionuclides on the haematopoietic system in man and animals are rarely seen. This is most commonly explained by supposing that the leukaemogenic precursor cell (so far unidentified) lies in a region of marrow generally beyond the range of α-particles emitted from bone. Alternatively, it has been proposed (Th76) that leukaemia is less likely to be induced than osteosarcoma in humans given radium because potentially leukaemogenic cells are sterilized by the amounts of α-irradiation causing osteosarcoma. To some extent this latter hypothesis has received recent experimental support since it has been shown that myeloid leukaemia is induced in CBA/H mice by injecting amounts of ^{224}Ra smaller than those required to give the maximum yield of osteosarcoma

343

(Hu84). The present experiment was designed to see whether this is also true in animals given ^{239}Pu.

It is generally accepted that ^{239}Pu is a bone surface seeker and that its toxicity can be attributed to this. In 3-month old CBA/H mice, however, the ^{239}Pu initially deposited on trabecular bone surfaces after injection is either rapidly buried by relatively uncontaminated bone or is resorbed equally quickly (Gr79). Either process reduces the irradiation of bone surface cells by ^{239}Pu α-particles causing the dose-rate to these cells to fall with time even though the plutonium persists in bone. It is known that ^{224}Ra (half-life 3.66 days) induces more osteosarcomas in mice if its total injected amount is protracted in time rather than given in a single injection (Mu78). Since all the plausible hypotheses advanced by the authors to explain their results depended on the short residence time of ^{224}Ra at bone surface it is possible that similar results may be obtained from ^{239}Pu given to 3-month old CBA/H mice. Accordingly, in the present experiment plutonium was administered either as a single injection or in sixteen injections spaced at 3.5 day intervals over eight weeks.

MATERIALS AND METHODS

^{239}Pu was obtained from Amersham International, England, as a solution of the element (99% ^{239}Pu, 1% ^{240}Pu -- other isotopes not detected) in 3M HNO_3.

This material was standardized against a ^{239}Pu standard (also obtained from Amersham International) by counting in a liquid scintillation mixture (Ke70) in a Packard Tricarb Model 3255 liquid scintillation spectrometer.

Solutions suitable for injection were prepared by diluting very small aliquots of the 3M HNO_3 solution (ca.50mg) with 1% trisodium citrate solution containing sufficient HNO_3 to bring the final solution to pH5. From experience it is known that solutions prepared this way pass unchanged through a 25 nm Millipore filter.

For the single injection experiment the injection solutions were prepared to contain 81.4, 244 or 814 Bq cm^{-3} and, for the multiple-injection experiment, to contain one-sixteenth these amounts. In each case dilutions were made with acidified 1% trisodium citrate solution.

The mice (CBA females with a mean age of 83.4±0.1 days at the first or only injection) were assigned by random selection to their injection groups. Those to be given ^{239}Pu were injected intraperitoneally with the appropriate injection solution. For the single injection experiment the mice were given 0.5 cm^3, but, for the multiple-injection experiment, the amount to be injected was calculated from the mean body mass of a subgroup of 25 animals and the volume injected adjusted accordingly. The animals given multiple injections were injected with sixteen aliquots spaced at 3.5 day intervals over eight weeks. The control animals for each experiment were given 0.5 cm^3 1% acidified trisodium citrate at the same time as the experimental animals were given ^{239}Pu.

The animals were provided with mouse nuts and water ad libitum until they died or were killed (see below). Apart from a close visual examination each day no routine ante-mortem procedures were applied. Radiographs were taken of anaesthetized animals with suspected bony lesions and tail vein blood smears were prepared from animals with suspected blood disorders.

Animals were killed by chloroform and exsanguination when at least one of the following criteria was satisfied.

1. The animal was seen to be suffering.

2. The animal was judged to be able to live for only one more day.

3. The animal was displaying specific signs, for example spleno-megaly with or without skin pallor.

All animals were radiographed as soon as possible after death.

In those animals which were killed blood samples were taken directly from the heart and examined for white and red cell numbers; a blood smear was also prepared and stained with Leishmann's blue to allow search for atypical white cells.

Samples of spleen, kidney, liver, sternum, lumbar vertebrae and left knee joint were routinely taken from each animal for sectioning. Other organs and tissues were taken for sectioning if seen to be abnormal at the post-mortem examination.

Most haematopoietic tumours suspected at autopsy (in recently dead animals) were transplanted into syngeneic hosts for confirmation. Occasionally osteosarcomas were transplanted by subcutaneous implantation.

The features of myeloid leukaemia and osteosarcoma as seen in tissues under the microscope were as described by Major (1979) and Loutit, Sansom and Carr (1976) respectively. Myeloid leukaemia is defined as a malignant condition arising in the granular cells of the haematopoietic tissues (bone marrow and splenic red pulp). The resulting condition is seen histologically as a gross excess of immature cells of the granular (and monocytic) series in sites of normal haematopoiesis with metastatic and invasive spread to abnormal sites (liver, kidney, connective tissue around bone) and to peripheral blood where cells atypical to blood may be seen in variable numbers.

Bones showing normal opacity to X-rays were often seen on spectioning to contain foci of cells clearly identifiable as early osteosarcomas. These observations, however, were not used as a basis for comparison between groups since not all bones were similarly examined. Osteosarcomas, for the purpose of comparison, therefore, are defined as those suspected by radiography and confirmed by histology.

RESULTS

Table 1 summarizes the animal data and shows the mean time intervals between injection and death. Except for the mice given 18.5 kBq kg^{-1} in a single injection, these values, for those animals given ^{239}Pu, could not be shown to be significantly different from the corresponding values for the control animals.

Table 1

Experiment details

^{239}Pu injected (kBqkg^{-1})	0	1.85	5.55	18.5
Single injection experiment				
Number of mice	36	38	39	40
Mean days injection to death	738±37	803±27	760±22	702±18
Multiple injection experiment				
Number of mice	45	43	45	42
Mean days injection to death	803±28	808±29	771±26	734±26

The numbers of mice in which myeloid leukaemia and osteosarcoma were diagnosed are shown in Table 2. All of these tumours are considered to be radiation-induced since their spontaneous occurrence in CBA/H mice has, so far, not been demonstrated for myeloid leukaemia and rarely so for osteosarcoma.

Table 2

Induction of myeloid leukaemia and osteosarcoma

^{239}Pu injected (kBq kg^{-1})	0	1.85	5.55	18.5
Single injection experiment				
Myeloid leukaemia No.	0	1	0	0
Mean days to death	–	795	–	–
Osteosarcoma No.	0	0	3	10
Mean days to death	–	–	814±13	677±43
Multiple injection experiment				
Myeloid leukaemia No.	0	1	2	1
Mean days to death	–	802	450±6	694
Osteosarcoma No.	0	1	3	12
Mean days to death	–	995	758±36	869±32

The yields of myeloid leukaemia were greater in those animals given ^{239}Pu in multiple injections although the numbers were too small to permit proper analysis. The incidences of osteosarcomas were unaffected by the mode of administration of ^{239}Pu.

DISCUSSION

Myeloid leukaemia has previously been diagnosed in mice given ten times as much ^{239}Pu as was given in the top group of the present experiment (SV81). However, the lesion was known to occur spontaneously in these mice (specific pathogen free ICR females); 17 of a group of 70 control animals developed the condition compared with 22 from 79 given 180 kBq ^{239}Pu. The authors claimed that the leukaemia occurred sooner in the ^{239}Pu-treated animals (age 459±19 days) than in the control animals (559±24 days).

Myeloid leukaemia has also been diagnosed in rats given ^{239}Pu as nitrate, one rat in a group of 22 given 109 kBq kg^{-1} in a single injection and 3 rats in a group of 19 given 111 kBq kg^{-1} in divided injections (Be65). Myeloid leukaemia does not occur spontaneously in these animals (Ta84).

Other haematopoietic tumours were diagnosed in CBA/H mice given ^{239}Pu (Lo78) but myeloid leukaemia was not seen.

The yields of osteosarcoma in the present experiment, for

equivalent amounts of ^{239}Pu, are similar to those obtained in other CBA/H females (Lo78) and also in CF1 mice (Fi62). The incidences of myeloid leukaemia are too small to permit a meaningful comparison to be made between yield and injected amount. However, since all of these leukaemias were induced by the injected ^{239}Pu, it can be said that myeloid leukaemia is induced in these mice by amounts of ^{239}Pu less than is needed for inducing a maximum yield of osteosarcoma.

The derivation of a leukaemogenic α-dose from these results may not be possible, however, from presently available information. Dose rate can be calculated with some precision since bones taken from animals bred from the same stock as those used in the present experiments have been analysed in several previous experiments (Gr81, Gr79). However, recent experiments in which myeloid leukaemia was induced in male CBA/H mice by ^{224}Ra (Hu84) indicate that there can be a long interval between the injection of ^{224}Ra and the diagnosis of leukaemia. The short half-life of ^{224}Ra (3.66 days) and the known biological loss of ^{224}Ra from mouse bones (unpublished experiments) combine to restrict the period over which more than 90% of the leukaemogenic dose was delivered to approximately 16 days following injection. The growth period of the tumour is not known but if it is assumed that the tumour is clonogenic with a doubling time of the order of one day, an estimate can be made of the time to reach a mass of 10% body mass assuming exponential growth. For a 20g mouse this period is approximately 30 days. Since the average period between injection and diagnosis in those mice was 485±43 days there is an interval of 450 days during which ^{224}Ra is absent from the bones; the stimulus, therefore, (third event -- Gr78) necessary to begin the development of the tumour did not appear to depend on the presence of the injected activity. The average interval between injection and diagnosis in the present experiment (638±79 days) is longer. It is not known therefore over what period the leukaemogenic dose was delivered in these animals since ^{239}Pu is present in mouse bones from injection to death (Ro67) and there is no experimental information available which favours the selection of any one period rather than any other during this interval. From the point of view of radiological protection, therefore, the value of the results of the present experiment are limited to demonstrating that, given the appropriate conditions, myeloid leukaemia can be induced by the presence of ^{239}Pu in bone. The calculation of the dose necessary for this to occur needs more information.

REFERENCES

Be65 Bensted, J.P.M., Taylor, D.M. and Sowby, F.D. (1965). The carcinogenic effects of americium-241 and plutonium-239 in the rat. Brit. J. Radiol. 38 920 - 925.

Br46 Brues, A.M., Lisco, H. and Finkel, M. (1946). Carcinogenic action of some substances which may be a problem in future industries. USAEC Report No. MDDC-145 July (1946).

Fi62 Finkel, M.P. and Biskis, B.O. (1962). Toxicity of ^{239}Pu in mice. Health Phys. 8 565 - 579.

Gr79 Green, D., Howells, G.R. and Thorne, M.C. (1979). Quantitative microscopic studies of the distribution and retention of ^{239}Pu in the ilium of the female CBA mouse. Int. J. Radiat. Biol. 36 499 - 511.

Gr81 Green, D., Howells, G.R. and Thorne, M.C. (1981). Morphometric studies on mouse bone using a computer-based image analysis system. J. Microsc. 122 49 - 58.

Gr78 Groer, P.G. and Marshall, J.H. (1978). A model for the induction of bone cancer by ^{224}Ra. In: Biological effects of ^{224}Ra, benefit and risk of therapeutic application. Edited by Muller, W.A. and Ebert, H.G. Published for the Commission of the European Communities by Martinus Nijhoff Medical Division The Hague/Boston. pp 201 - 209.

Hu84 Humphreys, E.R., Loutit, J.F., Major, I.R. and Stones, V.A. (1984). The induction by ^{224}Ra of myeloid leukaemia and osteosarcoma in male CBA mice. Int. J. Radiat. Biol. In Press.

Ke70 Keough, R.F. and Powers, G.J. (1970). Determination of plutonium in biological materials by extraction and liquid scintillation counting. Analyt. Chem. 42 419 - 421.

Li47 Lisco, H., Finkel, M. and Brues, A (1947). Carcinogenic properties of radioactive fission products and plutonium. Radiology 49 361 - 363.

Lo76 Loutit, J.F., Sansom, Janet and Carr, T.E.F. (1976). The Pathology of tumours induced in Harwell mice by ^{239}Pu and ^{226}Ra. In: The health effects of plutonium and radium. Edited by W.S.S. Jee The J.W. Press Salt Lake City, Utah pp 505 - 519.

Lo78 Loutit, J.F. and Carr, T.E.F. (1978). Lymphoid tumours and leukaemia induced in mice by bone-seeking radionuclides. Int. J. Radiat. Biol. 33 245 - 263.

Ma72 Mays, C.W. and Dougherty, T.F. (1972). Progress in the beagle studies at the University of Utah. Health Phys. 22 743 - 801.

Ma79 Major, I.R. (1979). Induction of myeloid leukaemia by whole-body single exposure of CBA male mice to X-rays. Br. J. Cancer 40 903 - 913.

Ma82 Major, I.R. and Mole, R.H. (1982). Myeloid leukaemia in X-ray irradiated CBA mice. Nature 272 455 - 456.

Mu78 Muller, W.A., Gossner, W., Hug, O. and Luz,A. (1978). Late effects after incorporation of the short-lived α-emitters ^{224}Ra and ^{227}Th in mice. Health Phys. 35 33 - 55.

Ne79 Nenot, J.C. and Stather, J.W. (1979). The toxicity of Plutonium, Americium and Curium. Published for the Commission of the European Communities by Pergamon Press, Oxford, England.

Ro67 Rosenthal, M.W. and Lindenbaum, A. (1967). Influence of DTPA therapy on long-term effects of retained monomeric plutonium: comparison with polymeric plutonium. Radiat. Res. 31 506 - 521.

Ro83 Rowland, R.E., Stehney, A.D. and Lucas, H.F. (1983). Dose-response relationships for radium induced bone sarcomas. Health Phys. 44 Suppl. 1 15 - 31.

Sp83 Spiers, F.W., Lucas, H.F., Rundo, J. and Anast, G.A. (1983). Leukaemia incidence in the U.S. dial workers. Health Phys. 44 65 - 72.

Sv81 Svoboda, V., Bubenikova, D. and Kotaskova, Z. (1981). Myeloid leukaemia in ^{239}Pu-treated mice. J. Cancer Res. Clin. Oncol. 100 255 - 262.

Ta84 Taylor, D.M. (1984). Personal communication.

Th76   Thorne, M.C. and Vennart, J. (1976). The toxicity of ^{90}Sr, ^{226}Ra and ^{239}Pu. Nature <u>263</u> 555 - 558.

Va73   Vaughan, J.M. (1973). The effects of irradiation on the skeleton. Clarendon Press, Oxford.

33

The Effect of Manganese Ingestion, Phosphate Depletion and Starvation on the Epiphyseal Growth Plate

B. ENGFELDT, A. HJERPE, F. REINHOLT, O. SVENSSON and B. WIKSTRÖM

In recent years there has been a growing interest in the biology and toxicology of manganese, mainly because of its importance as an occupational health problem (Me 81). Chronic toxicity is most often seen after inhalation of Mn fumes and is principally manifested by various neuro-psychiatric symptoms. Furthermore, like several other metal compounds, high-dose oral intake of Mn salts result in growth disturbances resembling vitamin D-deficiency rickets (Bl 38). However, the mechanisms involved are poorly understood. The aim of the present study was to compare the effect of Mn, phosphate depletion and starvation on the epiphyseal growth cartilage in young rats by applying stereological methods at the light microscopical level.

MATERIAL AND METHODS

Three-week old male Sprague Dawley rats were divided into groups with five animals in each and given 0 (control group), 1% and 2% (w/w) Mn added to a standard laboratory rat diet. One group of animals was given a diet with a very low content of phosphor (0.02%), and in order to detect a possible unspecific effect of malnutrition one group of animals was severely starved. After 25 days on the respective diets the animals were killed and samples were taken for determination of Mn in whole blood and cartilage by neutron activation analysis (Co 66), and Ca and P in serum by routine colorimetric methods. From each animal the upper part of one tibia

was cut into ten pieces, fixed in glutaraldehyde and embedded in
epoxy resin. From each block one semi-thin section was cut and from
each section one micrograph covering the whole growth plate was
taken. The total height of the plate was measured and the relative
volume fractions of the different zones of the plate was calculated
by point counting (We 79).

RESULTS AND DISCUSSION

Increasing doses of Mn in the diet resulted in decreasing
concentration of P in serum (Table 1). The rats that were given
2% Mn – an amount that on a molar basis exceeded the amount of P in
the food – developed severe hypophosphatemia and florid rickets.
These animals also showed an increased amount of Mn in blood and
cartilage. The animals that got 1% Mn in the diet developed slight
rachitic changes. The severity of the rachitic lesions, as judged by
the total height of the growth plate and the relative volume of the
hypertrophic zone (Table 2) was closely related to the decrease of P
in serum. Moreover, phosphate depletion per se also resulted in
rickets. Starvation, on the other hand, caused a decrease in the
total height of the plate and in the volume fraction of the
hypertrophic zone. Even though in Mn rickets other and more direct
effects cannot be excluded, the present data indicate that the most
important factor in this form of rickets is phosphate depletion
caused by the precipitation of insoluble $MnHPO_4$ in the intestine.
In this respect Mn rickets differs from another experimental model,
i.e. strontium rickets, in which the serum level of P remains
unaltered (Re 84). Thus it is likely that several different
pathomechanisms are involved when rickets is induced by adding
various metal ions to the diet.

SUMMARY

Manganese given orally to young rats resulted in rickets. By
characterizing the lesions by stereological methods, it was shown
that the severity of the lesions were dose-related. Florid rickets
was associated with a considerably decreased concentration of P in
serum. Our results indicate that the most important factor in the
development of Mn rickets is phosphate depletion due to intestinal
precipitation of insoluble $MnHPO_4$.

Table 1. Body weights and results of the analyses of Ca, P and Mn.

Mean ± SEM

Diet/ Group	Weight at sacrifice g	Calcium in serum mM	Phosphor in serum mM	Manganese	
				in serum	in cartilage ppm
Control	290±5	2.64±0.01	2.78±0.03	0.05±0.01	0.12±0.01
Mn 1%	138±6[1]	2.73±0.03	2.80±0.07	0.08±0.02	0.62±0.01[1]
Mn 2%	84±2[1]	2.71±0.05	0.36±0.07[1]	2.44±0.58[1]	11.63±1.90[1]
P 0.02%	109±5[1]	3.44±0.09	1.54±0.24[1]	-	-
Starved	108±3[1]	2.64±0.02	4.18±0.15[1]	-	-

[1]Different from the corresponding control value at a level of significance of $\alpha = 0.05$ (two-sided test).

Table 2. Results of the stereological analyses. Mean ± SEM

Diet/ Group	Total height of the growth plate μm	Resting zone V_v*	Prolifer-ative zone V_v*	Hyper-trophic zone V_v*	Calcifying zone V_v*
Control	333±18	0.100±0.006	0.356±0.012	0.377±0.008	0.167±0.006
Mn 1%	332±16	0.075±0.003	0.301±0.009	0.455±0.010[1]	0.173±0.006
Mn 2%	778±32[1]	0.032±0.014[1]	0.213±0.010[1]	0.635±0.016[1]	0.120±0.014
P 0.02%	516±29[1]	0.061±0.004[1]	0.351±0.013	0.498±0.013[1]	0.088±0.010[1]
Starved	197± 7[1]	0.098±0.006	0.400±0.005	0.281±0.003[1]	0.244±0.007[1]

*V_v = volume density i.e. volume of each zone relative to total growth plate volume.

[1]Different from the corresponding control value at a level of significance of $\alpha = 0.05$ (two-sided test).

REFERENCES

B138 Blumberg H, Shelling O and Jackson D A, 1938, The production of manganese rickets in rats, J. Nutrition 16, 317 - 324.

Co66 Cotzias C G, Miller S T and Edwards J, 1966, Neutron activation analysis: The stability of manganese concentration in human blood and plasma, J. Lab. Clin. Med. 67, 936-949.

Me67 Mena I, Marin O, Fuenzalida S and Cotzias G, 1967, Chronic manganese poisoning, Neurology 17, 1123-1129.

Me81 Mena I, 1981, Manganese. in Disorders of Mineral Metabolism, (Eds Bronner F and Cobern S W) Academic Press, pp. 233-270.

Re84 Reinholt F P, Hjerpe A, Jansson K and Engfeldt B, 1984, Stereological studies on the epiphyseal growth plate in strontium rickets with special reference to the distribution of matrix vesicles, J. Bone Joint Surgery, Accepted.

We79 Weibel E R, 1979, Stereological Methods for Biological Morphometry, Academic Press, New York.

34

Influence of External Irradiation on Sr Deposit in Bone

P. GERASIMO, R. DUCOUSSO and H. METIVIER

Simultaneous exposure to external irradiation and internal emitters can occur as a consequence of nuclear war, as well as following a sufficiently serious accident with a nuclear reactor. In both cases, some of population that might ingest ^{90}Sr could also be expected to receive substantial doses of external radiation. It is therefore of interest to study the effects of a combination of Sr and external irradiation in an animal model system.

The aim of this work is to show a difference in the retention by organism and skeleton, or in the cellular distribution of the cation, between irradiated and un-irradiated rats.

MATERIALS AND METHODS

CD/COBS male rats of 200gr purchased from Charles River France were irradiated at various doses, and injected intravenously with ^{85}Sr (370kBq). Animals were killed on different times after injection of Sr. Deposit of cation was studied in skeleton and in subcellular fraction of hepatic cells. Hypophysectomy and thyroidectomy were also performed.

All other details are described elsewhere (Ge 84).

RESULTS AND DISCUSSION

On the first day after irradiation, the dose of 9Gy produced a transitory increase of phosphate and calcium in serum, of about 20 percent. These data correlated with bone remodeling just after irradiation. We did not observe any significant modifications for the two other doses levels, 7, 5   and 4Gy.

After intravenous injection of strontium, Sr deposit was measured in skeleton of irradiated and un-irradiated rats (Table I). Kinetic studies with Sr, used like bone formation marker, demonstrated an apparent lack of correlation between Sr deposit and serum parameters, described previously.

TABLE I : Kinetic of strontium retention by skeleton

	Control	4 Gray	9 Gray
Time to reach saturation (minute)	20	20	20
Percent of injected Sr at saturation (1 hour)	52^+_-4	50^+_-4	53^+_-3

Calcium regulation at cellular levels is assured by mitochondria; osteocyte-like hepatocyte mitochondria concentrate calcium and strontium (Ma 73). Also we have used hepatic mitochondria, easier to isolate than osteocyte mitochondria to study Sr uptake. In toto irradiated animals we observed an large increase of Sr uptake in hepatic mitochondria (Fig.1). If we operated with thyroidectomised or hypophysectomised animals, the increase of Sr uptake was not really significant compared to controls (Fig.1). The same effect in observed if we used organ slices irradiated in vitro.

In all cases, similar results were obtained with ^{45}Ca.

Such observations lead us to think that a hormonal effect after irradiation is necessary for Sr and Ca uptake by mitochondria, probably through stimulation of hypothalamo-hypophysal hormones and thyroid hormones.

In conclusion, irradiation does not alter retention of Sr by skeleton. But on the other hand, irradiation produces changes of metabolism of Sr and Ca, at cellular scale, in mitochondria, probably by hormonal stimulation. Consequently we can expect,for survivors of such an irradiation, disturbance of alkaline earth cation metabolism in tissues and particularly in bones.

REFERENCES

Ge 84 Gerasimo, P. and Ducousso, R. (1984). Effet de l'irradiation sur la distribution subcellulaire du strontium dans le foie de rat in vivo et in vitro , C.R. Acad. Sc. Paris, <u>298</u>, 267-270.

Ma 73 Matthews, J.L. and Martin, J.H. (1973). Role of mitochondria in modulating calcium and phosphate . Physico-chimie et cristallographie des apatites d'intérêt biologique, Colloques Internationaux du CNRS, <u>230</u>, 150-155.

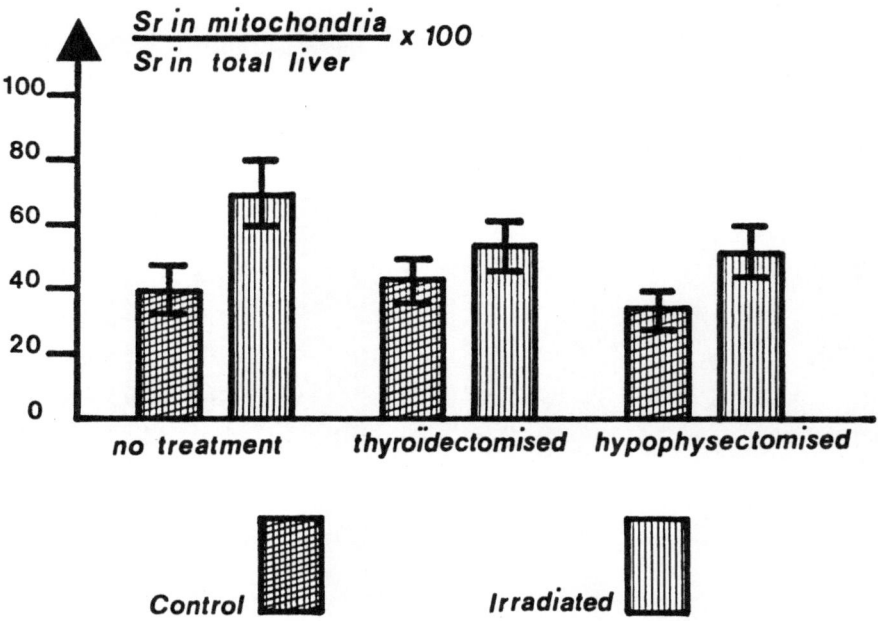

FIGURE 1 Uptake by mitochondria in control; thyroidectomised and hypophysectomised rats (injection of Sr, 20mn before sacrifice ; irradiation,9Gy, 1 day before of strontium). Vertical lines are S.E.M.

REFERENCES

Part 7
Trace Metals in Bone

35

The Variation with Flow-Rate of the Extraction of Bone-Seeking Tracers in Recirculation Experiments

P. TOTHILL, G. HOOPER, I. D. McCARTHY and S. P. F. HUGHES

INTRODUCTION

Bone blood flow is important, not only for the life and growth of bone itself, but also for the homeostasis in the body of several substances and the transport of all the materials that are the subject of this symposium. Its measurement is complicated by multiple arteries and veins and the presence of bone marrow. The main techniques that have been used are: (1) the clearance of "bone-seeking" tracers such as calcium, strontium and fluorine, (2) indicator fractionation using microspheres and (3) the washout of diffusible tracers such as iodo-antipyrine or xenon. All rely on radioactive labels and most are invasive, practicable only in experimental animals. Only the first has been attempted in man; its success requires that the extraction from blood by bone of a particular tracer is constant and this assumption has usually been made.

Before entering peri-vascular space en route to bone mineral any solute in plasma has to diffuse through the capillary endothelium. The Renkin theory of capillary permeability (Re59) predicts that only at low flows is there time for complete transfer of a diffusible solute before the distal end of the capillary is reached. At higher flows the extraction is diffusion-limited.

Evidence for the flow-dependence of extraction in bone has been provided by comparing the venous concentration of the tracer of interest with that of a non-permeable marker injected simultaneously

into the arterial supply of the bone. Using a perfusion of ^{99m}Tc
methylene diphosphonate (MDP) into the tibial nutrient artery of a
dog McCarthy et al showed that extraction decreased with increasing
flow (McC80,83). Such experiments are invasive and examine only a
part of the circulation to one bone. Schoutens et al provided
qualitative confirmation of the flow-dependence of the extraction of
^{45}Ca and ^{99m}Tc polyphosphate in recirculation experiments in rat
tibiae and femora by comparing clearances with flow measured by
microsphere uptake, heating and cooling the legs to promote flow
differences (Sc79). We reported similar findings in the rat skeleton
(To80,84a).

This presentation extends the clearance versus microsphere uptake
experiments to the dog, with better quantitation. The microsphere
technique used offers the best available method of measuring bone
blood flow in animals. We have reviewed its validity (To84b); some
minor doubts remain, as will be seen later.

METHODS

10 adult greyhounds with weights between 20 and 30 kg were
anaesthetised with pentabarbitone. Cannulae were inserted into left
carotid and tail arteries and attached to pumps to withdraw blood at a
known rate. The dogs were ventilated, the chest opened and cannulae
inserted into the left atria. After the pumps were started, ^{85}Sr as
strontium chloride was injected into the heart, followed by ^{113}Sn-
labelled microspheres, 15 μm in diameter (New England Nuclear
Corporation). In 2 of the animals Na^{18}F and in 2 others ^{99m}Tc MDP
were added to the ^{85}Sr injection. After 5 minutes the animal was
killed with an overdose of potassium chloride. The leg bones were
removed quickly to minimise the possibility of post-mortem migration
of ^{85}SrCl$_2$ (To78).

The periosteum was scraped off the bones, they were each cut into
4 segments and the diaphyseal marrow removed. Radioactivity of bones
and blood was measured in a large sample detector or well
scintillation counter as appropriate. Corrections were made for background, crossover between different energy channels and decay, and
measurements expressed as a proportion of the administered dose.
Counting statistics were better than 3% and for most samples the

number of microspheres in a specimen was no greater limit to precision, although bigger uncertainties applied for some segments in which flow was low.

Methods of calculation

The reference organ technique was used to obtain the cardiac output (CO) by dividing the pump rate by the proportion of the administered microsphere activity in the arterial blood. Blood flow (F) then came from CO multiplied by microsphere uptake in the bone. Specific flow was derived from F divided by bone weight.

Clearance of tracers from blood to bone was similarly obtained from bone activity x pump rate ÷ blood activity. The extraction ratio (E) was defined as C/F and was the net extraction in the 5 minute period between injection and death.

RESULTS

Mean results for whole bones are summarised in Table 1.

Table 1. Blood flows from microsphere distributions and ^{85}Sr clearances from bone uptake and blood concentration. Mostly n = 20. Means ± standard deviations.

	Blood flow (F) ml min^{-1}	Clearance of Sr-85 (C) ml min^{-1}	Extraction ratio, C/F	Specific flow ml min^{-1} 100 g^{-1}
Tibia	5.3 ± 3.4	4.1 ± 3.5	0.69 ± 0.16	5.1 ± 2.8
Femur	13.0 ± 7.8	6.2 ± 3.3	0.50 ± 0.07	10.9 ± 5.6
Radius + ulna	3.8 ± 2.6	2.6 ± 1.6	0.70 ± 0.08	4.9 ± 2.4
Humerus	14.3 ± 8.0	5.9 ± 2.8	0.46 ± 0.11	13.0 ± 6.2
Tibia marrow	0.34 ± 0.41	0.10 ± 0.13		8.6 ± 11.1
Femur marrow	1.79 ± 1.36	0.23 ± 0.15		28.0 ± 21.0
Humerus marrow	1.07 ± 0.73	0.12 ± 0.07		29.4 ± 18.6
Cardiac output	3974 ± 1746			

It can be seen that the blood flow to the proximal bone of each leg was much **higher** than that to the distal bone, the mean ratio of specific flows being 3.3 ± 0.9 for the forelegs and 2.3 ± 0.4 for hind legs.

The difference was maintained after normalisation for bone weight. Differences of [85]Sr clearance were less so that on average the extraction in the tibia was 1.38 times that in the femur, and in the radius plus ulna 1.52 times that in the humerus. There is a wide dispersion of flows and clearances and this finding is illustrated more clearly in Fig. 1, in which the extraction ratio (E) for [85]Sr is plotted against specific blood flow. This figure also illustrates the most important finding from these studies, of a diminution of extraction ratio as flow is increased.

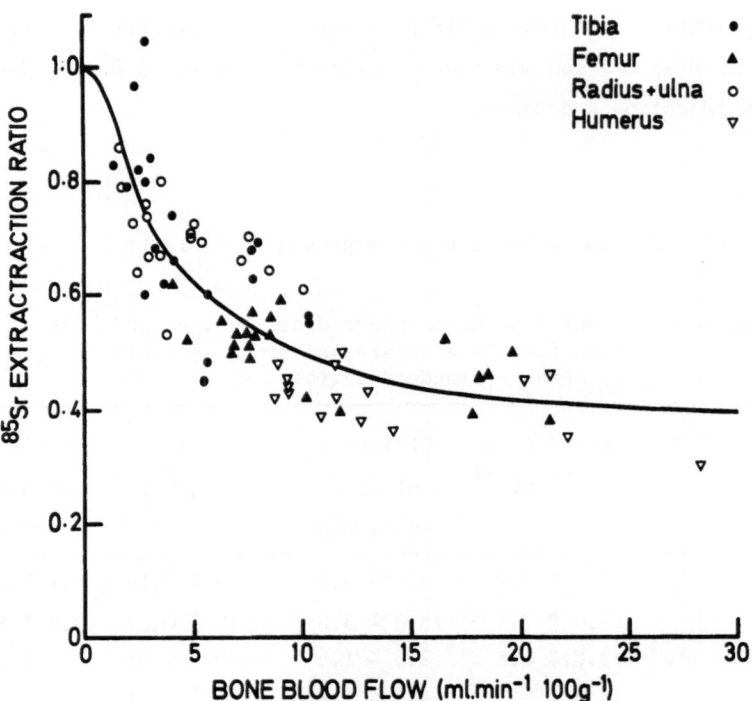

FIGURE 1   Variation of extraction ratio of [85]Sr with blood flow in dog leg bones.

As this result is in accordance with the Renkin theory of capillary permeability it was thought best to fit a regression line arising from that theory, which leads to the expression $PS = -F\ln(1-E)$, where P is the permeability and S the surface area of a capillary or set of capillaries, in the absence of back diffusion. It has been postulated that PS is constant if a given bone is perfused over a range of flow rates (McC83) and if so a plot of $-F\ln(1-E)$ against F would produce a horizontal line. Fig. 2 shows that our data cluster around a line, but that it is not horizontal. On the other hand it does not go through the origin, which would be the case if extraction did not change with flow. This intermediate finding is not surprising in view of the mixture of bones and animals and possible causes of blood flow differences. The technique gives a plausible and useful fit to the data.

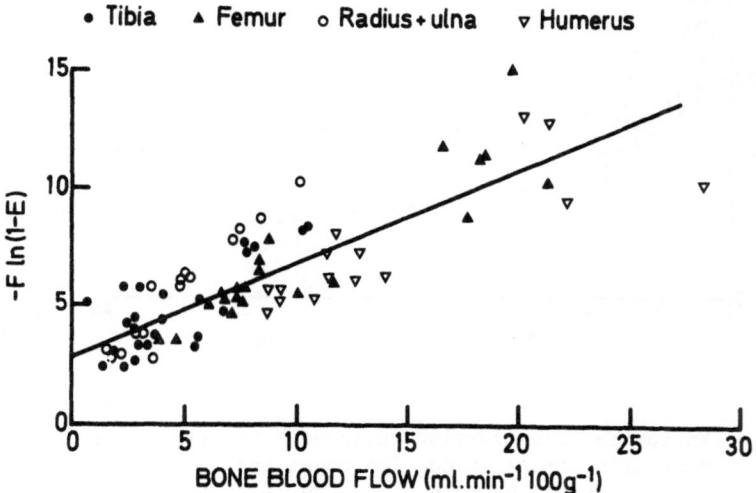

FIGURE 2   Function -Fln(1-E), derived from Renkin theory, plotted against dog leg bone blood flow (F).

Clearances, flows and extraction ratios were also calculated for each of the bone quarters, the centre two representing mostly the diaphyses and the end two the metaphyses. Extraction is plotted against flow in Fig. 3. Specific flows were in general lower in the cortical bone of the shafts and extraction lower for a given flow. In fact, the regression line fitted to the shaft data is closer to that expected with a constant product PS.

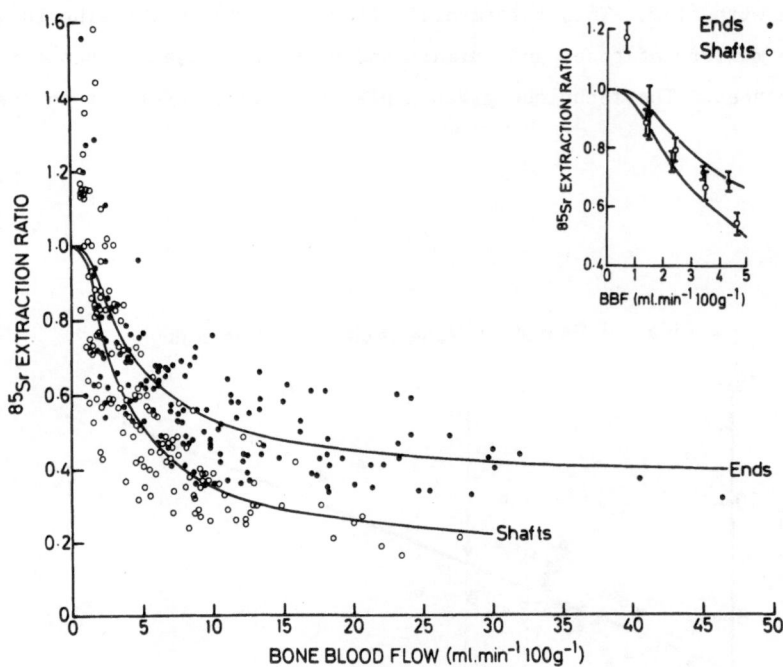

FIGURE 3   Variation of extraction ratio of ^{85}Sr with blood flow in
central sections of dog leg bones and in outer sections.
In the insert the mean values for each interval of 1 ml
min^{-1} 100 g^{-1} and their standard errors are plotted on an
expanded scale.

More limited data are available for ^{18}F and ^{99m}Tc MDP, and
extraction ratios for these two agents are plotted against flow in
Fig. 4. The regression line is that for ^{85}Sr. There is little
difference in behaviour between the three tracers; on average ^{18}F
extraction was slightly higher and ^{99m}Tc MDP extraction lower than
that for ^{85}Sr.

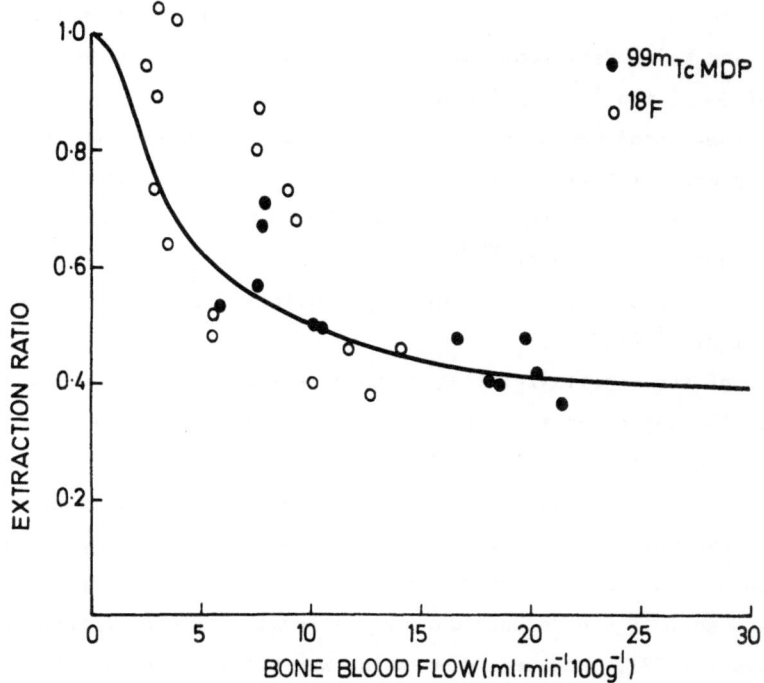

FIGURE 4   Variation of extraction ratios of ^{18}F and ^{99m}Tc MDP with blood flow in dog bones. The regression line from the [85]Sr data is superimposed.

DISCUSSION

Table 1 and Fig. 1 show that there was a wide range of bone blood flow, as determined by microsphere uptake, in different bones and dogs; this spread has provided the opportunity to examine the variations of extraction with flow rate without any interventions. The fact that the spread persists after normalising for bone weight demonstrates the folly of trying to predict total skeletal flow from measurements on a single bone, as has been frequently attempted.

Figs. 1 and 4 show that within each bone type and more particularly when all the results are combined, the extraction ratio for all three tracers falls with increasing flow from a value of near unity at low flows to about 0.4 at a specific flow of 30 ml min^{-1} 100 g^{-1}. The reduction is greater if only the bone shafts are considered (Fig. 3). The results confirm the data obtained with rats. Schoutens et al reported that clearances of $^{45}CaCl_2$ and ^{99m}Tc polyphosphate increased less quickly than bone blood flow, but did not quantitate extractions (Sc79). We found in similar experiments that the mean extraction of $^{85}SrCl_2$ and $Na^{18}F$ fell from more than one to about 0.6 at specific flows of 50 ml min^{-1} 100 g^{-1} (To84a).

The flow-dependence of extraction is consistent with theories of capillary wall diffusion. It also agrees with the results of nutrient artery perfusion experiments. For example, McCarthy and Hughes found that the net extraction of ^{99m}Tc MDP in 2.5 minutes in the dog tibia was 0.29 at a flow rate of 1.9 ml min^{-1}, 0.18 at 3.8 ml min^{-1} and 0.05 at 7.6 ml min^{-1} (McC83).

A few of the results relating to bone segments with very low flow rates in the dog experiments and many more of the rat results introduce some niggling doubts about the validity of the technique, as clearances were apparently higher than blood flows. An extraction greater than unity is clearly impossible. We identified a possible cause in some of the rat experiments, namely post-mortem migration of ^{85}Sr from soft tissue to bone during the lengthy time of cooking and dissection (To78). However, dissection was much quicker in the dog experiments and of the rat tibiae. It may be that such movements can occur in vivo, leading to higher concentrations of ^{85}Sr in bone than could be accounted for by transport in the blood, but we have no evidence on this possibility. Alternative explanations of impossibly high extraction ratios could come from a failure of microspheres to represent fully the blood entering bone. Prior trapping in a capillary bed (To80), unequal partition at junctions, as has been demonstrated in models (Of83), or arterio-venous shunting are all possibilities, but with no evidence implicating any of them. The underestimate of flow does not need to be very great to cause the anomalies. The addition of only 1 ml min^{-1} 100 g^{-1} to the segment flows would bring all the extractions below one.

These small doubts about validity are included as a caution and do not affect the main conclusions. Ignorance of the flow-dependence of extraction has led to a number of erroneous deductions. In early work Copp and Shim found that ^{85}Sr clearances were the same in dog tibia and femur and deduced that blood flows were also similar (Co65). Our measurements show that the specific flow to the femur is about twice

that to the tibia, the near equality of specific ^{85}Sr clearances being
modified by different extraction ratios. Wootton et al (Wo76)
developed a method of measuring total skeletal flow in man based on the
premise of an invariant 100% extraction of ^{18}F. We have demonstrated
the invalidity of the single passage experiments leading to this
deduction (To84c). Closer to the subject of this symposium, the same
assumption has led to doubtful conclusions about plutonium deposition
in bone (Hu77,82). In fact, the finding that extraction varies with
flow demonstrates that skeletal blood flow cannot be measured by the
clearance of any "bone-seeking tracer". Clearances of other diffusible
substances will be similarly related in a non-linear manner to blood
flow and this must be considered in the interpretation of bone uptake.

SUMMARY

The extraction of "bone-seeking" and all other diffusible tracers
depends on the rate of blood flow. The clearance by bone from blood
of such tracers cannot therefore be used to measure bone blood flow.

Specific blood flows and clearances differ considerably in different
parts of the skeleton.

REFERENCES

Co65   Copp D. H. and Shim S. S., 1965, Extraction ratio and bone
clearance of ^{85}Sr as a measure of effective bone blood flow , Circ.
Res. 16, 461-467.

Hu77   Humphreys E. R., Fisher G. and Thorne M. C., 1977, The
measurement of blood flow in mouse femur and its correlation with
^{239}Pu deposition , Calcif. Tissue Res. 23, 141-145.

Hu82   Humphreys E. R., Green D., Howells G. R. and Thorne M. C., 1982,
Relationship between blood flow, bone structure and ^{239}Pu deposition
in the mouse skeleton , Calcif. Tissue Int. 34, 416-421.

McC80   McCarthy I. D., Hughes S. P. F. and Orr J. S., 1980, An
experimental model to study the relationship between blood flow and
uptake for bone-seeking radionuclides in normal bone , Clin. Phys.
Physiol. Meas. 1, 135-143.

McC83   McCarthy I. D. and Hughes S. P. F., 1983, The role of skeletal
blood flow in determining the uptake of ^{99m}Tc-methylene diphosphonate
Calcif. Tissue Int. 35, 508-511.

Of83   Øfjord E. S. and Clausen G., 1983, Intrarenal flow of microspheres and red blood cells: skimming in slit and tube models , Am.
J. Physiol. 245, H429-H436.

Re59   Renkin E. M., 1959, Transport of potassium-42 from blood to
tissue in isolated mammalian skeletal muscles , Am. J. Physiol. 197,
1205-1210.

Sc79   Schoutens A., Bergmann P. and Verhas M., 1979, Bone blood flow
measured by ^{85}Sr microspheres and bone seeker clearances in the rat ,
Am. J. Physiol, 236, H1-H6.

To78   Tothill P. and MacPherson J. N., 1978, Post-mortem migration of
bone-seeking radionuclides in the rat and rabbit and its effect on
estimates of bone uptake , Clin. Sci. Mol. Med. 55, 221-223.

To80   Tothill P. and MacPherson J. N., 1980, Limitations of microspheres as tracers for bone blood flow and extraction ratio studies ,
Calcif. Tissue Int. 31, 261-265.

To84a   Tothill P. and Hooper G., 1984, Bone blood flow and extraction
ratios: microspheres and bone seekers , in: Proceedings of Third
International Symposium on Circulation in Bone (Edited by Hungerford
D. S. and Arlet J.) (Baltimore: Williams and Wilkens).

To84b   Tothill P., 1984, Bone blood flow measurement , J. Biomed. Eng.
(in press).

To84c   Tothill P. and Hooper G., 1984, Invalidity of single-passage
measurements of the extraction of bone-seeking tracers in rats and
rabbits , J. Orthop. Res. (in press).

Wo76   Wootton R., Reeve J. and Veall N., 1976, The clinical measurement of skeletal blood flow , Clin. Sci. Mol. Med. 50, 261-268.

36

Chromium Exchange in the Rat Skeleton

S. WALLACH and R. L. VERCH

INTRODUCTION

In a recent study of ^{51}Cr exchange in rats 9–18 months old it was noted that skeletal ^{51}Cr decreased by 30% compared to 2 month old control rats (Wa85). The present study was undertaken to study this aging phenomenon further by additional experimentation and to collate our prior experience with skeletal ^{51}Cr exchange in rats under pathologic and physiologic conditions.

METHODS

Male Sprague–Dawley rats weighing 200–500 g were obtained from Blue Spruce Farms (Altamont, NY, USA) and acclimatized to the animal facility for 14 days before the experiments were initiated. All rats received Wayne rat chow and tap water ad lib. Three days before sacrifice, each animal was injected intravenously with a tracer dose of trivalent ^{51}Cr of high specific activity (New England Nuclear Corp., Boston, MA, USA; 550 mCi per mg) which contained 1–2 μCi ^{51}Cr and 1.9–3.8 ng total Cr. The isotope was prepared for injection by dilution in rat serum so that 0.20 ml contained the desired tracer dose. Identical doses were delivered into 250 and 500 ml plastic bottles containing 1.0 ml of 22% bovine serum albumin per 100 ml and 1.4 mg $K_2Cr_2O_7$ per 100 ml. These served as 100% standards for the determination of total body ^{51}Cr using a rat whole body counter for rats weighing less than 400 g and a gamma camera for rats weighing above 400 g. The standards and rats were counted differentially at the ^{51}Cr peak (0.32 MeV) three days after ^{51}Cr injection. Immediately after determination of body ^{51}Cr content, all urine passed during the previous three-day period was collected and the rats were killed by exsanguination from the abdominal aorta under pentobarbital anesthesia (5 mg per 100 g BW). Serum and various tissues, including the left tibia, were taken and placed in counting vials for ^{51}Cr analysis in an automatic gamma well counter. Standards consisting of 1% of the injected dose were prepared and interspaced among the sample vials. The tissues were counted differentially at the 0.32 MeV peak. The serum and tissue data were expressed as percent injected dose per g or ml and as percent injected dose per tibia. The tibial data is detailed in this manuscript and the remainder of the data will be reported in a separate manuscript. The Student t Test for matched groups (two-tail) was used to determine statistical significance.

To define total and regional skeletal ^{51}Cr more closely, seven rats of varying sex, size and strain were sacrificed three days after ^{51}Cr injection as per the above protocol. The left tibia was removed for ^{51}Cr counting as above and the remainder of the viscera and most of the skin removed manually. The carcasses were then placed in vats containing 0.5 M NaOH for 4-5 days with two changes of NaOH during the procedure. After dissolution of all soft tissues, the bones were removed, rinsed thoroughly in tap water and air-dried. The bones were divided into the following anatomic groups: skull, upper extremity long bones, scapulae, body vertebrae, tail vertebrae, pelvis, femurs, and right tibia. Ribs, small bones of the extremities and other unidentifiable fragments were pooled as a miscellaneous group. All nine groups and the fresh dissected left tibia, which was not subjected to NaOH treatment, were counted in an automatic gamma well counter as per the above protocol.

RESULTS

Tibial ^{51}Cr exchange was negatively correlated with body weight as shown in Figures 1 and 2 in which the ^{51}Cr data are expressed as percent dose per g (r = 0.95) and percent dose per tibia (r = 0.86), respectively.

TABLE 1. Tibial ^{51}Cr Parameters Segregated According to Weight

| | | ^{51}Cr Content | |
	Mean Weight	Percent Dose/g	Percent Dose/Tibia
Group 1 (11)	323 ± 15	0.600 ± .033	0.383 ± .015
Group 2 (12)	474 ± 11*	0.264 ± .022*	0.242 ± .016*

Values are means ± SEM.
Parenthesis indicate number of animals in each group.
*p<.0005

Table 1 compares the tibial ^{51}Cr data in the 11 rats weighing 270 to 380 g (Group 1) with the 12 rats weighing 440 to 560 g (Group 2). The larger rats in Group 2 had a 37-56% lesser tibial ^{51}Cr content than Group 1 (p < 0.0005).

The total and regional skeletal ^{51}Cr data for individual rats are shown in Table 2 in order of increasing body weight. As noted previously (Wa85a), although there was greater body retention of ^{51}Cr with increasing weight, the increment was relatively small and did not exceed 35% despite increments in body weight beyond 100%. Skeletal weight accounted for 4-6% of body weight and skeletal ^{51}Cr for 12-17% of retained body ^{51}Cr. On a percent dose per g basis, a trend to declining skeletal ^{51}Cr content with increasing body weight was discernible among all anatomic portions of the skeleton. A 60-80% decrease in skeletal ^{51}Cr content (per g) was present in the male 560 g rat (No. 7) compared with the two female rats weighing less than 200 g (Nos. 1,2). The male rats weighing 280 - 380 g (Nos. 3-6) had intermediate values. The data were insufficient to determine whether the weight related decline in ^{51}Cr content (per g) was different in various parts of the skeleton. Inexplicably, there was no agreement or a fixed relationship between the ^{51}Cr content of the two tibias processed by the two different methods.

Using the range of values in Figure 1 as a "normal" relationship between weight and tibial ^{51}Cr content, a comparison has been made with the tibial ^{51}Cr data noted in previously published (Ja79, Ja81, Ka79, Li80, Wa83, Wa84, Wa85a) and unpublished experiments (Table 3, Figure 3). The mean tibial ^{51}Cr content for the intact rats in these experiments are shown as closed symbols in Figure 3 and fall within or close to the "normal" range. The single group of intact female rats fell slightly below this range.

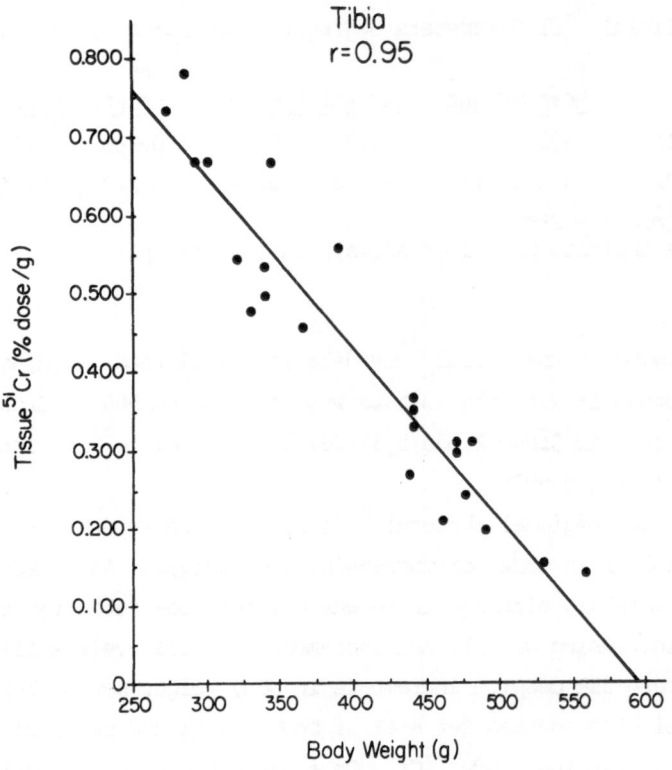

Figure 1:   Relation between tibial ^{51}Cr content and body weight
in male Sprague-Dawley rats 250-560 g BW. Tibial ^{51}Cr
is expressed as percent dose per g.

The effects of endocrine ablation and replacement on tibial ^{51}Cr
content are given in Table 4. Streptozotocin induced diabetes
mellitus caused a 15% decrease in tibial ^{51}Cr whereas endogenous
hyperinsulinemia induced by glucose feeding caused a 33% increase in
tibial ^{51}Cr. Insulin administration to the diabetic rats restored
tibial ^{51}Cr content to normal. Adrenal, hypophyseal and
thyroparathyroid ablation all increased tibial ^{51}Cr by 30-90% which
was not reversed by short term replacement with growth hormone,
thyroxine, parathyroid hormone or calcitonin. Neither ADH
deficiency nor pitressin replacement had an effect on tibial ^{51}Cr.

Since some of the endocrine ablated groups were of lower body
weight than the controls (although of comparable age), it is
possible that part of the increased ^{51}Cr was related to low body
weight. However, the tibial ^{51}Cr levels were higher than would be
expected from the "normal" relationship between tibial ^{51}Cr and body

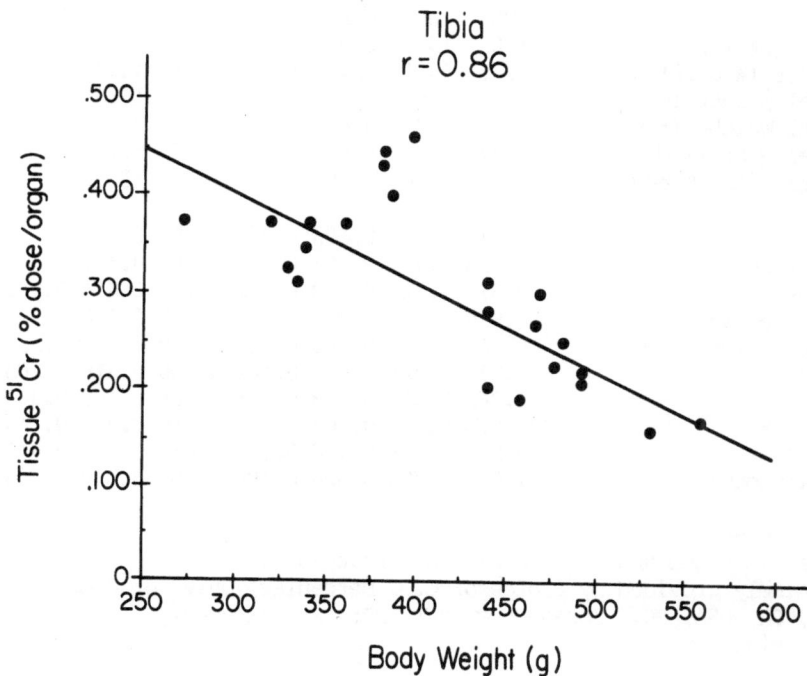

Figure 2:   Relation between tibial ^{51}Cr content, expressed as
              percent dose per bone, and body weight in male
              Sprague–Dawley rats 250–500 g BW.

weight indicated earlier in this report. Unfortunately, "normal"
data are not available below 250 g and the possibility that the
increase in tibial ^{51}Cr content in the endocrine ablated rats was to
some degree due to an upward inflection in the "normal" relationship
at low body weight cannot be eliminated.

Table 5 contains experimental data in rats subjected to Cr
deprivation and overload, LiCl administration, pregnancy and salt
loading. The significant changes in tibial ^{51}Cr observed in several
of these experiments appear to be due in part to weight differences
between the control and experimental groups and not to the
experimental conditions alone.

TABLE 2. Skeletal ^{51}Cr Content In Individual Rats

	Rat Number						
	1	2	3	4	5	6	7
Sex	F	F	M	M	M	M	M
Strain	BHE	BHE	BHE	BHE	SD	SHR	SD
Body Weight (g)	178	197	289	319	320	373	560
Body ^{51}Cr (% dose)	37.5	40.1	49.5	40.6	45.1	44.7	51.1
Skeletal Weight (g)	8.0	8.5	11.1	13.9	18.3	15.8	-
Skeletal Weight (% BW)	4.5	4.3	3.8	4.4	5.7	4.2	-
Skeletal ^{51}Cr (% dose)	6.37	6.99	6.91	5.91	7.54	5.13	-
Skeletal ^{51}Cr (% body ^{51}Cr)	17.0	17.4	14.0	14.6	16.7	11.5	-
Skull*	0.592	0.692	0.403	0.298	0.356	0.234	-
Upper Extremities*	0.718	0.927	0.606	0.373	0.481	0.371	-
Scapulae*	0.977	1.125	0.728	0.492	0.746	0.434	0.293
Body Vertebrae*	0.938	1.061	0.738	0.452	0.372	0.378	0.271
Tail Vertebrae*	0.561	0.732	0.598	0.348	0.459	0.307	0.132
Pelvis*	0.832	0.924	0.682	0.441	0.456	0.316	0.285
Femurs*	0.762	0.947	0.668	0.444	0.508	0.368	0.364
Tibia 1*,**	0.678	0.779	0.567	0.420	0.536	0.226	0.143
Tibia 2*	0.928	0.998	0.724	0.474	0.458	0.361	0.448
Miscellaneous*	1.052	0.703	0.620	0.490	0.301	0.380	0.359

*Percent dose/g
**Tibia dissected and counted without treatment with NaOH
BHE: Kindly provided by Professor C.D. Berdanier, Univ. of Georgia, Athens, GA, USA; SD: Sprague-Dawley; SHR: Spontaneously hypertensive rat

DISCUSSION

Atomic absorption spectrophotometric measurements of skeletal Cr, although fraught with technical problems, indicate that there are significant quantities of Cr in the skeleton. Recent Cr measurements in this laboratory indicated a mean value of 29.8 ± 4.1 (SEM) ng/g in fresh adult rat tibia compared to mean levels of 3-31 ng/g in soft tissues (Ve83). Rosholt and Hegarty (Ro81) have inexplicably reported values 200 fold higher in other rat bones using emission spectrography. In any case, the present and previous reports from this laboratory indicate that skeletal Cr is readily exchangeable with injected ^{51}Cr and the skeleton is a major concentrating organ for both stable and radioactive Cr.

Skeletal uptake of ^{51}Cr depends upon the size of the skeletal pool of stable Cr as well as its rate of exchange. It is therefore difficult to equate ^{51}Cr levels with stable Cr levels. Nevertheless, some data exist supporting Cr deficiency with increasing age and also with pregnancy (Wa85). The fact that

TABLE 3. Mean Tibial ^{51}Cr in Intact Rats of Varying Weight

Reference	Rat Strain	Sex	Mean Weight	Mean Tibial ^{51}Cr (Percent Dose/g)
Ja79	CD	M	155	1.51
Ja79	CD	M	185	0.94
Ka79	CD	M	225	0.76
Wa85a	CD	M	237	0.94
Ja79	CD	M	259	0.87
Wa83	BH	M	259	0.78
Li80	CD	M	260	0.74
Li80	CD	M	265	0.71
Li80	CD	M	270	0.72
Wa83	SD	M	281	0.65
Wa83	BH	M	285	0.63
Wa85b	WKY	M	289	0.77
Wa85a	SD	M	290	0.75
Wa84	SD	F	291	0.53
Wa83	SD	M	303	0.66
Wa85b	WKY	M	306	0.58
Wa85a	SD	M	320	0.75
Wa83	SD	M	322	0.46
Wa85a	SD	M	330	0.64
Ka79	CD	M	350	0.46
Ja81	CD	M	392	0.55
Ja81	CD	M	406	0.37
Wa85a	SD	M	465	0.33
Wa85a	SD	M	547	0.17
Wa85a	SD	M	562	0.24
Wa85a	CD	M	615	0.15

Each group contained 5-12 rats. CD: Charles River Breeding
Laboratories. SD: Sprague-Dawley (Blue Spruce Farms). BH:
Brattleboro heterozygote (Blue Spruce Farms). WKY: Taconic Farms.

decreases in ^{51}Cr uptake by the skeleton were seen in experimental
models of both these conditions suggests that decreased ^{51}Cr uptake
may in fact reflect Cr depletion from the skeleton.

The ^{51}Cr data in experimental insulin deficiency and in
hyperinsulinemia probably represent the combined effects of size and
exchangeability of the skeletal Cr pool. In previous publications
(Ka79, Wa83), soft tissue ^{51}Cr distribution data were presented
supporting a positive influence of insulin on tissue ^{51}Cr exchange.
Other studies (Wa85) have suggested that diabetes mellitus causes
Cr depletion. The present data showing reduced skeletal ^{51}Cr uptake

TABLE 4. Mean Tibial ^{51}Cr During Endocrine Ablation and Replacement
(Percent Dose/g)

Condition	Control	Experimental	Endocrine Replacement
Diabetes Mellitus (Ka79)	0.46	0.39*	0.44 (Insulin)
Glucose Feeding (Wa83)	0.46	0.61*	-
Adrenalectomy (Ja79)	0.87	1.12*	-
Hypophysectomy (Ja79)	1.51	2.03*	-
	0.94	1.76*	1.64 (GH + T$_4$)*
Thyroparathyroidectomy (Li80)	0.74	1.01*	-
	0.71	0.97*	1.02 (T$_4$)*
	0.72	0.93*	1.00 (PTH)*
			0.91 (CT)*
ADH Deficiency (Wa83)	0.78	0.87	-
	0.63	0.73	0.75 (Pitressin)

Values are means for 5-12 rats per group.
*p<.05-.001
Parentheses indicate published references.
GH: Growth hormone; T$_4$: L-thyroxine; PTH: Parathyroid hormone;
CT: Calcitonin; ADH: Antidiuretic hormone.

TABLE 5. Mean Tibial ^{51}Cr in Non-Endocrine Experiments

Condition	Control	Experimental
Cr Deprivation (Ja81)	0.37	0.41
Cr Overload (Ja81)	0.55	0.59
LiCl Administration (Wa83)	0.66	0.69
	0.65	0.53*
Pregnancy (Wa84)	0.53	0.26*
NaCl Loading (Wa85b)	0.63	0.54*
	0.77	0.58*

Values are means for 5-12 rats per group.
*p<.05-.001, see text for explanation.
Parentheses indicate published references or submitted manuscripts.

in insulin deficiency and increased uptake during endogenous hyperinsulinemia are compatible with a similar effect of insulin on the skeleton.

In contrast, the skeletal ^{51}Cr data obtained in other endocrine deficiency states are discordant with ^{51}Cr exchange data in soft tissues. Skeletal ^{51}Cr was significantly increased in adrenalectomized, hypophysectomized and thyroparathyroidectomized rats. In the latter two preparations, soft tissue ^{51}Cr exchange was decreased and replacement with either growth hormone (GH) or thyroxine (T$_4$) returned soft tissue ^{51}Cr exchange toward normal with no influence on the increased skeletal [51]Cr (Ja79, Li80). The explanations for the differing responses of the skeleton and soft tissues and the insensitivity of skeletal ^{51}Cr to hormonal replacement are unclear. Skeletal turnover is generally reduced in hypophysectomized and thyroparathyroidectomized subjects. Thus, the kinetics of skeletal ^{51}Cr exchange are not related to the overall turnover of the skeletal system in these instances.

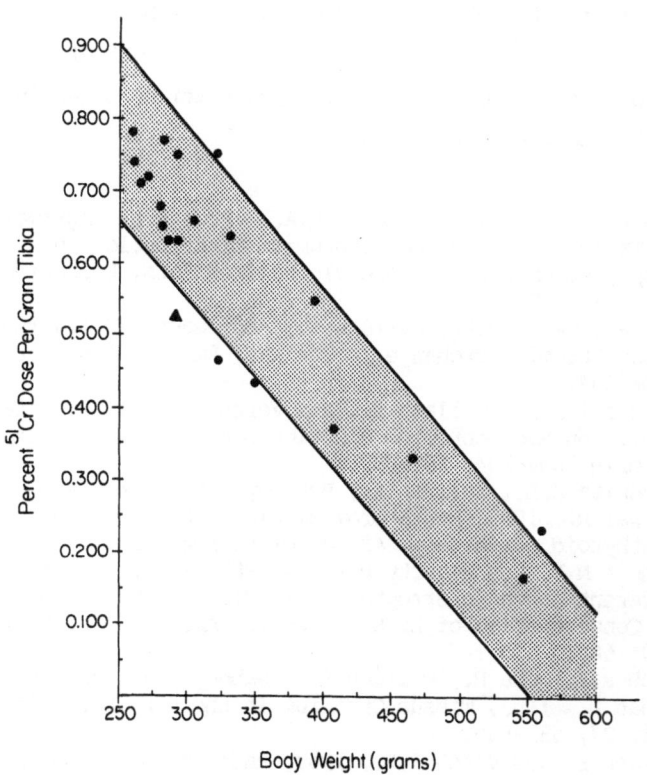

Figure 3:   Relation of mean tibial ^{51}Cr content observed in previous experiments summarized in Table 3 (●,▲) to range of tibial ^{51}Cr contents observed in the present experiments. The closed circles represent male rats and the closed triangle female rats.

SUMMARY

In summary, the skeleton appears to contain significant quantities of Cr which are readily exchangeable. Both aging and pregnancy decrease ^{51}Cr uptake by the skeleton and these phenomena probably result from Cr depletion from the skeleton rather than a primary decrease in Cr transport and exchangeability. Skeletal Cr exchange, however, appears to be under metabolic control of the endocrine system with insulin enhancing skeletal Cr exchange and the adrenal, pituitary and thyroparathyroid secretions decreasing Cr exchange, possibly by indirect mechanisms. Skeletal Cr exchange does not appear to depend on skeletal turnover. An assessment of the importance of skeletal Cr and of these observations regarding its kinetics will require further study.

REFERENCES

Ja79   Jain R., Wallach S., Peabody R.A., Verch R.L., Agrawal R., and Taylor R., 1979, Radiochromium Distribution in Hypophysectomized and Adrenalectomized Rats, Endocrinology 105, 1226-1229.

Ja81   Jain R., Verch R.L., Wallach S., and Peabody R.A., 1981, Tissue Chromium Exchange in the Rat, Am. J. Clin. Nutr. 34, 2199-2204.

Ka79   Kraszeski J.L., Wallach S., and Verch R.L., 1979, Effect of Insulin on Radiochromium Distribution in Diabetic Rats, Endocrinology 104, 881-885.

Li80   Lifschitz M.L., Wallach S., Peabody R.A., Verch R.L., and Agrawal R., 1980, Radiochromium Distribution in Thyroid and Parathyroid Deficiency, Am. J. Clin. Nutr. 33, 57-62.

Ro81   Rosholt M.N. and Hegarty P.V.J., 1981, Mineralization of Different Bones in Streptozotocin-Diabetic Rats: Study on the Concentration of Light Minerals, Am. J. Clin. Nutr. 34, 1680-1685.

Ve83   Verch R.L., Chu R., Wallach S., Peabody R.A., Jain R., and Hannan E., 1983, Tissue Chromium in the Rat, Nutr. Reports Intl. 27, 531-540.

Wa83   Wallach S. and Verch R.L., 1983, Radiochromium Conservation and Distribution in Diuretic States, J. Am. Coll. Nutr. 2, 163-172.

Wa84   Wallach S. and Verch R.L., 1984, Placental Transport of Chromium, J. Am. Coll. Nutr. 3, 69-74.

Wa85   Wallach S., 1985, Clinical and Biochemical Aspects of Chromium Deficiency, J. Am. Coll. Nutr., in press.

Wa85a   Wallach S. and Verch R.L., 1985, Radiochromium Distribution in Aged Rats, J. Am. Coll. Nutr., in press.

Wa85b   Wallach S. and Verch R.L., 1985, Radiochromium Conservation and Distribution During Osmotic Diuresis, J. Am. Coll. Nutr., in preparation.

37

Historical Changes of Trace Metals in Human Bones from France

Z. JAWOROWSKI, F. BARBALAT, C. BLAIN and E. PEYRE

INTRODUCTION

 During the past few decades a paradigm according to which man's
activity dangerously polluted the global environment and human
population with heavy metals dominated scientific thinking and public
opinion. This paradigm is based on a theoretical speculation which
states that the levels of Pb in man and in the environment were in
the past about 500 times lower than existing levels (Pa 65).
However, in a global scale study of temporal trends in concentration
of heavy metals in the glacier ice from the past few hundred years,
no detectable increase was found in the flows of Pb, Cd, Hg, V, U and
Ra-226 in to the global atmosphere (Ja 81). In the case of Pb the
existing evidence indicates that its contemporary level in human
bones is not much different than the prehistoric one and that in
European population this level decreased dramatically during the last
century (Table 1) due to improvements in hygiene conditions (Gr 75,
Ja 67).

 The heavy metals may enter the human body as natural input with
food, water and air, which depends mainly on the local geochemical
conditions and from the artificial sources in immediate (i.e. at

383

home and workplace) or more distant man's environment. The useful
information on the relative importance of these sources may be
provided by comparison of temporal changes of the levels of these
metals in human bones, which were changing in the past in relation to
the varying availability and use of particular metals and to the rate
of their anthropogenic dispersion in the environment.

In this paper we present the results of Pb, Cd and Zn
determination in ancient and contemporary human bones from France.
Some of the artificial sources of these metals in human body were not
existent in the past, but on the other hand others were more abundant
than now. We also determined the content of Ba and Mg which enter
the human body mainly with vegetarian and animal food, respectively.
Their environmental mobilization by man is similar to that of the
three other metals and their role as an immediate contaminant of man
is probably limited, but they, together with Ca, might be used as
indicators of long-term dietary or fossilization changes.

MATERIALS AND METHODS

Of a total of 180 human bone samples we studied 151 ancient and
29 contemporary bones. All ancient bones were parts of the limbs
except for 4 ribs and 3 vertebrae from Notre Dame de Paris. Among
contemporary human bones there were 11 vertebrae, 12 ribs, 1 femur
and 5 tibiae. All samples were collected in seven departments in
Northern, Central and Southern France. The ancient bones were
collected from graves at cemeteries exposed to percolating water
(Neolithic, Bronze Age, Roman and Merovingian), from a dolmen (Bronze
Age), from a cave (Bronze Age), and from ground burial sites and
underground crypts in churches and monasteries (Middle Ages and 18th
Century). The contemporary bones were collected by autopsy at
St Lois Hospital in Paris, from 18 persons aged 34 to 89 years, who
died between February and March 1984 (Table 2).

After collection the bones were sealed in polyethylene bags and
stored in a limited access laboratory with filtered air at positive
pressure. In a glove-box with filtered air, about 2 grams of bone
were ground from the internal wall of the medullary cavity, with
diamond drill. Before collecting the bone powder a 0.5 mm thick
surface layer was removed from the walls of the medullary cavity.

The medullary cavity was open at the moment of collecting the bone powder, so it was exposed only to the controlled atmosphere of the glove-box.

The contemporary bones were cleaned with stainless steel tools from periosteum, bone marrow and other soft tissues and then dried to a constant weight at 70°C. Then bone powder was prepared from tibiae and femora in the same way as in the case of ancient bones, only the spongiosa was collected from the central part of the body of the vertebrae and the ribs were ground in toto.

The powder bone was dried and then 500 mg samples were placed in clear-fused quartz beakers and wet ashed in Ultrapure Noratom or Suprapure Merck concentrated nitric and perchloric acids. The concentrations of Pb and Cd were determined by flameless atomic absorption spectrometry on a Varian AA spectrometer Model 875 using a graphite furnace GTA 95; Zn, Ba, Mg and Ca were determined by optical emission spectrometry, with inductively coupled plasma (ICP) source, Philips PV 8490 and detector Sopra IPS 1500. In several cases Pb was determined directly on the powdered samples by mass spectrometry, using Thompson THN 212 spark source mass spectrograph.

The lower limits of detection of Pb and Cd by atomic absorption spectrometry were 1.0 and 0.5 $\mu g\ g^{-1}$, and the mean analytical error, including calibration was $\pm$ 10%; for detection of Zn the lower limit was 2 $\mu g\ g^{-1}$, for Ba 0.1 $\mu g\ g^{-1}$, for Mg 0.1 $\mu g\ g^{-1}$ and for Ca 10 μg g^{-1}, and the mean analytical error was 5%; the detection limit for Pb by mass spectrometry was 0.1 $\mu g\ g^{-1}$ and the mean analytical error 50%.

RESULTS AND DISCUSSION
TISSUE DISTRIBUTION

It is well known that Pb levels differ greatly in various types of bone. A longitudinal gradient of Pb concentration in the human long bones from Roman period was observed earlier (Ah 81), as well as important differences between the concentrations of Pb and Zn in particular osteons of the same contemporary bones, and even between various regions of the same osteons (Li 81). Here we observed the variances between the content of metals at different depths in the walls of shafts of the ancient and contemporary long bones (Table 3).

The concentrations of Ba and Mg, which in contemporary bones are
rather homogenously distributed, in the ancient bones tend to differ
at particular depth from the surface. The content of Ca in the
modern long bones was usually higher in the deeper layers of the
shafts and lower near their surface. Both in modern and ancient
bones the content of Zn was higher in the external layers of the
bones than in the deeper ones. This effect is less clearly seen also
in case of Pb. The greatest difference is observed in case of Cd,
the concentration of which in the external layers of the shaft of
long bones was several times higher than in the deeper ones. These
data indicate that a concentration gradient of metals in cortical
bones forms during life, which can be altered or even reversed by
fossilization. It seems that the least influenced by this process
and least exposed to contamination part of the bone is at the inner
surface of the medullary cavity, near the center of the shaft,
between 0.5 to 4 mm below the surface of the cavity. We believe that
this is the best site for collecting the bone fragments for trace
analyses.

TEMPORAL CHANGES

The mean concentrations of Ca and Ba were slowly decreasing from
high values in the oldest bones to low contemporary levels (Table 4).
A similar trend was observed for concentrations of Ra-226 in human
bones from the past 1700 years (Ja 82), which was interpreted as
resulting from decrease in the consumption of cereals, which are
principal source of Ra-226 intake in European diet. A similar
interpretation might be offered for Ba (source vegetables) but not
for Ca. Higher concentration of Ba in external layers of ancient
bones than in the deeper layers suggests that fossilization processes
are probably responsible for the higher content of Ba in the old
bones, rather than the dietary changes; the same interpretation is
also valid for Ca.

Contrary to Ba and Ca, the concentration of Mg increased
steadily throughout the ages and is now about 4 times as high as in
paleolithic bones. We believe that this is an effect of post mortem
changes, such as the replacement of soluble Mg salts by much less
soluble Ca and Ba salts, rather than a change from a predominantly

vegetarian diet to one more rich in animal food.

The concentrations of Zn remained stable during the past few millenia and are now the same in contemporary bones as in Neolithic ones.

This is in contrast with the concentrations of Pb and Cd which changed dramatically during the past ages. The concentrations of Pb increased abruptly in the late Middle Ages to a level an order of magnitude higher than in Roman and Merovingian period, and then recently decreased to rather low contemporary level. It may appear from Table 1 that the dramatic decrease in the Pb level in Parisian population started at the end of the 18th century, but this is only an effect of the lack of 19th century samples. However, the data from other countries indicate that the high level of Pb in man persisted in Poland at least until the end of 19th century before dropping in the 20th century down to a near-prehistorical level (Ja 68), and in Denmark the high level of Pb in human bones was observed until the 1940s, and in 1972 dropped by about one order of magnitude (Gr 75). This indicates that the contemporary low Pb level in the skeleton of Europeans is a new phenomenon.

The high Pb content in human bones in the past seems to be associated with the use of this metal for innumerable household, medical and technical aims and coincides with the rise of Pb smelting in the late Middle Ages (Nr 78). The majority of these sources of contamination with Pb have disappeared from the immediate environment of contemporary man, which resulted in the present low Pb level in inhabitants of major European cities.

During the last century in the bones of French population, and probably also in other countries, the concentration of Cd increased by an order of magnitude. This is probably due to the extensive use of this metal for anti-corrosion plating, construction of batteries, production of pigments, plastic stabilizers, fungicides, bactericides, antiseptics, porcelain and glass coloring, copying papers, solders etc, (Nr 80), and not to an increase of Cd content in the atmospheric precipitation observed in Scandinavian and Alpine glaciers (Ja 81).

Table 1. COMPARISON OF PREHISTORIC, MIDDLE AGES TO 19TH CENTURY AND
CONTEMPORARY LEVELS OF Pb IN HUMAN BONES FROM VARIOUS COUNTRIES.
Ranges of concentrations in $\mu g\ g^{-1}$ dry weight.

Country	Prehistoric	Middle Ages to 19th century	Contemporary
Peru	0.1 - 2.7[a]	14.8 - 102[b]	
	0.06 - 1.9[c]		
Nubia	0.4 - 3.0[d]		
Denmark	0.2 - 1.1[e]	3.3 - 40.8[e]	0.2 - 8.8[d,e]
Sweden	10[f]	10 - 40[f]	
South Germany	0.1 - 8.1[c]	0.4 - 16.7[c]	0.3 - 19.3[c]
South Poland	0.4 - 7.5[b]	3.7 - 373[b]	0.4 - 36.7[b]
France	0.1 - 36.0[g]	2.5 - 280[g]	5 - 35.0[g]

a)Er-79; b)Ja-82; c)Dr-82; d)Gr-79; e)Gr-75; f)Ah-81; g)this work.

Table 2. SAMPLING. CEP - cemetery exposed to precipitation; CAV -cave; CHG - church or monastery ground burial; CHC church burial in coffins, crypts or sarphaguses; F - femur; T - tibia; H - humerus; U - ulna; Fi - fibula; R - rib; V - vertebra; M - metacarpal.

Age (years before present)	Site and type of burial			Departement	Number and type of samples
HUMAN BONES					
Neolithic 5600	Passy-sur-Yonne	(PAS)	CEP	Yonne	2 H,F
Bronze 3000	Grotte de l'Herm	(HER)	CAV	Ariège	1 U
	Dolmen in Aveyron	(DOL)	CEP	Aveyron	2 T,Fi
	Pincevent	(PIN)	CEP	Yonne	1 F
Roman 1600	Maule	(MAL)	CEP	Yvelines	20 F,H,T,U
	Chiragan	(CHI)	CHP	H.Garonne	1 F
Merovingian 1200-1500	Maule	(MAL)	CEP	Yvelines	22 T,F,H
	Sens	(SEN)	CEP	Yonne	23 T
Middle Ages					
800	Villeneuve Tolosane	(VIL)	CEP	H.Garonne	1 H
650	Muret	(MUR)	CHG	H.Garonne	6 F,T
400-600	N-D de Paris	(ND)	CHG	Paris	51 T,H,F,V,R
400-600	Maubuisson	(MAU)	CHG	Val d'Oise	13 T,Fi
18th Century 200	Toulouse	(TOU)	CHC	H.Garonne	8 H,T,F
Contemporary	Paris	(PAR)	-	Paris	29 V,F,T,R

Table 3. DISTRIBUTION OF METALS IN BONE STRUCTURE. In $\mu g\ g^{-1}$ (Ca in %) dry weight; CAV – sample collected from the surface of medullary cavity; EXT – sample collected from external surface of the shaft; 1, –2, –3, –4 – successive 2 mm thick layers; determined by mass spectroscopy; identification of bones Table 2.

No of sample and type of bone	Layer	Cd	Pb	Zn	Ba	Mg	Ca
NEOLITHIC							
G 1A H	CAV-1	0.17	1.4	138	75	265	33.0
	CAV-1	0.30	<0.1	142	62	485	33.7
G 2 F	CAV-2	0.15	<0.1	112	45	750	33.6
BRONZE AGE							
T H1 U	CAV-1	0.07	1.0	70	130	1225	23.9
T A1 T	CAV-1	0.10	36.0	108	71	1500	30.0
T A2 Fi	CAV-1	0.11	34.0	128	82	1500	28.1
P 1A F	CAV-2	0.20	0.1	114	50	760	28.0
ROMAN							
M 559 F	EXT-1	0.34	26.0	385	88	575	26.0
	CAV-1	0.12	16.0	115	300	700	21.8
MEROVINGIAN							
M 816 T	CAV-1	0.22	12.0	133	51	1015	32.7
	CAV-2	0.26	16.0	100	49	950	32.8
	CAV-3	0.15	16.0	100	52	909	32.4
MIDDLE AGES							
ND4-1 T	EXT-1	0.40	210.0	490	36	1200	25.1
	EXT-2	0.30	90.0	170	26	1300	25.3
	EXT-3	0.20	105.0	120	25	1380	25.4
	CAV-1	0.25	100.0	92	16	1120	24.6
CONTEMPORARY							
W 35 T	EXT-1	0.21	60.0	150	0.5	2970	25.5
	EXT-2	0.08	30.0	135	0.5	2835	24.7
	CAV-1	0.09	30.0	112	0.05	2925	22.6

Table 4. ARITHMETICAL MEAN AND RANGE OF CONCENTRATION OF METALS IN HUMAN BONES. In $\mu g\ g^{-1}$ (Ca in %) dry weight; standard deviation in parentheses; number of samples and identification of sites and bones in Table 2.

Years before present	Site	Cd	Pb	Zn	Ba	Mg	Ca
Neolithic 5600	PAS	0.20(0.07) 0.15–0.30	0.1–1.4	106(15) 112–138	57(14) 45–75	570(248) 265–780	35.0(1.9) 33.0–33.7
Bronze Age 3000	HER,DOL,PIN	0.12(0.05) 0.07–0.30	15(18) 0.1–36	108(22) 70–128	77(32) 50–130	1145(378) 740–1500	28.5(3.2) 23.9–32.5
Roman 1600	MAL,CHI	0.22(0.22) 0.09–0.50	8.6(5.3) 1.0–22	109(26) 70–180	35(19) 6–83	789(230) 240–1150	26.6(1.9) 21.8–30.7
Merovingian 1400	SEN	0.23(0.14) 0.06–0.60	6.4(8.9) 1.0–30	107(14) 84–138	78(23) 49–120	757(116) 575–1075	31.8(2.7) 25.8–37.0
Merovingian 1200–1500	MAL	0.17(0.10) 0.05–0.50	7.3(11) 1.0–41	115(27) 89–210	30(14) 12–63	824(234) 595–1570	32.7(3.0) 27.6–36.4
Middle Ages 500	MUR	0.16(0.11) 0.08–0.36	15(16) 2.5–40	122(20) 105–152	51(47) 9–128	1933(388) 1300–2400	29.8(2.8) 27.6–33.3
400–600	ND	0.21(0.15) 0.05–0.54	91(67) 13.5–280	131(60) 60–365	16(12) 3–60	1330(402) 400–2270	25.7(1.8) 19.0–30.7
400–600	MAB	0.16(0.07) 0.07–0.25	82(32) 50.0–152	108(9.1) 95–125	10(4) 5–19	2661(545) 1680–3750	26.7(1.1) 25.0–28.6
18th century 200	TOU	0.18(0.11) 0.06–0.37	61(31) 14.0–105	118(21) 100–155	22(8) 10–33	1681(417) 1350–2500	28.1(2.5) 25.0–31.2
Recent	PAR,SAR	2.20(2.20) 0.07–8.0	16.9(10.1) 5.0–35	126(21) 78–170	2.7(3.9) 0.5–15	2460(347) 1230–3015	18.5(3.4) 7.3–22.6

CONCLUSIONS

Content of Cd and Zn did not change in the old bones due to
fossilization processes. On the other hand these processes are
probably responsible for an increase of Ba and Ca in older samples
and for a decrease of Mg and Pb in very ancient bones.

The Pb level in human bones from France increased largely in the
late Middle Ages, reaching extremely high levels in some samples.
This was due to sources of contamination in man's immediate
environment at home and workshop. Majority of these sources
disappeared in 20th century, which resulted in a decrease of Pb
content in contemporary Europeans by one order of magnitude. This
indicates that the effects of improved hygiene conditions surpassed
the effects of the recent man-made emission of Pb into the
atmosphere. This is not surprising as the flow of Pb into the global
atmosphere from all anthropogenic sources is only about 7% of the
natural flow, i.e. less than its long-term natural fluctuation
(Ja 81).

The concentration of Cd in the bones of Europeans increased
during the last few decades by an order of magnitude above the
pre-industrial level. This is due to an increase in use of this
metal, the production of which in Europe was in 1970s more than 100
times higher than before World War I (Nr 80), rather than due to
dispersion of Cd in the atmosphere, as the man-made contribution to
its flow into the global atmosphere is only about 0.5% of the natural
input (Ja 81).

REFERENCES

Ah81 Ahlgren, L, Christoffersson, J O and Mattson, S, (1981). Lead
    and barium in archeological Roman skeletons measured by
    nondestructive x-ray fluorescence analysis. In: D K Smith,
    C Barrett, D E Leyden and K Pradecki (Eds), Advances in X-ray
    Analysis, Vol. 24 pp. 337-382.

Dr82 Drasch, G A, (1982), Lead burden in prehistorical, historical
    and modern human bones. Sc. Total Environ. 24, 199-231.

Er79 Ericson, J E, Shirahata, H and Patterson, C C, (1979), Skeletal
    concentrations of lead in ancient Peruvians. New Engl. J. Med.
    300, 546-551.

Gr75 Grandjean, P, (1975), Lead in Danes, Historical and toxicological studies. Environmental Quality and Safety, Suppl. Vol. 2, Academic Press, New York.

Gr79 Grandjean, P, Nielsen, O V and Shapiro, I M, (1979), Lead retention in ancient Nubian and contemporary populations. J. Environ. Pathol. Toxicol., 2, 781-787.

Ja67 Jaworowski, Z, (1967), Stable and radioactive lead in environment and human body. Report NEIC-RP-29, Nuclear Energy Information Center, Warsaw.

Ja68 Jaworowski, Z, (1968), Stable lead in fossil ice and bones. Nature, 217, 152-153.

Ja81 Jaworowski, Z, Bysiek, M and Kownacka, L, (1981), Flow of metals into the global atmosphere. Geochim. Cosmochim. Acta, 45, 2185-2199.

Ja82 Jaworowski, Z, and Bilkiewicz, (1982), Are heavy metals and radium in man related to emission from coal burning? In: Health Impacts of Different Sources of Energy. IAEA, Vienna, pp. 159-167.

Je76 Jeanmaire, L, Patti, F, Gros, R, Cappellini, L, Garcet, M and Laporte, J, (1976), Teneurs en plomb d'os humains provenant de la région Parisienne. Report CEA-R-4800, Centre d'Etudes Nucléaires Fontenay-aux-Roses.

Li81 Lindh, U, (1981), The nuclear microprobe applied to bio-environmental studies. Nucl. Instr. Meth., 181, 171-178.

Nr78 Nriagu, J O, (1978), Properties and the biological cycle of lead. In: Nriagu, J O (Ed.), The Biogeochemistry of Lead in the Environment, Part A. Elsevier, Amsterdam.

Nr80 Nriagu, J O, (1980), Human influence on the global cadmium cycle. In: Nriagu, J O (Ed.), Cadmium in the Environment, Part I. John Wiley and Sons, New York.

Pa65 Patterson, C C, (1965), Contaminated and natural lead environments of man. Arch. Environ. Health, 11, 344-363.

38

Some Aspects of Lead Uptake by the Bones

C. A. BAUD, S. BANG, C. KRAMAR, D. LACOTTE, H. J. TOCHON-DANGUY and J. –M. VERY

A skeleton dating from the Medieval period was recovered from a lead coffin buried in the underground of the St. Peter's cathedral in Geneva. A particularity of this skeleton was a chalky white coat partly spotting the surface of the cranio-facial bones. Fragments of the frontal bone were studied by means of microradiography (Ph65), electron probe microanalysis (Ca72), infra-red spectrophotometry (Kl70), X-ray diffraction (Bh70) and electron microscopy (Fe81).

The microradiographs show a radio-opaque deposit in the bone surface layers, infiltrating through vascular channels and lacuno-canalicular systems into the underlying bone tissue. The X-ray Pb $L\alpha$ images show the topographic distribution of lead, corresponding exactly to that of the radioopaque deposit.

The infra-red spectrum of the chalky white substance is typical of a well crystallized Pb-apatite structure: the assigned PO_4^{3-} ion frequencies are 1050 and 990 cm^{-1} for the ν_3 mode, 579 and 548 cm^{-1} for the ν_4 mode. The X-ray diffraction pattern is characteristic of lead hydroxyapatite; a and c crystallographic parameters, respectively 9.894 and 7.660 Å, are compatible with such an apatite. Crystal size

and/or perfection, evaluated by measuring the width of the
X-ray diffraction lines, is above that of bone mineral
along c axis: $\beta(002) = 0.082$.

Electron micrographs show a subsurface alteration of
the bone structure, composed of tangled crystals and
aggregates. High resolution electron micrographs exhibit
well formed crystals, with a regular lattice pattern and
little or no evidence of defects.

The results of these observations show that :
- lead from the environment is taken up by dead bone (see
  also Wa81);
- lead hydroxyapatite is formed at the expense of bone
  calcium hydroxyapatite by a dissolution-recrystalliza-
  tion process.

REFERENCES

Bh70 Bhatnagar V.M., 1970, The preparation, X-ray and
infra-red spectra of lead apatites , *Archs oral Biol*.<u>15</u>,
469-480.

Ca72 Carroll K.G., Needleman H., Tuncay O.C. and Shapiro
I.M., 1972, The distribution of lead in human deciduous
teeth , *Experientia* <u>28</u>, 434-435.

Fe81 Featherstone J.D.B., Nelson D.G.A. and Mc Lean J.D.,
1981, An electron microscope study of modifications to
defect regions in dental enamel and synthetic apatites ,
Caries Res. <u>15</u>, 278-288.

Kl70 Klee W.E. and Engel G., 1970, I.R. spectra of the
phosphate ions in various apatites , *J. Inorg. Nucl. Chem*.
<u>32</u>, 1837-1843.

Ph65 Philipson B. and Lindström B., 1965, Microradiographic determination of lead in mineralized tissues ,
Histochemie <u>5</u>, 250-259.

Wa81 Waldron H.A., 1981, Postmortem absorption of lead by
the skeleton , *Am. J. Phys. Anthropol*. <u>55</u>, 395-398.

39

Lead Accumulation in Rat's Bone in Relation to Age

M. BLANUŠA, Dj. BREŠKI and M. CIGANOVIĆ

INTRODUCTION

Lead in bone gives the best picture of past lead exposure, since 90%
of lead in the body is deposited in bones with a very long biological
half-time. The aim of this study was to establish a correlation
between bone lead level and the level of lead in the oral dose in
rats of different age.

METHODS

Different doses of lead chloride (50, 500, 1500, 3500, 5000 and
7500 ppm of lead) were given to adult rats in drinking water for four
weeks. The animals, four months of age (females weighing about 180 g
and males about 260 g), were divided into groups of 4-10 animals each.
At the end of four weeks the rats were killed, their right femurs
were dissected and dry ashed at 450°C. Lead was determined by flame
atomic absorption spectrophotometry (Varian, AA-375). Some additional
animals at lead doses of 1500 and 3500 ppm, were mated and exposure
was continued through pregnancy and lactation. Their newborns and
11 day-old pups were killed by exsanguination. The same animals were
mated for the second time after 13 weeks of exposure to lead. The
exposure continued through pregnancy and lactation. After the newborns and 11 day-old pups from the first and second mating were
killed, their carcasses were treated and analysed for lead using the
same technique as for femurs.

RESULTS

After four weeks of exposure to lead, a linear correlation between the lead concentrations in femurs (y) and the concentration of lead in drinking water (x) was calculated (Table 1). The correlation coefficient (r) was 0.963 and a and b of the line (y=a+bx) were 4.29 and 0.029 respectively. Lead levels obtained in the carcasses of the newborn and lactating 11-day old animals from the first and second mating on two different levels of lead in drinking water are presented in Table 2. The difference between bone lead levels in pups

Table 1. Lead in femurs of adult rats exposed to lead in drinking water for 4 weeks

Lead level (µg/ml)	Sex	No of animals	Lead in femurs (µg/g wet weight)
50	female	5	0.9 ± 0.2 *
500	female	4	32.2 1.9
1500	female	10	47.1 2.8
1500	male	9	50.0 2.5
3500	female	9	114.0 4.4
3500	male	10	97.3 5.5
5000	female	5	160.7 5.9
7500	female	5	229.8 6.5
7500	male	10	225.9 14.6

*Results are presented as arithmetic means ± standard error of the mean.

Table 2. Lead in carcasses of newborns and 11 day-old pups from the first and second mating

Lead level (µg/ml)	Age (days)	First mating No of animals	First mating Lead (µg/g)	Second mating No of animals	Second mating Lead (µg/g)
1500	0	30	0.48 ± 0.03*	25	0.82 ± 0.04
1500	11	30	4.4 0.1	27	5.2 0.3
3500	0	40	1.7 0.1	30	3.9 0.4
3500	11	40	9.6 0.4	30	9.6 0.5

*Results are presented as arithmetic means ± standard error of the mean.

on two doses was highly significant. The length of parents' exposure, which was 9 and 18 weeks for the first and second mating respectively, did not influence the body burden of lead in newborn or lactating animals.

CONCLUSION

The results show a linear and highly significant correlation between oral lead dose and femur lead level in adult animals. Lead concentrations in the carcasses of newborn and 11-day old pups were also dependent on the level of lead their parents received in drinking water.

40

The Autoradiographic Method for Lead-210 Quantitative Determination

J. DONIEC

The method was developed for determination of lead-210 concentration on endosteal and periosteal surfaces and diffuse activity in the compact bone (tibia and femur from rabbit). A solid state nuclear track detector (cellulose acetate) was used for quantitative autoradiography of alpha particles originating from polonium-210, the daughter of lead-210 (beta decay).

The outline of lead-210 measurement was:
- exposure of the bone slide on photographic plate, optical density measurements,
- exposure of the same slide on nuclear track detector, track density measurements,
- calculation of optical density corresponding to polonium-210 alpha particles emission,
- subtraction of calculated optical density from polonium to get the lead concentration.

The method was calibrated with plaster of Paris standards containing lead-210 and/or polonium-210. Several correction factors were taken into consideration.

The method can be also applied to the autoradiography of the mixture of radionuclides: one with alpha decay, the other, beta decay.

The Autoradiographic Method for Lead-210 Quantitative Determination

J. DONIEC

Microdistribution of Lead-210 in the Rabbit's Osseous Tissue

J. DONIEC and M. TRZCINKA-OCHOCKA

The kinetics of lead-210 (administered intravenously as nitrate) microdistribution in the shaft of tibia and femur of male Chinchilla-like rabbits, aged 12 months was investigated. Lead-210 concentration in growing parts of periosteum and endosteum and in compact bone was measured by autoradiographic method.

Up to the second day after injection the lead transport velocity from plasma to micro-areas in growing parts of the bone is 25 times higher than for calcium and the velocity of lead transport to non-growing area in compact bone is three times higher than calcium. This confirms osteotropic properties of lead and suggests that the mechanism of mineral building has a strong influence on the lead deposition velocity.

Microdistribution of Lead-210 in the Rabbit's Osseous Tissue

J. DOLEŽAL and M. DRÁBKOVÁ-SCHÖCK

42

Lead in Human Bones and Teeth at the Part-Per-Million Level

M. V. STACK

INTRODUCTION

Present evidence on the relation between neuropsychological deficit
and lead levels in mineralised tissues is equivocal, and attention
continues to be given to analyses of mature primary teeth (Ma83,Sm83).
It is usual to base such surveys on analyses of a reference material
suitable for quality control (St82).

COMMENTS

Table 1 indicates that 5 - 15% of tooth lead values may be expected
to be below 1.5 ppm in urban environments; the mean percentage in six
southern Norwegian counties lies within this range; however, 20 - 40%
of values are low in six northern counties(Fo78). Higher proportions
of low lead values (55 - 80%) occur in surveys of archaeological bone
(Dr82, Sh80). The highest proportions refer to surveys of fetal bone
(Ba69, Ba81), few lead levels exceeding 1.5 ppm.

SUMMARY

A survey of recent analytical data on lead levels in bone and tooth
samples shows that, under favourable conditions, values not much exceeding 1 ppm should be found for the minority of shed teeth of the
primary dentition, most values being within the range of 2 - 5 ppm.
Much greater proportions of low values are seen in surveys of fetal
and archaeological material.

405

Table 1. Percentages of lead concentrations within six ranges (ppm):
Archaeological, developing and mature specimens (bone/tooth)

Author/ MRC DU	Specimens	(N)	Lead concentration ranges (ppm)						Centuries before present
			0-1½	1½-3	3-4½	4½-6	6-7½	7½-9	
Dr82	Femur	(36)	55	33	3	6	3		38 - 25
Dr82	Femur	(41)	81	12	5	0	2		12 - 11
Sh80	Temporal bone	(26)	68	28	0	4	0		19 - 12
Ba81	Fetal tibia	(44)	84	14	0	2			
Ba69	Fetal femur	(27)	85	13	0	3			
MRC	Fetal teeth	(50)	31	37	24	4			(dentine)
Ma83	Decid.teeth	(136)	15	33	26	12	3	11	
Sm83	Decid.teeth	(82)	6	31	36	21	6	1	
MRC	Decid.teeth	(107)	5	29	31	18	13	5	
Ha84	Decid.teeth	(55)	12	42	25	11	5	2	(dentine)
Concentration ranges:			0-3	3-6	6-9	9-12	12-15	15-18	(ppm)
Ha84	Decid.teeth	(45)	21	27	19	16	7	2	(enamel)

Author codes as in references: MRC DU refers to MRC Dental Unit work
Ha84 data represent means for groups of teeth from Helsinki & Kuopio

REFERENCES

Ba69 Barltrop D., 1969, "Transfer of Lead to the Human Fetus" in:
Mineral Metabolism in Paediatrics (Edited by Barltrop D. and Burland
W.L.), pp. 135-151 (Oxford & Edinburgh: Blackwell).
Ba81 Barry P.S.I., 1981, "Concentrations of Lead in the Tissues of
Children" Br. J. industr.Med. 38, 61-71.
Dr82 Drasch G.A., 1982, "Lead Burden in Prehistorical, Historical
and Modern Human Bones" Sci. total Environment 24, 199-231.
Fo78 Fosse G. and Justesen N.-P.B., 1978, "Lead in Deciduous Teeth
of Norwegian Children" Archs environ. Hlth 33, 166-175.
Ha84 Haavikko K., Anttila A., Helle A. and Vuori E., 1984, "Lead
Concentrations of Enamel and Dentine of Deciduous Teeth of Children
from Two Finnish Towns" Archs environ. Hlth 39, 78-84.
Ma83 Marecek J., Shapiro I.M., Burke A., Katz S.H. and Hediger M.L.,
1983, "Low-Level Lead Exposure in Childhood Influences Neuropsycho-
logical Performance" Archs environ. Hlth 38, 355-359.
Sh80 Shapiro I.M., Grandjean P. and Nielsen O.V., 1980, Lead Levels
in Bones and Teeth of Children in Ancient Nubia: Evidence of both
Minimal Lead Exposure and Lead Poisoning" in: Low Level Lead Exposure
(Edited by Needleman H.L.), pp. 35-42 (New York: Raven Press).
Sm83 Smith M., Delves T., Lansdown R., Clayton B. and Graham P., 1983,
"The Effect of Lead Exposure on Urban Children: The Institute of Child
Health/Southampton Study" Devel.Med. Child Neurol. 25, Suppl. 47.
St82 Stack M.V. and Delves H.T., 1982, "Tooth-Lead Analysis:An Inter-
laboratory Study" in: Collaborative Interlaboratory Studies in Chemical
Analysis (Edited by Egan H. and West T.S.). pp. 115-118 (Oxford & New
York: Pergamon Press).

43

Comparative Study of the Chemical Behaviour of Trace Elements in Dental Enamel

V. VERNOIS, N. DESCHAMPS, A. BOULAY and M. GOLDBERG

Dental enamel is a very particular biological structure. There is a major difference between enamel and the mineralized tissues because of the limited growth period of enamel. The evolution of this structure is largely dependent on exterior phenomenon. Among the different factors, the environmental make up influences the chemical composition of enamel.

The biological behaviour of this structure can be studied using the variations of its chemical composition. In such a study, a systematic analysis and an examination of incorporation phenomena were carried out on a human population and on an animal model.

The different human dental samples came from five ancient necropolises staggered from the first to the nineteen century. Some archeological studies have been carried out on each necropolis. The interest of such a model is that the population were of a rural sedentary origin and were buried in situ. The chemical analysis of spring water and vegetation allows the establishment of environmental chemical profiles. A series of dental samples has been taken from a contemporary population to control the stability of enamel composition during a long period of burial.

The animal model is a dynamic method of following a chemical element from absorption to the incorporation in the mineralized dental structures.

I. Material and Methods

Human experimentation.

A total of 150 enamel samples (30 mg) have been taken from the teeth of individuals in the five ancient necropolis and in the contemporary population. In certain cases, several teeth from the same individual have been analysed. In the results, values obtained from temporary teeth and permanent teeth have been separated.

Enamel samples have been stored in cadmium containers (10 mm thickness irradiated under a neutron flux (10^{13} n.cm^{-2}.s^{-1}) for 12 days. Under these experimental conditions, the only chemical separation necessary is that of sodium due to its high concentration in the samples of dental enamel (1). These separations were carried out by the method of mineral exchange in acid conditions (2).

As, Au, Br, Ca, Co, Cu, Eu, La, Mn, Na, P, Sb, Sr, U, W and Zn concentrations have been determined under such conditions.

The large geographic differences between populations and the age variation amongst individuals within each one affect the mean results.

The concentration values obtained for all the individuals examined have been compared using the following two methods :
- a statistical analysis based on the correlation matrix (3) which permits the comparison of all elements across the entire sample,
- a comparison between the variation of the values of each element in each of the six populations based on the minima-maxima ratio method.

In order to check the absence of structural defects on the samples from the ancient necropolises' populations, microscopic investigation hav also been carried out using a scanning electron microscope.

II. Results and Discussion

The mean values obtained on each human population represent a scale of values but cannot be used to compare the results, because of the large spread of standard deviation which gives unacceptable confidence limits for most of the results (Table I).

PERMANENT TEETH : MEAN VALUES

	As	Au	Br	Ca %	Co	Cu
VIEIL-TOULOUSE	0.04 ± 0.05	N.S.	0.6 ± 1	29 ± 3	0.2 ± 0.04	1.6 ± 0.4
VENERQUE	N.S.	N.S.	0.9 ± 0.8	27 ± 9	0.2 ± 0.1	1.8 ± 0.7
MONTLAUR	N.S.	N.S.	1.1 ± 4	29 ± 5	0.3 ± 0.08	1.7 ± 0.5
MAIRAC	N.S.	0.03 ± 0.01	0.9 ± 0.7	26 ± 3	-	2.3 ± 1.2
LADERN	0.15 ± 0.3	N.S.	0.04 ± 0.04	28 ± 2	0.3 ± 0.09	2.2 ± 0.4
MODERN TEETH	N.S.	N.S.	0.5 ± 0.8	30 ± 1	0.2 ± 0.06	2.3 ± 0.5

	Eu	La	Mn	Na %	P (PO4) %	Sb
VIEIL-TOULOUSE	N.S.	N.S.	1.5 ± 3	0.6 ± 0.2	12 ± 5	0.02 ± 0.04
VENERQUE	N.S.	N.S.	1.5 ± 3	0.6 ± 0.2	15 ± 5	0.014 ± 0.01
MONTLAUR	N.S.	N.S.	1.7 ± 2	0.5 ± 0.2	16 ± 7	0.02 ± 0.05
MAIRAC	N.S.	N.S.	1.7 ± 0.5	0.5 ± 0.2	9 ± 4	0.007 ± 0.002
LADERN	N.S.	N.S.	2.1 ± 2	0.6 ± 0.3	14 ± 4	0.015 ± 0.012
MODERN TEETH	N.S.	N.S.	1.1 ± 1	0.7 ± 0.3	17 ± 5	0.012 ± 0.01

	Sr	U	W	Zn
VIEIL-TOULOUSE	60 ± 20	N.S.	N.S.	65 ± 30
VENERQUE	45 ± 10	N.S.	N.S.	30 ± 20
MONTLAUR	70 ± 40	N.S.	N.S.	80 ± 20
MAIRAC	40 ± 10	N.S.	N.S.	85 ± 20
LADERN	35 ± 5	N.S.	N.S.	90 ± 30
MODERN TEETH	60 ± 30	N.S.	N.S.	110 ± 20

DECIDUOUS TEETH : MEAN VALUES

	As	Au	Br	Ca	Co	Cu
MONTLAUR	N.S.	N.S.	7.6 ± 6	23 ± 6	N.S.	1 ±
LADERN	0.06 ± 0.05	0.03 ± 0.01	0.1 ± 0.06	30 ± 3	0.2 ± 0.03	1.8 ±
MODERN TEETH	N.S.	0.02 ± 0.04	14 ± 14	19 ± 3	N.S.	1.3 ±

	Eu	La	Mn	Na	P	Sb
MONTLAUR	0.01 ± 0.07	N.S.	4.8 ± 2	0.5 ± 0.2	15 ± 2	0.01 ±
LADERN	0.006 ± 0.004	0.06 ± 0.03	4 ± 3	0.8 ± 0.05	16 ± 2	0.025 ±
MODERN TEETH	N.S.	N.S.	0.8 ± 0.5	0.4 ± 0.05	11 ± 2	0.07 ±

	Sr	U	W	Zn
MONTLAUR	35 ± 10	N.S.	N.S.	60 ± 15
LADERN	25 ± 4	N.S.	N.S.	75 ± 10
MODERN TEETH	25 ± 4	N.S.	N.S.	75 ± 10

Table I

However, the correlation matrix method allows comparison of all the results, their analysis and interpretation being carried out via a correlation graph (Figure 1). Only those elements, because they can be correlated between the different populations, are shown since this type of analysis excludes concentration values that present an excessive variation between populations.

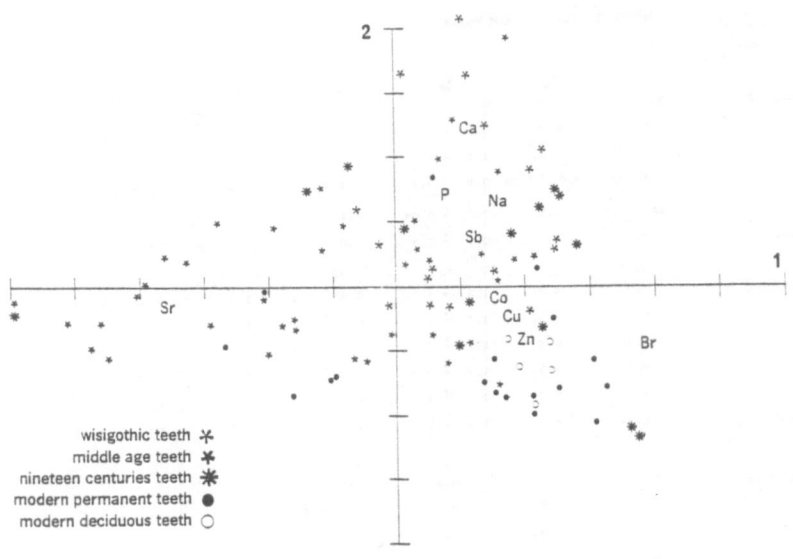

Figure 1

This analysis permits the definition of two constitutive groups of
elements present in dental enamel :
- the elements associated with the major constituents of the mineral
  structure : calcium, phosphorus as well as sodium and antimony,
- the copper-zinc-cobalt group associated with the organic phase of
  enamel at the origin of its major biological reactions.

Strontium is in opposition to these two groups and undoubtedly plays
a special role at the interface between them.

The analysis of the minima-maxima ratio diagrams (Figure 2) shows that
the spread of the results is relatively small in comparison to the majority
of the elements which appear on the correlation graph. For the other
elements, the comparisons have been established between each ancient
necropolis population and the modern control population.

Two groups of elements can therefore be isolated:
- the elements which have a spread of results that is almost always
  constant across the different populations: Mn, Br, Au and W,
- the elements for which the spread of results varies in relation to

the population and its environmental chemical profile : As, Eu, La and U.

In the first group, the result spread depends on the dental sample studied. The variations observed are therefore a result of the physiopathological condition of the enamel of each tooth.

In the second group, the dispersion of the results is linked to the individual from which the sample was taken. The variations are therefore dependent on the interaction between the individual and his environment (nutritional sources).

This phenomenon can be verified by the animal studies using an element of the same chemical group as those found in the human population (rare earths) (6).

As a chloride, dysprosium does not go through the intestinal wall (7) (Table II). However, it is incorporated in the dental zones which are present in the buccal cavity.

The comparative study of the buccal fraction of the incisors (continuous growth) and the molars (interrupted growth) shows that the ratio between incorporated and absorbed dysprosium is similar irrespective of the entry route (Table III). The distribution of dysprosium in the molar groups throughout the animal studies (Figure 3) confirms the hypothesis that a metabolism exists for the elements of this chemical series. The incorporation is therefore associated with an active transfer due to a metabolic process.

In conclusion, the results show the importance of oligoelements in dental enamel.

In relation to the environmental chemical profile, the incorporation of oligoelements in dental enamel is definitely dependent on the presence of biological systems. The modifications these systems undergo are certainly at the origin of physiopathological changes in dental enamel and probably play an important role in carious phenomenon.

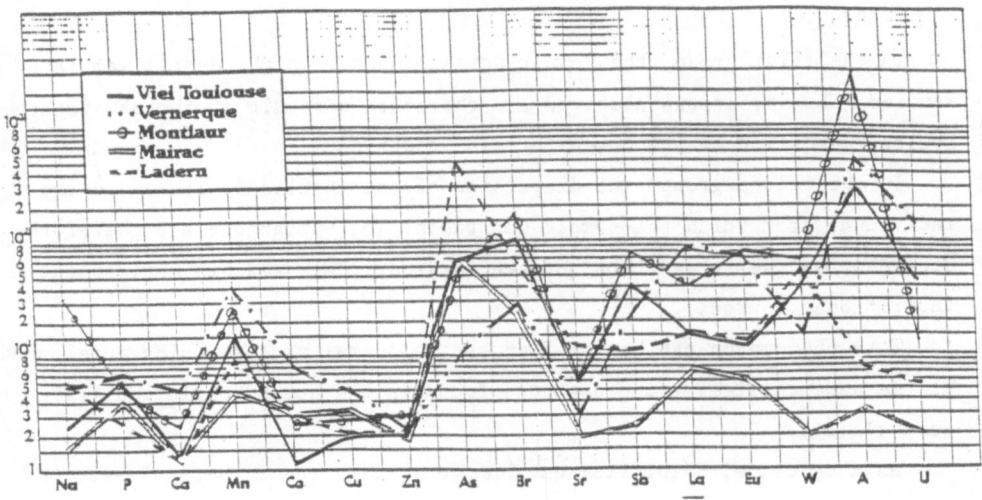

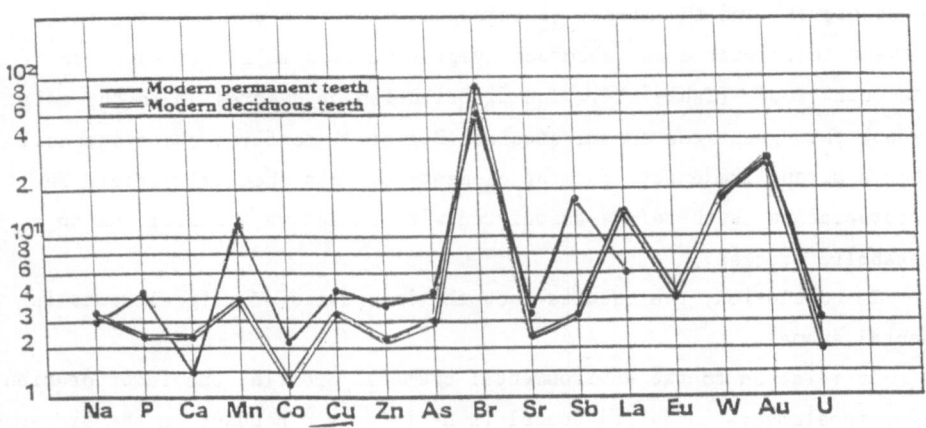

Figure   2

TABLE II Injection by drinking water

Ref. animals	A	B	C	D	E
Mass of Dysprosium absorbed during 32 days (mg)	21	13	11	8	10
Dy absorbed/g animal weight (μg/g)	56.7	35.9	28.7	26.1	24.7
LOWERS INCISORS					
Buccal zone	8.3	5.5 ± 1.1	9.1 ± 1.4	10.4 ± 0.3	3.4 ± 0.5
Maturation zone	$<10^{-3}$	$<10^{-3}$	$<10^{-3}$	$<10^{-3}$	$<10^{-3}$
Edification zone (μg/g)	$<10^{-3}$	$<10^{-3}$	$<10^{-3}$	$<10^{-3}$	$<10^{-3}$
MOLARS (μg/g)	26.5 ± 3.5	30.1 ± 1.8	11.7 ± 6.7	11.0	17.0
FEMURS (μg/g)	$<10^{-4}$	$<10^{-4}$	$<10^{-4}$	$<10^{-4}$	$<10^{-4}$
LIVERS (μg/g)	$<10^{-3}$	$<10^{-3}$	$<10^{-3}$	$<10^{-3}$	$<10^{-3}$

Table II Intravenous injection

Ref. animals	1	2	3	4	5	6	7	8	9	10
Mass of Dysprosium absorbed during 32 days (mg)	32	29	28	25	16.2	16.2	13	13	6	6
Dy absorbed/g animal weight (μg/g)	83.1	74.5	72.8	68.9	42.3	42.3	41.5	43.8	15.7	15.7
LOWERS INCISORS										
Buccal zone	33.3 ± 2.5	15.5	37.6 ± 2.6	16.0 ± 3.1	22.7 ± 1.4	34.3	47.3 ± 2.6	33.6 ± 1.1	36.6 ± 3.8	34.5
Maturation zone	44.3 ± 4.2	26.5	43.2 ± 3.9	19.2 ± 1.1	39.3 ± 1.9	46.3	68.3 ± 0.2	51.3 ± 0.8	46.1 ± 1.9	42.6
Edification zone (μg/g)	58.5 ± 4.7	44.1	66.1	34.8 ± 1.9	48.4 ± 0.7	51.8	75.0	58.6	51.1 ± 25.7	50.7
MOLARS (μg/g)	16.6	28.2	34.7	23.3	19.8	12.8	19.6 ± 4.5	17.5 ± 5.8	10.9	9.4
FEMURS (μg/g)	Not analysed	Not analysed	66.4 ± 3.9	65.1	Not analysed	Not analysed	94.0 ± 51.1	71.5 ± 8.3	Not analysed	Not analysed
LIVERS (μg/g)	4750	2400	2900	3500	3650	2780	2140	1700	720	Not analysed

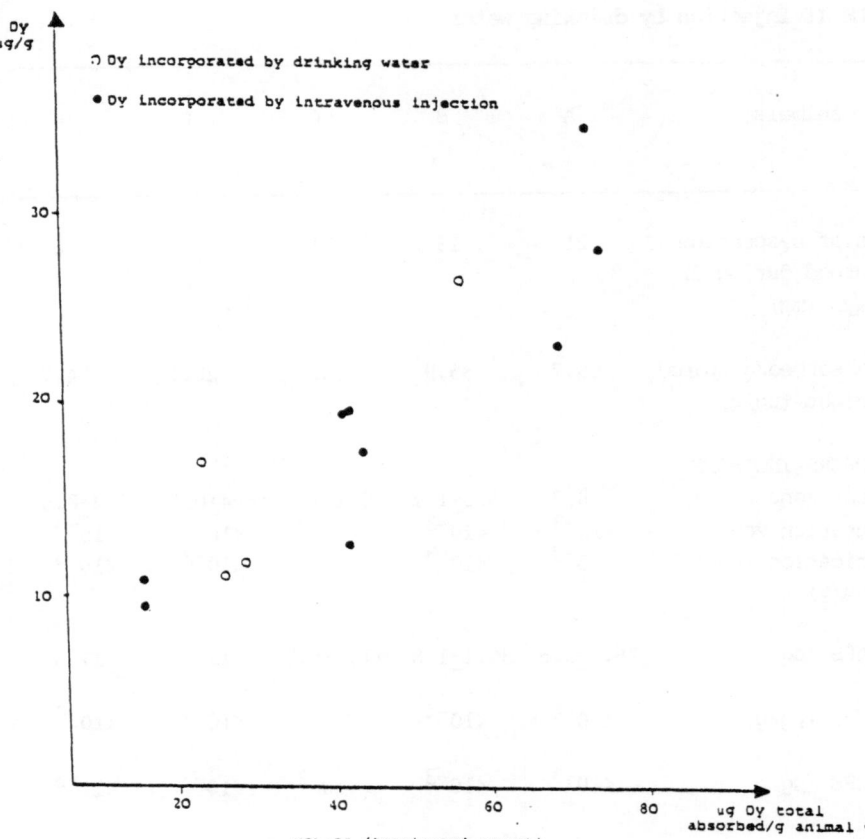

DISTRIBUTION OF DYSPROSIUM CONCENTRATION IN FUNCTION OF THE
DIFFERENT INCORPORATION MODES

Figure 3

Table III

Dy incorporated/Dy absorbed/g animal weight	INTRAVENOUS INJECTION										INGESTION BY DRINKING WATER				
Ref. animals	1	2	3	4	5	6	7	8	9	10	A	B	C	D	E
Mass of dysprosium absorbed (mg)	32	29	28	25	16	16	13	13	6	6	21	13	11	8	10
LOWERS INCISORS															
Edification zone	0.7	0.2	0.5	0.5	1.1	1.2	1.8	1.3	3.3	3.2	—	—	—	—	—
Maturation zone	0.5	0.4	0.4	0.3	0.9	1.1	1.7	1.2	2.9	2.7	—	—	—	—	—
Buccal zone	0.4	0.6	0.9	0.2	0.5	0.8	1.1	0.8	2.3	2.2	0.2	0.2	0.3	0.4	0.2
MOLARS	0.2	0.4	0.5	0.3	0.5	0.3	0.5	0.4	0.6	0.6	0.5	0.8	0.4	0.4	0.6

References

1. Deschamps N., Vernois V., Calza F. : J. Radioanal. Chemistry 70
    n° 1 - 2, 109–116 (1982).

2. Girardi F., Pietra R., Sabbioni E. : Rapport Euratom EUR 4287 E.

3. Jaffrezic H., Joron J.L., Treuil M. : J. Radioanal. Chemistry 69
    n° 1 - 2, 235–238 (1982).

4. Losee F.L., Cutress T.W., Brown R. : Caries Res. 8, 123–134 (1974)

5. Steinnes E., Dahm S., Furseth R. : Acta Odontol. Scand. 32,
    125–129 (1974).

6. Vernois V., Deschamps N., Revel G., Septier D., Goldberg M. : J. Biol.
    Buccale 10, 135–145 (1982).

7. Weiss G.B. : Annu. Rev. Pharmacol. 14, 343 (1977).

Part 8
Metabolism and Effects of Stable Elements

Part 8

44

Ultrastructural Study of Bone and Small Intestine Cells in Lead-Intoxicated Rats

G. SILVESTRINI and F. BONUCCI

Lead poisoning is one of the oldest known intoxications and is rather frequent also in our modern era, chiefly because lead use in industrial processes has increased. Lead encephalopathy, peripheral neuritis, anaemia, and the presence of nuclear inclusion bodies in epithelial cells of kidney tubules are well known, whereas the changes induced by the element in bone and intestine remain unclear.

Adult rats have been intoxicated by the administration of lead with drinking water with the main aim of studying the changes induced by the element in bone, where it is incorporated in calcifying matrix (Sc64), and in the small intestine, where it penetrates the epithelial cells during its absorption.

MATERIAL AND METHODS

Twenty adult white rats, feeding on a standard diet, were supplied for 20 days with drinking water containing lead (50 mg lead acetate in 250 ml of water, renewed every day). Five rats who drank normal water were used as controls. The animals were killed under ether anaesthesia by perfusion with a 1:1 solution of 2% glutaraldehyde and 4%

paraformaldehyde buffered at pH 7.2 with cacodylate buffer. Small specimens of tibial epiphyses, costochondral junctions, and small intestine were taken immediately after death and soaked for 2 hours in the same solution used for perfusion. They were successively post-fixed in 1% osmium tetroxide buffered as above, and embedded in Araldite. Semithin sections were examined under the light microscope after staining with Azure II - Methylene blue or the von Kossa method. Ultrathin sections were examined under the electron microscope either unstained or after staining with uranyl acetate and lead citrate.

RESULTS

Bone tissue

The histological picture of tibial and costal trabecular bone of lead-poisoned animals was similar to that of controls. Osteoblasts were not numerous and were cytologically normal. Osteocytes appeared unchanged. The number of osteoclasts was moderately increased: small, deeply stained inclusion bodies were recognizable in the nuclei and cytoplasm of many of them (inset, Fig. 1).

Under the electron microscope, the calcified matrix, whose degree of calcification was not modified, was bordered by flat, "lining" cells and by osteoblasts. These showed developed granular endoplasmic reticulum and Golgi apparatus and apparently were like the osteoblasts of controls. The thin osteoid border consisted of loosely arranged, uncalcified collagen fibrils and contained many small, roundish, vesicle-like structures surrounded by a membrane (Fig. 2). Part of them were in contact with, or contained small aggregates of needle-shaped crystals; others contained very small (from 10 to 20 nm), intrinsically electron-dense granules (Fig. 2). These granules were visible also in unstained sections. Similar vesicles were present also in the osteoid border of controls, but

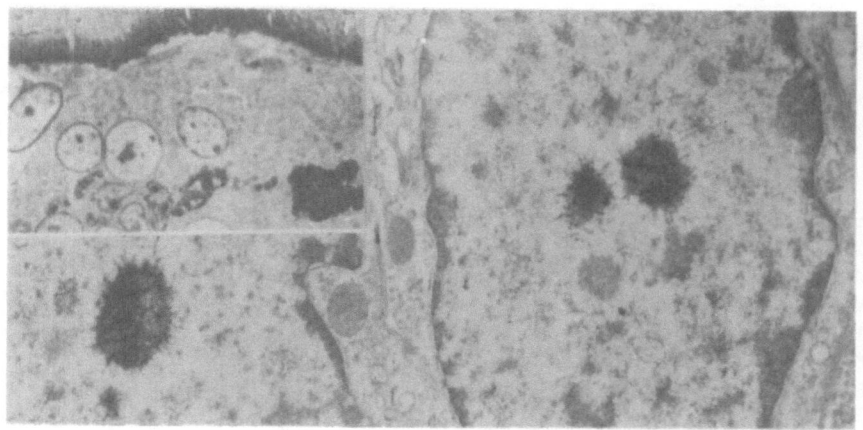

Fig. 1 - Inclusion bodies of osteoclasts of lead-poisoned rats: they appear as deeply stained granules under the light microscope (inset; see also that part of the nuclei are shrunken; bone matrix above. x 750) and as roundish structures with protruding filaments under the electron microscope; x 18,000.

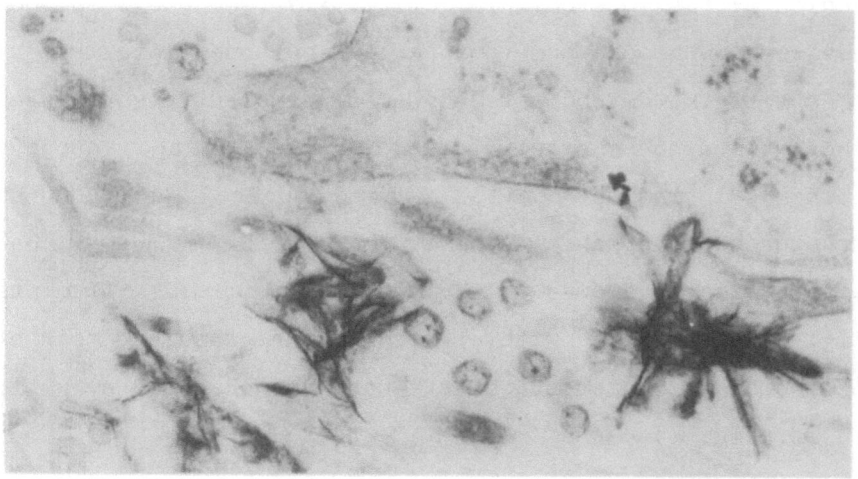

Fig. 2 - Detail of the osteoid border of lead intoxicated rats. Note small extracellular vesicles which contain electron-dense granules. Early aggregates of crystals are also present; x 75,000.

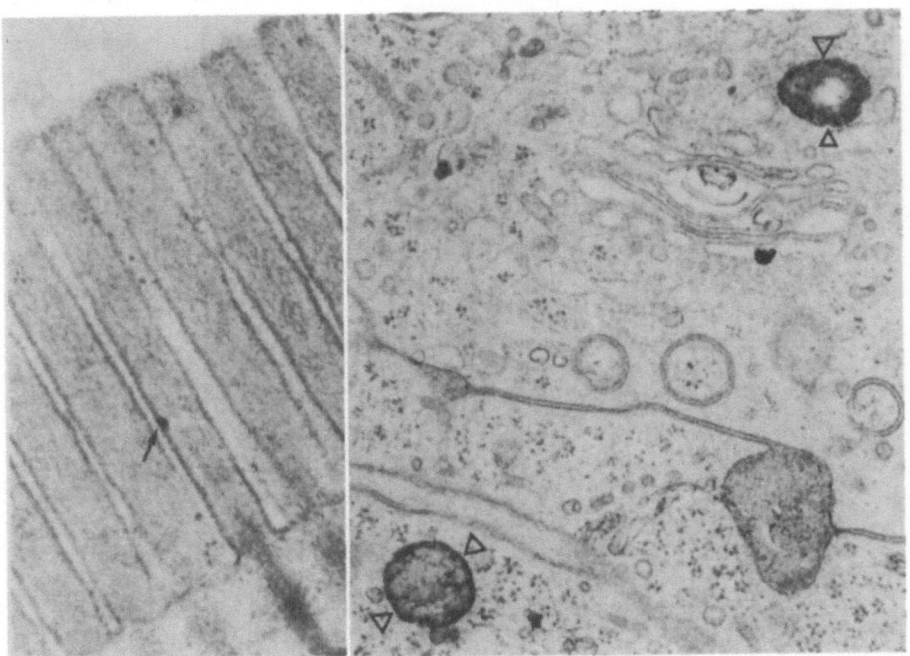

Fig. 3 - Left: detail of the microvilli of intestinal epithelial cell; arrow points to an electron-dense granule.
Right: part of the cytoplasms of two adjacent epithelial
cells; both contain electron-dense granules within vacuoles (arrowheads); other granules are contained in an ex-
pansion of the intercellular cleft. x 72,000 and x 10,000.

they were much more numerous in lead-poisoned rats.

Part of the osteoclasts showed a normal ultrastructure;
others contained characteristic intranuclear and intracy-
toplasmic inclusion bodies. These appeared as roundish
structures of variable diameter (mean 0.5 μm) which characteristically showed protruding peripheral filaments
(Fig. 1) often mixed with electron-dense granules. Most of
the nuclei of these osteoclasts were shrunken and pyknotic
(inset, Fig. 1).

Small intestine

The histological picture of the small intestine of intoxicated rats was the same as that of controls. Under the
electron microscope, the ultrastructure of the epithelial

cells appeared unchanged. However, very small, intrinsically electron-dense granules were present in some of them.
Part of these granules were placed just over the membrane
of the microvilli (Fig. 3), which were otherwise unchanged, part were localized in cytoplasmic vacuoles containing
an amorphous, slightly electron-dense material (Fig. 3),
and others were collected in expansions of the intercellular clefts below the terminal bar (Fig. 3).

DISCUSSION

The presence of inclusion bodies in nuclei and cytoplasm of osteoclasts is the most evident change in bone of
lead-intoxicated rats. The presence of these bodies in
osteoclasts had already been reported in pigs, puppies
and rats with spontaneous or experimental lead poisoning
(Hs73, Va74, Bo83). Moreover, the electron-probe analysis
of the inclusion bodies had shown the presence of lead in
them (Bo83). The present investigation confirms that even
a brief administration of lead induces the appearance of
the inclusion bodies in osteoclasts, and shows that they
consist of aggregates of filaments and granules. Their ultrastructure is practically the same as that of the inclusion bodies which can be found in the epithelial cells of
the renal tubuli (Be61, Go70, Mo73) and it is possible
that inclusions of osteoclasts and of renal cells have the
same structure and composition. Unfortunately, the effect
of lead on cell function and metabolism remains largely
unknown and consequently the genesis of the inclusion bodies is not understood. Their formation probably requires
a high intracellular concentration of the element, as suggested by the fact that they do not form in osteoblasts,
where the lead transport (from blood vessels to calcifying

matrix) probably occurs quickly, and are present in osteoclasts, where lead accumulation is favoured by the continuous resorption od lead-containing bone matrix. It has
been shown that the formation of the inclusion bodies is
inhibited by cycloheximide, which indicates that protein
synthesis is required for their biogenesis (Ch75),and that
they contain non-histonic, acidic proteins (Ri68, Mo73,
Bo83) and glycidic molecules (Bo83). The gradual accumulation of lead in the osteoclast probably induces a derange-
ment of its metabolic activity, as shown by shrinkage and
pyknosis of nuclei. At this stage of nuclear degeneration
the osteoclast breaks away from the bone matrix and probably dies (Bo81).

Small vesicles are present between the uncalcified collagen fibrils of the osteoid border of lead intoxicated
rats. They are similar to, although usually smaller than,
the "matrix vesicles" which are present at the calcification front in calcifying cartilage, bone and mantle dentine (Bo84a). These vesicles seem to be formed by exocytosis
from the osteoblasts (Bo84b) and contain one or several
intrinsically electron-dense granules. In this respect,
they are completely similar to vesicles of dentine of lead
injected rats (Oz81), whose granules contain lead.Although
the electron-probe analysis of the bone vesicles of lead-
intoxicated rats has not been completed, their close similarity with the vesicles of dentine suggests that their
granules also contain lead. It may be speculated that
both in dentine and in bone the intravesicular granules
represent early aggregates of inorganic material, extruded
from the osteoblasts and odontoblasts into the extracellular space. The observation that the vesicles are more numerous in the bone of lead-intoxicated rats than of con-

trols suggests that their formation is accelerated by the necessity of reducing an excessive intracellular concentration of lead. In other words, the process of vesicle formation and granule accumulation in them could be an exaggeration of that by which the osteoblasts extrude Ca ions into the osteoid border during normal calcification. In fact, small, usually single electron-dense granules can be found in some of the vesicles present in the osteoid border of controls (Bo84b).

Granules similar to those found in osteoblast vesicles are present in epithelial intestinal cells. Although it is not possible to state with certainty that they contain lead, their similarity with the granules in bone, and their lack in the intestinal cells of controls support this possibility. The ultrastructural results seem to show that lead is initially linked to the membrane of the microvilli, introduced into the cytoplasm, collected in cytoplasmic vacuoles, shifted to the peripheral membrane and finally collected in expansions of the intercellular cleft to be carried into the blood vessels. These results do not completely explain the mechanism by which lead is transported through the epithelial cells of the small intestine; however, they suggest that it is the same process of active transport which leads to intestinal absorption of calcium and other ions.

REFERENCES

Be61   Beaver D.L., 1961, The ultrastructure of the kidney in lead intoxication with particular reference to intranuclear inclusions , Am. J. Pathol. 39, 195-208

Bo81   Bonucci E., 1981, New knowledge on the origin, function and fate of osteoclasts , Clin. Orthop. 158,

252-269

Bo84a Bonucci E., 1984, Matrix vesicles: their role in calcification , in: Dentin and dentinogenesis (Linde A., ed.), CRC Press, Boca Raton, v. 1, pp 135-154

Bo83   Bonucci E., Barckhaus R.H., Silvestrini G., Ballanti P., Di Lorenzo G., 1983, Osteoclast changes induced by lead poisoning (saturnism) , Appl. Pathol. 1, 241-250

Bo84b Bonucci E., Silvestrini G., 1984, Electron microscope investigations on the origin of matrix vesicles in bone ,in: Endocrine control of bone and calcium metabolism (Cohn D.V., Potts J. T. Jr., Fujita T., eds.), Elsevier Science Publ., Amsterdam, pp 414-417

Ch75   Choie D.D., Richter G.W., Young L.B., 1975, Biogenesis of intranuclear lead-protein inclusions in mouse kidney , Beitr. Pathol. 155, 197-203

Go70   Goyer R.A., May P.M., Krigman M.R., 1970, Lead and protein content of isolated intranuclear inclusion bodies from kidneys of lead poisoned rats , Lab. Invest. 22, 245-251

Hs73   Hsu F.S., Krook L., Shively J.N., Duncan J.R., Pond W.G., 1973, Lead inclusion bodies in osteoclasts , Science 181, 447-448

Mo73   Moore J.F., Goyer R.A., Wilson M., 1973, Lead inclusion bodies solubility, amino acid content, and relationship to residual acidic nuclear proteins , Lab. Invest.29, 488-494

Oz81   Ozawa H., Yamada M., Yamamoto T., 1981, Ultrastructural observations on the location of lead and calcium in the mineralizing dentine of rat incisors , in:Matrix vesicles (Ascenzi A., Bonucci E., De Bernard B., eds.), Wichtig, Milan, pp 179-187

Ri68   Richter G.W., Kress Y., Cornwall C.C., 1968, Another look at lead inclusion bodies , Am. J. Pathol. 53, 189-217

Sc64   Scheiman-Tagger E., Brodie A.G., 1964, Lead acetate as a marker of growing calcified tissues. A modified method , Anat.Record 150, 435-439

Va74   Van Mullem P.J., Stadhouders A.M., 1974, Bone marking and lead intoxication. Early pathological changes in osteoclasts , Virchows Arch. Abt. B 15, 345-350

Acknowledgments: This investigation has been carried out with the financial support of Consiglio Nazionale delle Ricerche e Ministero della Pubblica Istruzione.

45

Aluminium Fluoride Inter-Relationships in Renal Failure

M. GIBSON, I. M. HOUSE, B. KELLY, J. KWAN and V. PARSONS

While using neutron activation analysis for estimating fluoride in uraemic bone we discovered appreciable quantities of aluminium in bone, particularly from patients living in the Newcastle area.[1] This finding was confirmed and linked to an indolent type of fracturing osteomalacia[2] in this area. Other complications include dialysis encephalopathy,[3] uraemic neuropathy,[4] microcytic anaemia,[5] and suppression of parathyroid hormone secretion.[6] Many of these symptoms can be reversed by the use of aluminium free dialysate water[7] and by the administration of desferrioxamine.[8]

Very little work has been carried out on the nature of the aluminium salts involved in the toxic process, although evidence has shown a selective laying down of aluminium in bone mineralising sites,[9] suggesting that aluminium is linked to hydroxapatite formation, either as a calcium aluminate or as a fluoroapatite. The presence of fluoride and silica in uraemic sera has been separately described[10,11] raising the possibility of a fluorosilicate compound. At first it appeared that fluorine could be laid down without aluminium as occurred in uraemic bone from Birmingham, an area with fluoride added to the water which was not high in aluminium (see Table 1), but when a mass plot of bone aluminium content against fluoride was made from all three areas (allowing for calcium content of bone) a linear or curvilinear relationship was found (see figure 1).[12] This relationship could have been a spurious one and so we set up to

427

study the effects of fluoride administration (20 to 40 mg of sodium fluoride orally a day) on the concentrations of aluminium in the plasma of patients on regular dialysis.

METHODS

Fluoride was measured using an ion specific electrode[10] and aluminium by atomic absorption spectrophotometry method.[13] Samples were taken prior to dialysis on a series of patients on regular dialysis therapy using water with a low aluminium content (<70 μmol/l) and low fluoride content (<1 ppm). No attempt was made to limit normal fluoride intake from tea and other oral sources.

RESULTS

Table 1. Ionic composition of bone from uraemic patients in London (L), Birmingham (B), Newcastle (N), and from normal patients (NL) without renal failure (%±SD)

	NL	L	B	N
Ca %	34.1±3.0	36.1±2.6	31.2±4.6	31.3±2.4
F %	0.21±0.1	0.35±0.16	0.47±0.2	0.48±0.24
Al %	0.036±0.02	0.081±0.09	0.158±0.1	0.90±1.57

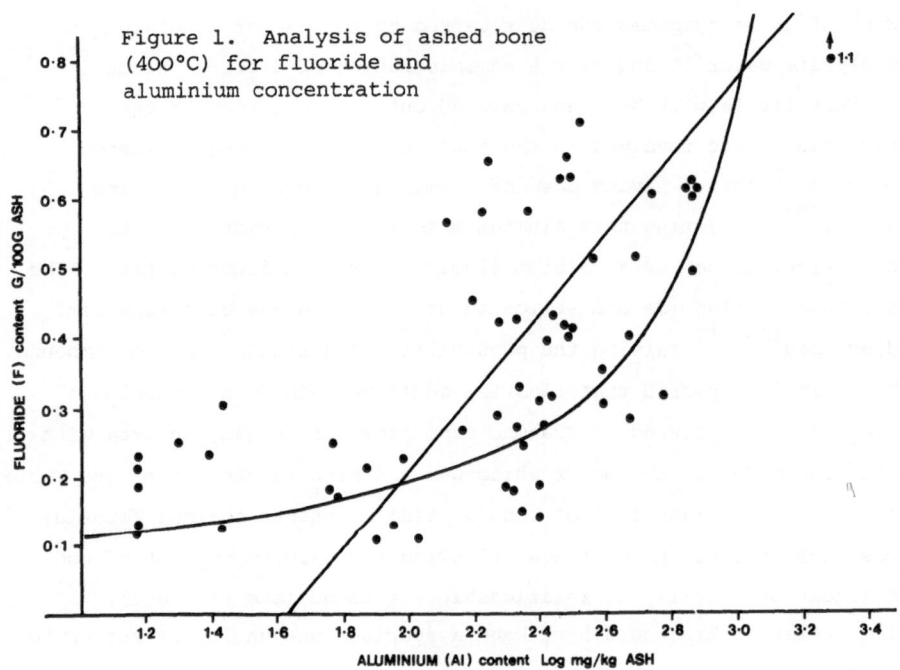

Figure 1. Analysis of ashed bone (400°C) for fluoride and aluminium concentration

Table 2. Changes in plasma F^- and Al^{---} in controls (no NaF) and those given 10-40 mg NaF daily for two weeks, remaining on oral $Al(OH)_3$

	Alµg/l	Fµg/l	%Al	%F change
Controls				
MB	120→70	120→110	-42%	-8%
JD	55→40	80→75	-27%	-6%
AN	20→25	40→30	+25%	-25%
SMCT	60→60	90→50	0%	-44%
HO	60→45	100→70	-25%	-30%
KA	55→40	90→60	-27%	-33%
WM	25→25	90→75	0%	-17%
MT	100→150	150→130	-30%	-13%
Given 10 mg NaF				
RG	55→85	85→95	+55%	+12%
JG	20→45	110→95	+125%	-14%
PT	15→45	180→70	+200%	-61%
JA	120→50	100→90	-58%	-10%
VB	20→50	130→100	+150%	-23%
DT	340→430	100→130	+26%	+30%
Given 20 mg NaF				
FL	150→135	60→75	-10%	+25%
OP	70→95	160→100	+36%	-37%
JC	40→50	100→80	+25%	-20%
JM	55→30	100→100	-45%	-0%
FM	140→130	100→50	-7%	-50%
IA	30→25	65→50	-17%	-23%
Given 40 mg NaF				
DB	120→65	100→380	-46%	+280%
SI	190→130	100→80	-32%	-20%
MA	100→50	160→	-50%	-
LJ	50→40	75→50	-20%	-33%
JS	20→15	80→210	-25%	+162%
BJ	50→40	370→250	-20%	-33%

DISCUSSION

One of the immediate problems that emerged from this study was the fluctuating concentrations of aluminium and fluoride in the pre-dialysis samples of the control groups, reflecting inherent difficulties of single measurements at low levels near the detection levels of both ions, and this must be taken into consideration when the results of fluoride administration are discussed. The next variable was the compliance of the patients in their aluminium hydroxide ingestion, and its timing with the fluoride and food intake. Within the gut there must be a series of dissociations between calcium, phosphate, fluoride and aluminium salts. Aluminium salts could equally well interact in the bowel lumen with administered fluoride, food phosphate and the calcium load at that time, both from exogenous sources and from endogenous secretion. Using desferrioxamine as a chelator of aluminium, the first result is seen in a mobilisation of aluminium from bone and a rise in circulating measurable aluminium for several weeks before a fall.[14] Using only 10 mg NaF, five out of six patients showed a rise in aluminium concentrations after two weeks and falls or modest rises (within the control group range)of fluoride, in keeping with our previous findings on giving fluoride to patients with renal failure.[10] We interpreted this as fixation of fluoride in bone which had been stimulated to turn over faster under the influence of a small increment of fluoride concentration. With larger doses of fluoride ten out of twelve patients showed consistent falls in aluminium concentration with variable changes in fluoride concentration. Where these changes are taking place is difficult to ascertain, but it is recorded that increasing the aluminium intake impairs the absorption of fluoride[15] and the urinary excretion of fluoride.[16] The urinary excretion of fluoride in these patients is minimal and the ions must be deposited in soft tissues and bone.

CONCLUSION

Aluminium and fluoride are both deposited in bone or uraemic patients, especially in those exposed to water ingested or used in dialysate containing these ions. Extra loads of aluminium given as aluminium hydroxide or fluoride given as sodium fluoride are deposited in either soft tissues or bone. It is suggested that these two ions interact in the gut and bone to form complex salts which interfere with the absorption and deposition of calcium and phosphate. Further research must be given to the potential hazard of exposing patients to both ions indiscriminately.

REFERENCES

1. Parsons V., Davies C., Goode C. et al. (1971). Aluminium in bone from patients with renal failure. Brit.Med.J., iv, 273-275

2. Ward M.K., Feest T.G., Ems H.A. et al. (1978). Osteomalacic dialysis osteodystrophy. Lancet, I, 841-845

3. Alfrey A.C., Legendre G.R., Kaehny W.D. (1976). The dialysis encephalopathy syndrome. Possible aluminium intoxication. New Eng.J.Med., 294, 184-188

4. Eno A.I. (1982). Uraemic neuropathy. Correlations between electroneurographic parameters and serum levels of PTH and Al. European Neurology, 21, 396-402

5. Short A.I.K., Winney R.J., Robson J.S. (1980). Reversible microcytic anaemia in dialysis patients due to aluminium intoxication. Proc. EDTA, 17, 226-233

6. Cannata J.B., Briggs J.D., Junor B.J.R. et al. (1980). Effect of acute aluminium overload on calcium and PTH metabolism. Lancet, I, 501-503

7. Platts M., Goode G.C., Hislop J.S. (1977). Composition of domestic water supply and the incidence of fractures and encephalopathy in patients on home dialysis.

8. Ackrill R., Ralston A.J., Day J.P. et al. (1980). Successful removal of aluminium from a patient with dialysis encephalopathy. Lancet, II, 692-693

9. Maloney N.A., Ott S.M., Alfrey A.C. et al. (1982). Histological quantitation of aluminium in iliac bone from patients with renal failure. J.Lab.Clin.Med., 94, 206-216

10. Parsons V., Choudhury A.A., Wass J.A.H. et al. (1975). Renal excretion of fluoride in renal failure and after renal transplantation. Brit.Med.J., 1, 128-130

11. Dobbie J.W., Smith M.J.B., Abdullah R.A.S. (1981) Silicon and the kidney. Proceedings VIII Int. Congress Nephrology. Athens. 1030-1034. S.Karger, Basel.

12. Parsons V., Kerr D.N.S., Ellis H. et al. (1980). Aluminium and fluoride in three geographically different renal units. Q.J.Medicine, 196, 514

13. Clarkson E.M., Luck V.A., Hynson W.V. et al. (1972). The effect of aluminium hydroxide on calcium phosphorus and aluminium balances etc. Clin.Sci., 43, 514-513

14. Malluche H.H., Smith A.J., Abreo K. et al. (1984). The use of deferoxamine in the management of aluminium accumulation in bone in patients with renal failure. New.Eng.J.Med., 311, 140-144

15. Spencer H., Kramer L., Norris C. et al. (1980). Effect of aluminium hydroxide on fluoride metabolism. Clin.Pharmacol.Therap., 28, 529-535

46

Evaluation of Different Techniques Used to Determine Aluminium in Patients with Chronic Renal Failure

W. J. VISSER, F. L. VAN DE VYVER, A. H. VERBUEKEN, P. D' HAESE, A. B. BEKAERT, R. E. VAN GRIEKEN, S. A. DUURSMA and M. E. DE BROE

INTRODUCTION

The patient with chronic renal failure (CRF) is at considerable risk for aluminum accumulation, especially when undergoing chronic dialysis. The main sources of aluminum are:

- aluminum contaminating the dialysate (Pl77); this aluminum passes the dialyzer membrane
- aluminum-containing phosphate binders administered to decrease the serum phosphate levels (Ka77).

Furthermore, renal function impairment impedes effective elimination of aluminum, which is normally excreted by the kidneys (Go79).

Tissue accumulation of aluminum may cause malfunction of some organs. Thus, the association between elevated cerebral aluminum concentrations and dialysis encephalopathy seems reasonably well established. Also, a causal relationship between a characteristic type of osteomalacia occurring in CRF and aluminum accumulation in bone has been suggested by the confrontation of bone aluminum concentrations and bone histology in animal and human studies (El79). Recently, it has been proposed that microcytic hypochromic anemia (El78), and disturbed parathyroid gland secretion (Mo83) may be due to excessive aluminum accumulation.

Aluminum accumulation and resulting toxicity can be prevented and treated. In fact, aluminum sources may be eliminated to a large extent in most cases and aluminum can be effectively removed from the body by the aluminum chelating agent desferrioxamine (Desféral). The adminis-

433

tration of desferrioxamine to patients with debilitating aluminum-induced osteomalacia (AIOM) results in evident clinical improvement within a few weeks and regression of osteomalacia on bone histology within a few months (Ma84).

These considerations clearly demonstrate the need for reliable methods enabling both the evaluation of the amount of aluminum which is accumulated in the body, as well as the early diagnosis of AIOM.

The procedures used in this study were:

- electrothermal atomic absorption spectrometry (ETAAS) for the measurement of serum and bone aluminum concentrations (DH84);
- histology and histomorphometry of un-decalcified bone sections
- laser microprobe mass analysis (LAMMA) for the localization of aluminum in bone at the light microscopic level (Ve84).

The choice of serum and bone samples is evident: serum is a readily obtainable biological material and the bone is the major storage organ of aluminum in CRF. Also, bone biopsy specimens are taken routinely in our CRF patients.

PATIENTS AND METHODS

Patients

Fifty patients with severe renal failure were studied. Fifteen of them did not require dialysis treatment (serum creatinine level 6.2±2.7mg/dl, mean±SD). Twenty-seven were treated with maintenance hemodialysis with single passage of dialysate (60±46 months). Eight patients underwent longterm closed-circuit hemodialysis with regeneration of the dialysate using a REDY^R sorbent cartridge (58±33 months).

Samples

Duplicate transiliac bone biopsy specimens were taken 2cm beneath the anterior part of the iliac crest using a trephine of 7mm diameter. One specimen was used for histology, the other for ETAAS. After coagulation and centrifuging, serum samples for aluminum determination were transferred to polystyrene tubes with tightfitting polyethylene caps (Biolab, Limal, Belgium).

ETAAS

These methods have been described more extensively elsewhere (DH84) and may be summarized as follows. All materials were tested as potential sources of contamination. Serum samples were diluted 1:3 with double-distilled water. After determination of the wet weight, the bone

sample for ETAAS was transferred to a polystyrene tube with a polyethylene cap. The bone samples were subjected to nitric acid destruction in quartz Kjeldahl flasks, Teflon bombs or Teflon tubes. For the
actual measurements, a model 372 atomic absorption spectrometer with
an HGA-500 graphite furnace and an AS-40 auto-sampler were used (injection volume 20µl). Graphite tubes were un-coated. All instruments were
from Perkin-Elmer Corp. (Norwalk, CT, USA). Direct and standard-ad-
ditions methods were used.

Histology

Histologic and histomorphometric investigation of the second bone biopsy sample was performed after 24hr fixation in Burkhardt's solution
(Bu66) and subsequent transfer to absolute methanol. After dehydration,
the specimens were embedded in plastic. Un-decalcified, 4µm-thick bone
sections were cut with a Jung K microtome. Sections were stained according to Goldner for descriptive histology. Using tri-ammonium aurin
tricarboxylate (Aluminon[R], BDH, Poole, UK), aluminum deposits were
made visible. Aluminum deposits at the trabecular circumference were
evaluated with histomorphometry. Using a grid consisting of successive
semi-circles (Me76), the fraction of the trabecular boundary where red
lines were found, was expressed as a fraction of the total boundary
line (Al%).

LAMMA

The LAMMA consists of a dual laser system and a time-of-flight mass
spectrometer. A low-powered red helium-neon laser indicates the subcellular region to be analyzed, and a collinear powerful Q-switched neo-
dymium-YAG (Yttrium-Aluminum-Garnet) laser provides a high-power pulse,
which is able to vaporize and ionize a selected area of a few square
micrometers of the histological section. The latter is viewed with a
binocular microscope. After the perforation, the positive and negative
ions so created are moved into the mass spectrometer in order to produce a complete mass spectrum for each laser pulse (Ve84). Un-stained,
un-decalcified, 2µm-thick, plastic-embedded bone sections were used.

Statistical analysis

Spearman rank correlation coefficients (R_s) were used to study the
relationships between the parameters of serum and tissue aluminum.

RESULTS

Significant correlations were found between serum and bone aluminum
concentrations (FIG. 1) and between Al% and bone aluminum concentrations (FIG. 2).

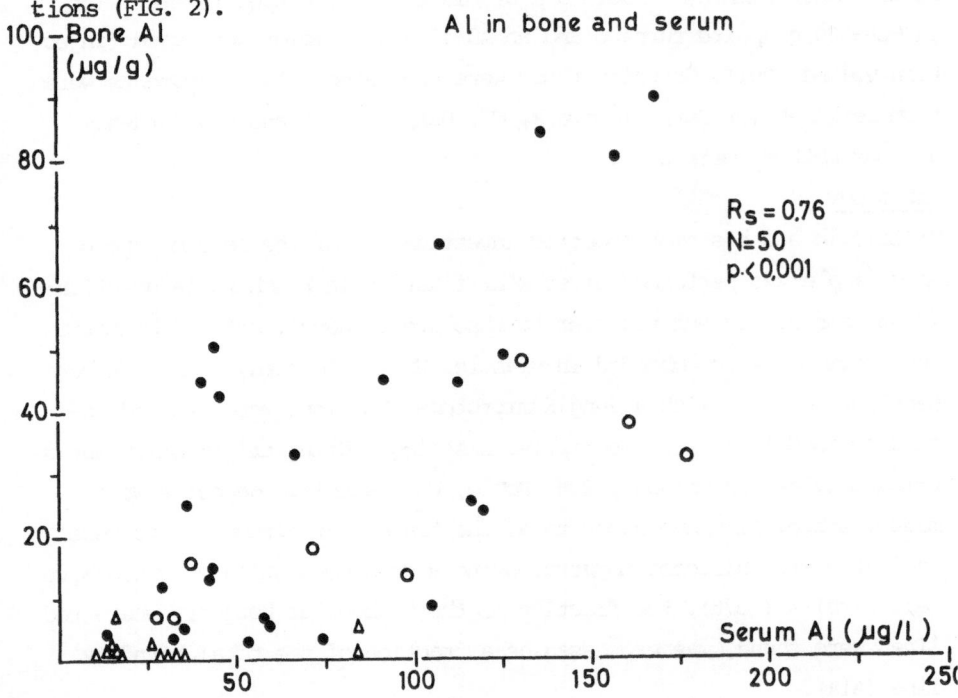

● conventional dialysis (n= 27)
○ redy dialysis (n = 8)
△ non dialyzed (n =15)

FIGURE 1   Relationship between serum and bone aluminum concentrations.
Reference values for serum aluminum: 2.0±0.4µg/g; for bone
aluminum: <1µg/g.

It appears from FIG. 1, that all patients with positive Aluminon-staining at the osteoid/calcified-bone boundary (OCBB) showed bone aluminum
concentrations of 30µg/g or more.

LAMMA investigations of unstained bone sections confirmed the presence
of aluminum at the OCBB in patients presenting red lines at Aluminon-
staining (Ve84). In 2 cases, purple instead of red lines were seen at
the OCBB after Aluminon-staining. LAMMA spectra of these purple lines
showed both aluminum as well as iron. Thus, in cases of purple lines
aluminum appears to be present at the OCBB, but the Al% cannot be determined. Consequently, such patients were not considered for establishing the relationship presented in FIG. 2. Furthermore, some patients presented brownish bone marrow cells at Aluminon-staining. Here

also, LAMMA confirmed the concomitant presence of aluminum and iron
(Va84b).

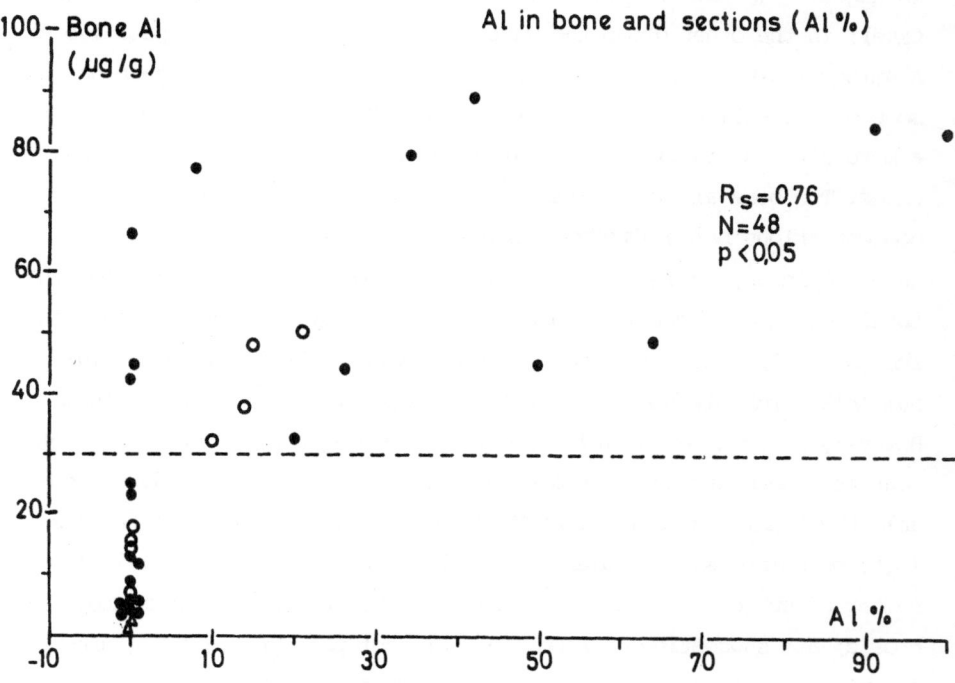

FIGURE 2   Relationship between the histochemical measure of aluminum
           present at the OCBB (Al%) and bone aluminum concentrations.

DISCUSSION

Although a significant correlation exists between serum and bone aluminum concentrations, the former do not provide reliable estimates of
the latter (FIG. 1). It is conceivable that serum aluminum levels mere-
ly reflect on-going aluminum loading and give little indication of total aluminum body load.

A significant correlation was observed between Al% (the histomorphometric measure of stainable aluminum at the OCBB) and bone aluminum
concentrations (FIG. 2). The existence of this correlation is explained in part, by the fact that all cases with aluminum levels of 30µg/g
or less showed none or negligible stainable aluminum. When only clearly Aluminon-positive patients were considered, (Al%>1), a less significant correlation between Al% and bone aluminum levels was observed
(R_s=0.57, P<0.05, N=13). The "30µg aluminum/g bone line" apparently

delimits 2 groups of patients: in the one group the Aluminon-staining is negative (3 patients with Al% <1 or =1 were considered to be negative); in the other group the vast majority of patients is positive at Aluminon-staining. The observation of a negative Aluminon-staining in some of the patients belonging to the latter group, is probably due to a more diffuse distribution of aluminum throughout the bone in these cases. The bone aluminum distribution in patients with bone aluminum concentrations below 30µg/g is unknown.

In our opinion, bone aluminum values are fairly representative for the total amount of aluminum accumulated in the body, because the bone is the major aluminum storage organ in CRF (De84). Stainable bone aluminum (Al%) probably bears less relationship with total body aluminum. However, it is an essential element in the diagnosis of AIOM. In fact, routine bone histological stainings (e.g. Goldner's stain) do not enable the final diagnosis of AIOM. Although some histological features (e.g. osteoidosis, irregularly distributed osteoid, a relatively low number of cubic i.e. active osteoblasts, and the absence of marrow fibrosis) are suggestive of AIOM, they are not pathognomonic. Aluminon-staining is indispensable for establishing the diagnosis.

LAMMA is a sensitive technique, which enables to localize aluminum in un-decalcified bone sections, even in some Aluminon-negative patients. It is also a valuable aid in validating the histochemical results. Furthermore, the technique may be useful when histochemical results are doubtful. For example, in cases where Aluminon-staining showed purple lines at the OCBB and/or brownish cells in the bone marrow, LAMMA has demonstrated the concurrent presence of iron and aluminum (Va84b). The question whether iron alone (i.e. in the absence of a significant amount of aluminum) yields purple lines or brownish marrow cells at Aluminon-staining, is currently under investigation with LAMMA. In patients with concomitant aluminum and iron overload, LAMMA has demonstrated the concurrent deposition of both elements, not only in the bone, but also in lysosomes of Kupffer cells and hepatocytes (Va84a, Ve84).

Bone histomorphometry is indicated whenever successive biopsies of the same patient are available. Thus, the effect of therapeutic measures may be evaluated (e.g. desferrioxamine treatment, Ma84).

SUMMARY

In patients with chronic renal failure (CRF), aluminum may accumulate
in the skeleton causing aluminum-induced osteomalacia (AIOM). Since
preventive measures may be taken to avoid further aluminum accumulation, and since aluminum can be removed from the body by desferrioxamine, it is essential to have at hand, methods for evaluating body
aluminum load, and for establishing the diagnosis of AIOM.

In 50 cases of CRF, serum and bone aluminum concentrations were determined using electrothermal atomic absorption spectrometry (ETAAS). Furthermore, un-decalcified bone sections were studied using histology,
histomorphometry of aluminum deposits, and laser microprobe mass analysis (LAMMA).

A highly significant correlation was found between serum and bone aluminum concentrations (R_s=0.76). However, serum aluminum values of individual patients were inadequate in estimating bone aluminum concentrations. It is suggested, that the serum aluminum concentration is a parameter of on-going aluminum loading, whereas the bone aluminum level is
a measure of the amount of aluminum stored in the bone (the major storage organ for aluminum in CRF), and therefore is an index of the total
amount of aluminum accumulated in the body.

A highly significant correlation was also found between the histomorphometric estimate of stainable aluminum at the osteoid/calcified bone
boundary (OCBB) and the bone aluminum level (R_s=0.76). The former parameter was designated Al%. When the Aluminon-negative patients were
excluded (Al% <1 or =1), the correlation was less significant (R_s=0.57,
P<0.05, N=13). All patients showing bone aluminum concentrations below
30µg/g were negative at Aluminon-staining.

Although routine bone histology may suggest AIOM, a positive Aluminon-
staining is essential for making the diagnosis..

REFERENCES

Bu66 Burkhardt R., 1966, Technische Verbesserungen und Anwendungsbereich
der Histo-Biopsie von Knochenmark und Knochen. Klin.Wochenschr. 44,
326-334.

De84 De Broe M. E., Van de Vyver F. L., Bekaert A. B., et al., 1984,
Correlation of serum aluminum values with tissue aluminum concentrations. Contrib. Nephrol. 38, 37-46.

DH84 D'Haese P., Van de Vyver F. L., Bekaert A. B., De Broe M. E., 1984, The measurement of aluminum in serum, blood, urine, and tissues of chronic hemodialyzed patients by use of electrothermal atomic absorption spectrometry. Clin. Chem., submitted.

El78 Elliott H. L., Macdougall A. I., Fell G. S., 1978, Aluminium toxicity syndrome. Lancet 1, 1203.

El79 Ellis H. A., McCarthy J. H., Herrington J., 1979, Bone aluminium in haemodialysed patients and in rats injected with aluminium chloride: relationship to impaired bone mineralisation. J. Clin. Pathol. 32, 832-844.

Go79 Gorsky J.E., Dietz A.A., Spencer H., Osis D., 1979, Metabolic balance of aluminum studied in six men. Clin. Chem. 25, 1739-1743.

Ka77 Kaehny W. D., Hegg A. P., Alfrey A. C., 1977, Gastrointestinal absorption of aluminum from aluminum-containing antacids. N. Engl. J. Med. 296, 1389-1390.

Ma84 Malluche H. H., Smith A. J., Abreo K., Faugere M.-C., 1984, The use of deferoxamine in the management of aluminum accumulation in bone in patients with renal failure. N. Engl. J. Med. 311, 140-144.

Me68 Merz W. A., 1968, Die Streckenmessung an gerichteten Strukturen im Mikroskop und ihre Anwendung zur Bestimmung von Oberflächen-Volumen-Relationen im Knochengewebe. Mikroskopie 22, 132-142.

Mo83 Morrissey J., Rothstein M., Mayor G., Slatopolsky E., 1983, Suppression of parathyroid hormone secretion by aluminum. Kidney Int. 23, 699-704.

Pl84 Plachot J.-J., Cournot-Witmer G., Halpern S., et al., 1984, Bone ultrastructure and x-ray microanalysis of aluminum-intoxicated patients. Kidney Int. 25, 796-803.

Pl77 Platts M. M., Goode G. C., Hislop J. S., 1977, Composition of the domestic water supply and the incidence of fractures and encephalopathy on home dialysis. Br. Med. J. 2, 657-660.

Va84a Van de Vyver F. L., Vanheule A. O., Verbueken A. H., et al., 1984, Patterns of iron storage in patients with severe renal failure. Contrib. Nephrol. 38, 153-166.

Va84b Van de Vyver F. L., Verbueken A. H., Visser W. J., Van Grieken R. E., De Broe M. E., 1984, Localisation of aluminium and iron by histochemical and laser microprobe mass analytical techniques in bone marrow cells of chronic haemodialysis patients. J. Clin. Pathol. 37, 837–838.

Ve84 Verbueken A. H., Van de Vyver F. L., Van Grieken R. E., et al., 1984, Ultrastructural localization of aluminum in patients with dialysis-associated osteomalacia. Clin. Chem. 30, 763–768.

47

Evaluation of the Role of Aluminium on the Bone Histomorphometry of Uremic Patients

J. L. SEBERT, A. FOURNIER, P. LEFLON, M. A. HERVE, A. MARIE,
J. GUERIS and M. GARABEDIAN

INTRODUCTION

Since the report by Ward et al (Wa 78), suggesting that aluminium may be a major factor of bone disease in dialyzed patients, evidence has accumulated in support of this hypothesis. It has been particulary shown that aluminium accumulates in bone of uremic patients, especially at the mineralization front (Co 81), and can induce the development of vitamin D resistant osteomalacia. Most cases of histologically proved osteomalacia have been reported in heavily intoxicated patients, exposed to contaminated dialysis water, presenting with symptoms including fractures and encephalopathy (Pi 80, Ho 82). Beside these well demonstrated cases of florid osteomalacia, due to severe aluminium intoxication, little is known about the bone effects of mild aluminium overload. In this study we evaluated the bone aluminium content and toxicity in uremic patients on chronic hemodialysis or hemofiltration with mild aluminium overload mainly induced by aluminium-containing gels prescribed to control serum phosphate.

MATERIAL AND METHODS

20 uremic patients (14 males, 6 females), aged 52 $\pm$ 15 (SD) years underwent iliac bone biopsy after double tetracycline labeling. They had been on chronic hemodialysis (12 patients) or hemofiltration (8 patients), 3 times weekly, for 28 $\pm$ 15 months and had no symptom of bone disease. Aluminium concentration was less than .3 μmol/l in the dialysate and ranged from .15 to .60 μmol/l in the substitution

443

fluid for hemofiltration. Aluminium hydroxide was given to 17 patients
in order to control plasma phosphate, and the total cumulative dose they
received ranged from 100 to 6 400 g. 6 patients were treated with
25 OH D_3 (5 - 30 μg/day) and 2 were treated with 1α OH D_3 1 μg/day.

Quantitative bone histomorphometry was carried out on undecalcified,
5 μm thick sections, using Zeiss integrated eye - pieces. The following
parameters were measured on Goldner Stained sections : osteoid volume
(OV) expressed in % trabecular bone volume; osteoid surface (OS) in
% trabecular surfaces; osteoid thickness index (OTI) calculated as
the ratio $\frac{OV}{OS}$ x 100 (Me 77); osteoblastic surface (OBL.S.) defined
as osteoid surface covered by plump osteoblasts; active resorption surface (ARS) defined as the % trabecular bone surface occupied by
Howship lacunae with close osteoclasts. The following dynamic parameters
of bone remodeling were derived from fluorescence study of unstained
sections : Tetracycline - labeled surface (Lab.S.) defined as the %
extent of single and double labeled surfaces; mineral appositional rate
(App. Rate); bone formation rate at tissue level (BFR) calculated
as App. Rate x Lab. S. In addition, the presence of aluminium was looked
for on sections stained with Aluminon[R].

Aluminium content of bone and plasma : The bone concentration of aluminium was determined on a second bone sample taken during the same biopsy procedure. Aluminium was measured in plasma and bone by inductively
coupled plasma emission spectrometry using a JOBIN YVON Elemental Analyzer JY 38 P. The upper limit of the normal range of plasma aluminium
concentration was .3 μmol/l with a detection limit of .15 μmol/l. Normal values for aluminium bone concentration, obtained from 7 non-uremic
corpses were .068 $\pm$ (SD) .036 μmol/g of fresh bone tissue.

Biochemical and hormonal parameters : Plasma calcium, phosphate and alkaline phosphatases were measured using a TECHNICON autoanalyzer.

Plasma parathyroid hormone (PTH) was measured by radioimmunoassay
using an antiserum specific of the mid-region of the molecule. Normal
range was 80 - 220 pg/ml. Vitamin D metabolites were measured by radio-
competition after previous lipidic extraction of the plasma and purification by chromatography on a Sephadex LH 20 column followed by a second high pressure liquid chromatography. The normal range of D metabolites was : 6 - 30 ng/ml for 25 OH D, 1 - 3 ng/ml for 24.25 $(OH)_2 D_3$
and 20 - 60 pg/ml for 1.25 $(OH)_2$ D.

Statistical methods :

In order to study the potential link between the various bone histomorphometric parameters and the biochemical and hormonal factors, 2 statistical methods were successively used : 1) the least squares simple linear regression analysis, 2) a multidimensional analysis combining polynominal evaluation and matricial discriminant analysis (Le 83).

The linear regression analysis shows the apparent link between 2 variables whereas the concomitant influence of the other parameters has not been eliminated. The combination of polynominal evaluation and matricial discriminant analysis allows one to point out the specific link between an explained variable(here one of the histomorphometric parameters) and each of the explanatory variables (here aluminium and the other biochemical parameters) independently of the influence of the others. The multidimensional analysis was performed on a COMMODORE 8000 computer using programs of the university of PARIS VII and of the institute of Technology of COMPIEGNE. This multidimensional analysis leads to the determination of the D^2 coefficient of MAHALANOBIS which represents the proper influence of each explanatory variable on a given explained one. This coefficient ranges from -1 to +1 according to the sign of the relation.

RESULTS

Bone histology : 8 patients had pure hyperparathyroidism : they had increased active resorption surfaces, and no evidence of a mineralization defect as shown by normal to high labeled surfaces and mineral appositional rates. These patients had high bone turnover with high bone formation rates. 8 patients had increased bone resorption coupled with decreased mineral appositional rate. These patients had hyperparathyroidism but low bone formation rates. The remaining 4 patients had low-normal bone resorption but had decreased labeled surfaces and mineral appositional rates in spite of increased osteoid surfaces. These patients had low bone turnover with low bone formation rate. No patient had true osteomalacia since in no case was the osteoid thickness index increased.

As shown in figure 1 osteoblastic surfaces were strongly correlated with active resorption surfaces (r = .86), labeled surfaces (r = .82), mineral appositional rate (r = .79) and bone formation rate (r = .87). Only 2 patients had traces of stainable aluminium at the interface of mineralized and unmineralized bone.

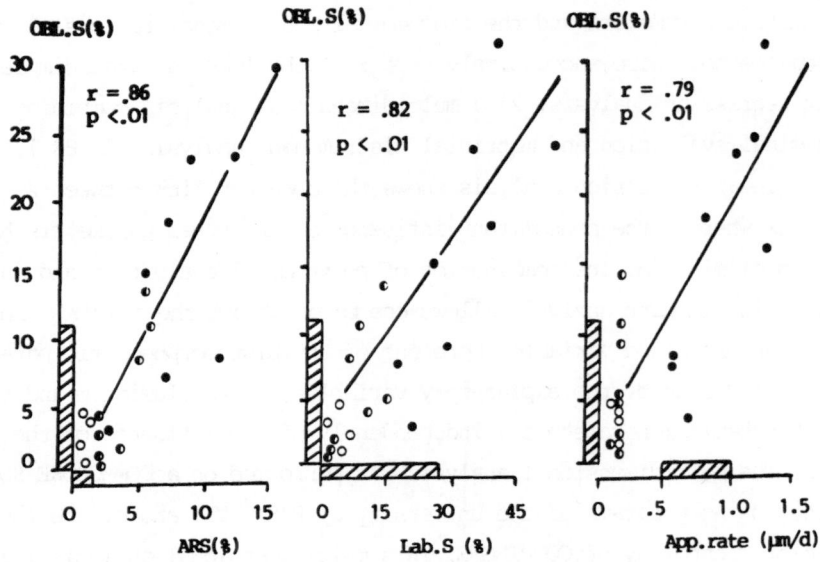

FIGURE 1 : Correlations between osteoblastic surfaces (OBL.S) and :
ARS (active resorption surface), Lab.S (extent of labeled
surface), App.Rate (mineral appositional rate).
Symbols indicate : (●) patients with pure hyperparathyroidism, (o) patients with low mineral appositional rate and
normal resorption, (◐) patients with both hyperresorption
and low mineral appositional rate.

Biochemistry : Bone aluminium was increased in all patients with a
mean value of .59 ± .44 µmol/g about 10 times higher than the mean value of .068 ± .036 µmol/g obtained in non-uremic controls. Plasma aluminium was increased in 17/20 patients with a mean value of 1.94 ± .44
µmol/l. The 3 patients with normal plasma levels were those who did not
receive oral aluminium hydroxide. Plasma and bone aluminium concentrations were significantly correlated (r = .59, p < .02). Bone aluminium correlated with the total cumulative dose of aluminium hydroxide
(r = .59, p < .02) but not with the duration on dialysis.

The mean plasma level of 25 OH D was 14.3 ± 11.8 ng/ml and only
5/20 patients had values under the lower limit of the normal range.

The 2 patients who were taking 1α OH D_3 had increased levels of
1.25 (OH)$_2$ D. When these 2 patients were excluded, the mean plasma level of 1.25 (OH)$_2$ D was 24.2 ± 17 (pg/ml), a value located in the lower
part of the normal range. Plasma 24.25 (OH)$_2$ D was in the normal range
in all cases and correlated with plasma 25 OH D (r = .52).

Plasma PTH was increased in all but one patient. Plasma PTH did not correlate with plasma calcium (r = .15) but there was a trend for a positive correlation between PTH and phosphate (r = .36, p < .10). 6 patients had increased alkaline phosphatase activity.

Table 1. Linear correlations between biochemical and histological data

	PTH		Alkaline phosphatase	
	r	p	r	p
OV	.33	NS	.42	.05
OS	.12	NS	.33	NS
OTI	.43	.05	.34	NS
OBL.S	.69	<.01	.75	<.01
ARS	.65	<.01	.60	<.01
Lab.S	.60	<.01	.53	<.05
App.Rate	.58	<.01	.61	<.01
B.F.R.	.61	<.01	.66	<.01

As shown in table 1, PTH and alkaline phosphatases correlated with many parameters of bone remodeling. At contrast, there was no significant correlation between bone or plasma aluminium and any of the histological parameters.

Results of the multidimensional analysis are presented in table 2. When the influence of all the other simultaneously measured biochemical factors was eliminated, negative relations were found between either bone or plasma aluminium and the histological parameters of bone formation and mineralization, including osteoblastic surfaces, mineral appositional rate and bone formation rate.

DISCUSSION

The major bone histomorphometric features of these patients on chronic hemodialysis or hemofiltration were hyperparathyroidism and low bone formation which were either seen alone or in association. True osteomalacia combining low mineral appositional rate and increased osteoid thickness giving evidence of a delay between apposition and mineralization was, at contrast, totally absent. Even more, the osteoid thickness was independent of a mineralization defect but appeared to be dependent on the degree of hyperparathyroidism as shown by the positive correlation between PTH and osteoid thickness index. It has been shown that matrix apposition is faster than mineral apposition in the early

stages of the forming phase of the bone remodeling unit and this can
contribute to increase the osteoid seam width, even if mineralization
is normal (Pa 80). Since PTH increases bone turnover, PTH excess could
then increase the mean osteoid seam width only by increasing the fraction number of newly forming units of faster appositional potential.
The observed relationship between PTH and osteoid thickness could so be
entirely due to increased bone turnover in the total absence of a mineralization defect.

Table 2. Effects of bone and plasma aluminium on bone remodeling,
assessed by multidimensional analysis.

	Bone Aluminium		Plasma Aluminium	
	D^2	p	D^2	p
OV	.44	<.05	.51	<.05
OS	.47	<.05	.63	<.05
OTI	.13	NS	.28	NS
OBL.S	-.47	<.05	-.62	<.01
ARS	.27	NS	.29	NS
Lab.S	-.07	NS	-.10	NS
App.Rate	-.39	<.05	-.31	NS
BFR	-.39	<.05	-.22	NS

D^2 is the D^2 coefficient of MAHALANOBIS which measures the proper influence on histological parameters of bone and plasma aluminium, independently of the other simultaneously measured biochemical factors including PTH, D metabolites, calcium and phosphate.

In spite of a total absence of true osteomalacia, our patients had
proved aluminium overload, as judged by elevated concentrations of aluminium in bone and plasma. In the absence of significant contamination
of dialysis water and substitution fluids, this aluminium overload appeared to be due to the use of oral phosphate binders as suggested by
the positive correlation found between bone aluminium content and the
total cumulative dose of aluminium hydroxide. Neither plasma nor bone
aluminium correlated with the histological parameters of osteoid accumulation. A positive correlation between bone aluminium and osteoid
volume has been recently reported in dialysed uremic patients but was
limited to patients with severe osteomalacia and was not observed in
patients with pure hyperparathyroidism or mild bone disease (Ho 82).
Although bone aluminium concentration was increased in all patients,
only 2 of them had traces of stainable aluminium on histological examination. This is in contrast with other reports showing a high degree

of correlation between the histochemical staining method and the direct
measurement of bone aluminium by atomic absorption spectrometry (Ot 82).
But, there again, it appeared that, if nearly all osteomalacic patients
had large amounts of stainable aluminium most patients with prevailing
hyperparathyroidism had little or none. The striking absence of histological osteomalacia and of stainable aluminium in the bone biopsies
of our patients could therefore be due to a milder degree of aluminium
overload. In fact, these patients were asymptomatic and had not been
severely exposed to aluminium contamination. However, when the influence of the other biochemical factors was eliminated by means of the multidimensional analysis a negative relationship was found between plasma or bone aluminium and both osteoblastic surfaces and mineral appositional rate. This is in agreement with a recent report showing that
short-term administration of aluminium in the rat does not cause osteomalacia but decreases bone formation (Go 84). Mild aluminium over- .
load, mainly due to aluminium containing phosphate binders, not severe
enough to cause osteomalacia, could therefore decrease osteoblastic
population and activity and reduce bone formation in uremic patients.

SUMMARY

The aluminium overload and its possible bone toxicity were evaluated in 20 asymptomatic uremic patients on chronic hemodialysis or
hemofiltration, who had not been exposed to significant aluminium contamination by dialysate water or substitution fluid, but had been
treated with aluminium hydroxide.

Histological examination of undecalcified bone sections showed : pure hyperparathyroidism in 8 patients, low bone formation without increased osteoid thickness in 4 and a mixture of the 2 in the remaining patients. No patient had true osteomalacia with increased osteoid
thickness. Only 2 patients had traces of stainable aluminium. In contrast, bone aluminium content measured by atomic emission spectrometry was increased in all patients and correlated with plasma aluminium and with the total cumulative dose of aluminium hydroxide.

The effects of bone and plasma aluminium on bone histology was evaluated by means of a multidimensional analysis which allowed to eliminate the influence of the other simultaneously studied biochemical
and hormonal factors including PTH, D metabolites, calcium and phosphate. A negative relationship was found between plasma or bone alu-

minium and osteoblastic surfaces (p < .01), mineral appositional rate and bone formation rate (p < .05). These results indicate that mild aluminium overload, not severe enough to cause osteomalacia decreases osteoblastic population and activity, and reduces bone formation in uremic patients.

REFERENCES

Co 81 COURNOT-WITMER G., ZINGRAFF J., PLACHOT J.J., ESCAIG F., LEFEVRE R., BOUMATI P., BOURDEAU A., GARABEDIAN M., GALLE P., BOURDON R., DRUEKE T., BALSAN S. 1981. "Aluminium localization in bone from hemodialyzed patients : relationship to matrix mineralization". Kidney Int. 20, 375-385.

Go 84 GOODMAN W.G., GILLIGAN J., HORST P. 1984. "Short - term aluminium administration in the rat. Effects on bone formation and relationship to renal osteomalacia". J. Clin. Invest., 73, 171-181.

Ho 82 HODSMAN A.B., SHERRARD D.J., AlFREY A.C., OTT S., BRICKMAN A.S., MILLER N., MALONEY N.A., COBURN J.W. 1982. "Bone aluminium and histomorphometric features of renal osteodystrophy". J. Clin. Endocrinol. Metab., 54, 539-546.

Le 83 LEFEVRE J. 1983. "Introduction aux analyses statistiques multidimensionnelles. Masson. PARIS.

Me 77 MEUNIER P., EDOUARD C., RICHARD D., LAURENT J. 1977. "Histomorphometry of osteoid tissue. The hyperosteoidoses" In MEUNIER P., (Ed). Bone Histomorphometry, ARMOUR-MONTAGU, Paris, 249-262.

Ot 82 OTT S.M., MALONEY N.A., COBURN J.W., ALFREY A.C., SHERRARD D.J. 1982. "The prevalence of bone aluminium deposition in renal osteodystrophy and its relation to the response to calcitriol therapy". N. Engl. J. Med. 307, 709-713.

Pa 80 PARFITT A.M., VILLANUEVA A.R., MATHEWS C.H.E., ASWANI S.A. 1980. "Kinetics of matrix and mineral apposition in osteoporosis and renal osteodystrophy. Relationship to rate of turnover and to cell morphology". Metab. Bone Dis. and Rel. Res. 2 suppl., 213-219.

Pi 80 PIERIDES A.M., EDWARDS W.G.Jr., CULLUM U.X.Jr., Mc CALL J.T., ELLIS H.E. 1980. "Hemodialysis encephalopathy with osteomalacic fractures and muscle weakness". Kidney Int. 18, 115-124.

Wa 79 WARD M.K., FEEST T.G., ELLIS M.A., PARKINSON I.S., KERR D.N.S., 1978. "Osteomalacic dialysis osteodystrophy : evidence for a water-borne aetiological agent, probably aluminium". Lancet,i, 841-845.

48

In Vitro Modelling of the Role of Aluminium in Inducing Osteomalacia in Dialysis Patients

N. C. BLUMENTHAL, A. L. BOSKEY and A. S. POSNER

INTRODUCTION

Osteomalacia renal osteodystrophy in patients on long-term hemodialysis has been associated with aluminum accumulation in bone (Ho82).
Aluminum has been shown to be localized at the mineralization front
in dialysis osteomalacia, suggesting it as a possible cause of this
disorder. Animal models of aluminum-induced osteomalacia have been
demonstrated which mimic the clinical disease (Go, in press, Ch83).
In addition, recent work has shown that aluminum had an inhibitory
effect on mineralization in organ cultures of embryonic chick bone
(Mi84). It has been demonstrated that aluminum exerts a significant
physical chemical effect on the formation and growth of crystalline
hydroxyapatite (HA) in three <u>in vitro</u> test systems thought to be analogous to biological mineralization (Bl84). This earlier study suggested that aluminum interfered with HA production in these different
systems by acting as a surface poison blocking nucleation and/or
growth sites on ACP and HA surfaces.

Subsequent work has shed further light on the mechanism of interaction of aluminum with the <u>in vitro</u> formation and growth of HA which
gives more understanding of the etiology of aluminum associated osteomalacia.

METHODS

The effect of a series of $AlCl_3$ concentrations, ranging from 0.00 to
10.0 mM aluminum, was studied in three test systems: (a) direct hy-

451

droxyapatite (HA) precipitation, (b) transformation of amorphous calcium phosphate (ACP) to HA and, (c) growth of HA seed crystals. In
these experiments aluminum was added in solution at the beginning
prior to any HA formation.

The specific conditions in each system were:

(a) Direct HA precipitation: 5 ml of reaction solution, 2.79 mM Ca
as $CaCl_2$, 1.87 mM PO_4 as Na_2HPO_4 (No ACP precursor).

(b) ACP transformation: 100 mg ACP in 100 ml reaction solution.

(c) HA crystal growth: 15 mg poorly-crystallized HA (previously
prepared at room temperature) in 100 ml of solution, 1.55 mM Ca as
$CaCl_2$, 1.07 mM PO_4 as Na_2HPO_4.

In addition, several experiments were designed to study the uptake
of aluminum by ACP and HA. ACP was synthesized with aluminum in the
preparative solution in order to determine the extent to which the
metal is incorporated with the amorphous phase. Two different amounts
of aluminum chloride were added to the calcium chloride solutions,
0.500 and 1.000 mM aluminum, respectively, which were subsequently
mixed with the dibasic sodium phosphate in order to precipitate ACP
(B172). After ACP formation the slurries were filtered on medium
sintered glass, the solid ACP was lyophilized and the filtrates were
stored for aluminum analysis.

Poorly crystallized HA, previously prepared at room temperature,
was exposed to various aluminum concentrations, 0.025, 0.050, 0.100,
0.250, 0.500, 0.750, 1.000 mM aluminum, respectively, by stirring
slurries of the HA in aluminum chloride solution at room temperature
and pH 7.4 for 1 hour. The slurries were then filtered on medium
sintered glass and the filtrates stored for aluminum analysis. All
aluminum analyses reported here were done by atomic absorption spectrophotometry at the laboratory of Dr. Jack W. Coburn at the V.A.
Wadsworth Hospital, Los Angeles, California. The amount of aluminum
that was bound to the ACP and HA in the above experiments was determined by taking the difference between the total amount in the initial reaction solution for each run and the amount that remained in
solution in the filtrate.

In this study two types of HA formation systems were used: (a) the
transformation of ACP to HA and, (b) the growth of HA on HA seed
crystals. Aluminum free (control) ACP and the two ACP samples copre-

cipitated with different amounts of aluminum were allowed to trans-
form to HA and the conversion rates recorded using 30 mg of ACP sus-
pended in 30 ml of reaction solution. HA crystal growth experiments
were carried out with aluminum-free (control) HA seeds and with HA
seeds previously exposed to various amounts of aluminum and the growth
rates were compared. The experimental conditions here were 15 mg of
HA seeds in 100 ml of solution that was 1.55 mM in Ca from $CaCl_2$ and
1.07 mM in PO_4 from Na_2HPO_4.

In addition, two experiments were performed where aluminum (from
$AlCl_3$) was added to the reaction solutions during the transformation
period when ACP converts to HA and during the time when HA growth was
taking place on HA seeds. The change in HA formation rate after aluminum addition was recorded for both systems. All experiments were
carried out at 37°C in 0.15M NaCl in a pH-Stat which maintained the
pH at 7.4 by automatic addition of 0.1M NaOH. A humidified nitrogen
gas atmosphere was maintained over the well stirred reaction solution
throughout each experiment. The amount of NaOH added as a function
of time is proportional to the extent of HA formation and/or growth
in all test systems (Bo73).

RESULTS

Aluminum delayed the formation and growth of HA in all of the systems
studied. In all experiments aluminum had no effect on the elapsed
time from mixing of reagents to the initial formation of HA (the induction time). Fig. 1 shows the dose related reduction in the rate
of transformation of ACP to HA of ACP coprecipitated in the presence
of 0.500 mM and 1.000 mM aluminum, respectively as compared to the
aluminum free control. Not shown is a similar dose related reduction
in the ACP to HA transformation rate where aluminum is added in solution prior to HA formation. Fig. 2 illustrates the dose related reduction in the rate of HA crystal growth, as compared to the aluminum
free control, by HA seed crystals that were pretreated with solutions
of varying aluminum concentrations. Not shown is a similar dose related reduction in HA seeded growth rate when different amounts of
aluminum were added in solution prior to any HA formation. Also, in
the direct precipitation of HA aluminum exerted a dose related effect
on the HA formation rate.

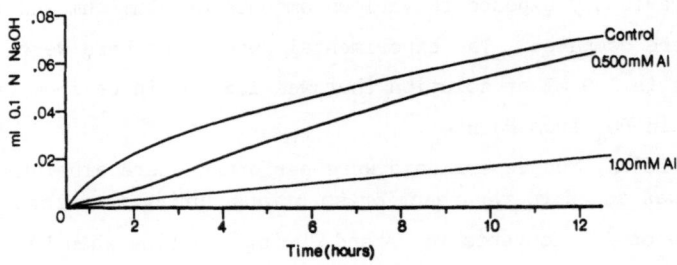

REDUCTION OF ACP-HA CONVERSION RATE BY ALUMINUM COPRECIPITATED WITH ACP

FIGURE 1

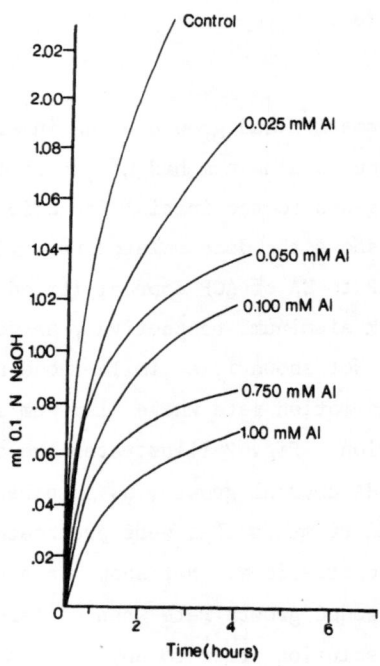

REDUCTION OF GROWTH RATE OF HA SEED CRYSTALS PRETREATED WITH ALUMINUM

FIGURE 2

When aluminum was added in solution during the period of transformation of ACP to HA and during the period of growth of HA on seed
crystals there was an immediate and significant decrease in the HA
formation rate in each system. Fig. 3 illustrates the uptake of aluminum on HA crystals as a function of the aluminum concentration in
solution. Not shown in Fig. 3 is data that indicates that where ACP
was coprecipitated with 0.500 mM and 1.000 mM aluminum, essentially
all of the metal originally in the reaction solution binds to the ACP.

ADSORPTION OF ALUMINUM ON SURFACE OF HA SEED CRYSTALS

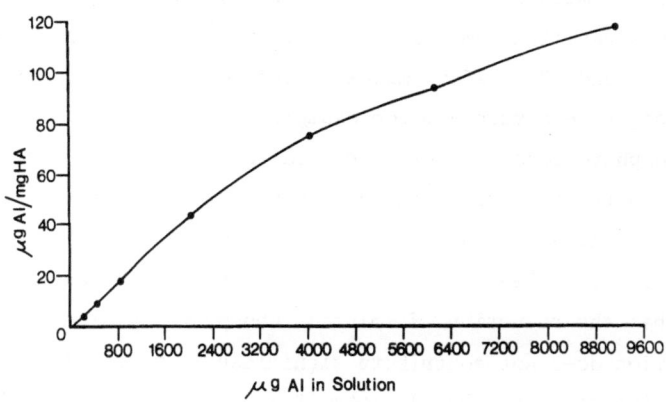

FIGURE 3

DISCUSSION

The results in this paper show clearly that aluminum binds to a significant extent to ACP and HA in vitro. This lends support to an
earlier suggestion that aluminum binds to and poisons growth sites
on the surface of HA and/or ACP, thereby, interfering with HA formation in seeded growth and ACP to HA systems (B184). In this previous
study aluminum was added in solution at the beginning, prior to any
HA formation, and aluminum uptake on HA or ACP was not measured.

The dose-related effect of aluminum on HA formation seen in Figures 1 and 2 is similar to the effect that was observed when aluminum was placed in solution before HA formation in the same test systems. This parallel behavior undoubtedly arises from the adsorption
of aluminum from solution onto the ACP or HA in the previous study,
in an amount that approximately corresponds to the aluminum concen-

tration in solution. The aluminum uptake results in the present paper show a decrease of HA formation rate that parallels increased
amounts of aluminum bound to ACP or HA.

Pretreating HA and ACP with aluminum in this work did not alter
the induction time for HA formation which also agreed with earlier
results where no effect was observed (B184). Again, this is probably
true because aluminum in solution in the previous study resulted in
adsorption of the metal on ACP or HA at the beginning of the experiment which, in effect, made the systems similar to the pretreated
systems discussed here. Further support for this comes from the results where the immediate decrease in HA formation rate in the two
test systems after aluminum addition indicates the rapid binding of
aluminum to HA and ACP. If aluminum interfered with any part of the
HA nucleation process such as, for example, the aggregation of calcium and phosphate ions to form a critical nucleus, there would be
an increase in the induction time of the reaction. Aluminum apparently acts on the early HA crystals and/or on the surface of ACP
after the initial nucleation events have occurred. In addition, it
was shown that the reduction of solution phosphate by aluminum phosphate formation does not contribute significantly to the inhibition
of HA formation or growth by aluminum (B184). The results in Figure 3
show that the uptake of aluminum on HA begins to decrease as the aluminum concentration in solution increases, which suggests that the
HA surface is probably becoming crowded with aluminum at higher concentrations.

From this work it is reasonable to conclude that as the aluminum
concentration in the serum of a patient on renal hemodialysis rises,
an increasing amount of the metal will be rapidly bound to the surface of newly formed bone apatite crystals, thereby, slowing their
subsequent growth. Also, if an ACP-like phase is the initially deposited mineral in the calcification process, then in a patient with
elevated serum aluminum levels the ACP precursor will bind to the
aluminum, slowing its transformation to bone apatite crystals. The
significant binding of aluminum to HA shown here explains the localization of the metal observed at the mineralization front in patients
with aluminum-associated osteomalacia. The aluminum concentrations
which reduced ACP transformation and HA crystal growth were in the

0.25 to 0.50 mM range as found in the serum of dogs with experimentally induced aluminum osteomalacia (Go, in press). The micromolar
aluminum levels which suppressed direct HA precipitation are not
much higher than the aluminum serum concentrations found in humans
with dialysis osteomalacia (Ho82). While there may be aluminum induced cellular changes in osteoblast and/or osteoclast function, the
in vitro findings of this study definitely suggest a significant
physical chemical effect on apatite proliferation in vivo by aluminum binding to HA and/or ACP. These results could well explain, in
part, aluminum associated osteomalacia.

ACKNOWLEDGEMENT

This work was supported by NIH Grant 18412 and a grant from the
Gebbie Foundation. The author is grateful to Ms. Theresa A. Herbert
who rendered valuable technical assistance to this project on a
Cornell University Medical College Summer Research Fellowship Program. This is publication 181 from the Laboratory of Ultrastructural Biochemistry.

SUMMARY

Aluminum was shown to bind to a significant extent to hydroxyapatite (HA) and to amorphous calcium phosphate (ACP) in vitro, which
sheds new light on the etiology of aluminum associated osteomalacia
observed in some patients on hemodialysis. Direct HA precipitation,
seeded HA crystal growth and transformation of ACP to HA were slowed
by aluminum binding to HA and ACP, respectively. All HA formation
experiments were done in a pH-Stat at 37°C, pH 7.4 in 0.15M NaCl.
The decrease in HA formation rate in all systems was proportional to
the amount of aluminum bound to HA or ACP, with no effect on the
induction time from mixing of reagents to initial HA formation.
Aluminum probably poisons growth sites on the surface of ACP and HA.
The results of this study explain the localization of aluminum observed at the mineralization front in patients with aluminum associated osteomalacia. Finally, the in vitro findings reported here
definitely suggest a significant physical chemical effect on apatite
proliferation in vivo by aluminum binding, which could explain, in
part, aluminum associated osteomalacia.

REFERENCES

B172 Blumenthal N.C., Posner A.S., Holmes J.M., 1972, Effect of preparation conditions on the properties and transformation of amorphous calcium phosphate, Mat. Res. Bull. 7, 1181-1190.

B184 Blumenthal N.C. and Posner A.S., 1984, In vitro model of aluminum-induced osteomalacia: Inhibition of hydroxyapatite formation and growth, Calc. Tiss. Int. 36, 439-441.

Bo73 Boskey A.L. and Posner A.S., 1973, Conversion of amorphous calcium phosphate to microcrystalline hydroxyapatite: a pH-dependent, solution-mediated solid-solid conversion, J. Phys. Chem. 77, 2313-2317.

Ch83 Chan Y.L., Alfrey A.C., Posen S., Lissner D., Hills E., Dunstan C.R., Evans R.A., 1983, Effect of aluminum on normal and uremic rats: tissue distribution, vitamin D metabolites and quantitative bone histology, Calcif. Tiss. Int. 35, 344-351.

Go(in press) Goodman W.G., Henry D.A., Ronald H., Nudelman R.K., Alfrey A.C., Coburn J.W., Parenteral aluminum administration in the dog. II. Induction of osteomalacia and effect on vitamin D metabolism, Kidney Int.

Ho82 Hodsman A.B., Sherrard D.J., Alfrey A.C., Ott S., Brickman A.S., Miller M.L., Maloney N.A., Coburn J.W., 1982, Bone aluminum and histomorphometric features of renal osteodystrophy, J. Clin. Endo. Metab. 54, 539-546.

Mi84 Miyahara T., Hayashi M., Kozuka H., 1984, The effect of aluminum on the metabolism of embryonic chick bone in tissue culture, Toxicol. Lett. 21, 237-240.

49

Is Osteomalacia of Renal Osteodystrophy due to Al Intoxication? An Experimental Study in the Rat

P. MOCETTI, P. BALLANTI, C. DELLA ROCCA, S. COSTANTINI, R. GIORDANO, A. IOPPOLO, A. MANTOVANI, D. STASOLLA and E. BONUCCI

INTRODUCTION

High Aluminum concentration found in bones of hemodialyzed uremic patients has been described as the major responsible for the development
of renal osteodystrophy (ROD) with severe osteomalacia. Histochemical
(Ma82) and physical methods (Co81) have shown Al presence mainly at
the mineralization front suggesting that the element has a specific
action in inhibiting the calcification process. However, the occurrence of high Al concentration in bone of hemodialyzed patients whose ROD
has prevalent hyperparathyroid changes rises several doubts about its
role in the induction of osteomalacia. To study the actual influence
of Al on bone mineralization, it has been administered to normal rats.

MATERIALS AND METHODS

45 male Wistar rats have been injected intraperitoneally with $AlCl_3$
aqueous sterilized solution (7.4 mg/week) (E179) and sacrificed after
9,12,13 weeks of treatment. 15 rats were kept as controls and injected
with physiological solution. Al content in serum, ribs and tibiae was
detected by atomic absorption spectroscopy. Rib and tibia specimens
were fixed in 4% paraformaldehyde buffered at pH 7.2 and embedded in
Araldite without decalcification. About 3 μm thick sections were stained using the Aluminon histochemical method specific for Al. About 1 μm
thick sections were stained with Azure II-Methylene blue for histomorphometric analysis performed on ribs and the epiphyseal ossification
center and metaphyseal trabeculae of the tibiae.

RESULTS

Atomic absorption spectroscopy showed that the three groups of treated animals, compared to controls, had a statistically significant increase of Al content in serum (1.05 ± 0.27, 1.07 ± 0.19, 1.21 ± 0.32
vs. 0.07 ± 0.01, 0.01 ± 0.005, 0.01 ± 0.008 ppm), ribs (131 ± 19,

153 $\pm$ 19, 169 $\pm$ 42 vs. 4$\pm$1, 13 $\pm$ 2, 6 $\pm$ 2 ppm) and tibiae (121 $\pm$ 20, 164 $\pm$ 15, 177 $\pm$ 49 vs. 2 $\pm$ 1, 3 $\pm$ 0.1, 3 $\pm$ 0.3 ppm). Moreover , Aluminon staining was positive in all treated rats along the whole mineralized trabecular perimeter. Histomorphometric results of Osteoid Volume (OV), Osteoid Surface (OS), Thickness Index of Osteoid (TIO), showed slightly enhanced values in treated rats; OV significantly increased in epiphyseal ossification center of the tibiae of group 2, OS in the epiphyseal bone of the tibiae of groups 1 and 2, and TIO in the epiphyseal ossification center of tibiae of group 2. Active Osteoid Surface (AOS) was significantly decreased in ribs of groups 1 and 2 and tibial metaphyseal trabecular bone of group 2.

DISCUSSION

The remarkable dispersion of osteoid histomorphometric values even within the same group of treated rats (Ba83) shows that Al has not a constant inhibitory effect on the mineralization process in normal rats. The results suggest that Al intoxication by itself is not the main responsible for the induction of osteomalacia. A decrease of AOS shows a probable Al inhibitory effect on osteoblastic activity (Li82).

SUMMARY

Intraperitoneal injection of Al to normal rats does not induce constant and sensible changes of the istomorphometric parameters of the trabecular bone. Al intoxication alone is not able to induce osteomalacic changes in normal rats.

REFERENCES

Ba83 Ballanti P., Mocetti P., Della Rocca C., Costantini S., Giordano R., Ioppolo A., Mantovani A., Stasolla D. and Bonucci E., 1983, Aluminum intoxication and osteomalacia in renal osteodystrophy , Min. Metab. Res. in Italy, 4, 139-142.

Co81 Cournot-Witmer G., Zingraff J., Plachot J.J., Escaig F., Lefèvre R., Boumati P., Bourdeau A., Garabédian M., Galle P., Bourdon R., Drüeke T. and Balsan S., 1981, Aluminum localization in bone from hemodialyzed patients: relationship to matrix mineralization ; Kidney Int., 20, 375-385.

El79 Ellis H.A., Mc Carthy J.H. and Herrington J., 1979, Bone aluminium um in haemodialysed patients and in rats injected with aluminum chloride: relationship to impaired bone mineralization , J. Clin. Path., 32, 832-844.

Li82 Lieberberr M., Grosse B., Cournot-Witmer G., Thil C.L. and Balsan S., 1982, In vitro effects of aluminum on bone phosphatases: a possible interaction with bPTH and vitamin D_3 metabolites , Calc. Tiss. Int., 34, 280-284.

Ma82 Maloney N.A., Ott S.M., Alfrey A.C., Miller N.L., Coburn J.W. and Sherrard D.J., 1982, Histological quantitation of aluminum in iliac bone from patients with renal failure , J. Lab. Clin. Med., 99, 206-216.

Index

Key words index with page numbers

461

marrow
  cell radiosensitivity 5, 6
  stem cells 6
  volume 26
matrix vesicles 44
mercury 37
methylene diphosphonate 2, 35
microdosimetry 24
microradiography 38
mineral homeostasis 12
mitrochondria 4
morphology 3
morphometry 12, 18, 26, 30, 46, 47
myoglobin 4

neptunium 17
neutron activation analysis 45
niobium 17
non-neoplastic lesions 31

osteoblast 44
osteocalcin 1
osteoclasts 30, 44
osteoid
  surface 30, 47, 49
  thickness 49
  volume 47, 49
osteomalacia 45, 46, 47, 48, 49
osteonectin 1
osteoporosis 10, 12, 30
osteosarcoma 16, 24, 29, 31, 33
  location 16, 31

parathyroids 36
partitioned clearance model 11
pathogenesis 29
periosteal area 26
peritrabecular fibrosis 31
peteosthor 29
phosphate depletion 33
phosphoproteins 1
phosphorus 43
placental transfer lead 39
plasma emission spectrometry 47
plutonium 3, 7, 13, 16, 17, 18, 19, 20,
    21, 22, 23, 24, 25, 26, 27, 31, 32, 35

bone half time 20
burial 27
in cortical bone 17, 18
distribution 26
distribution in man 13
fallout 20
in human bone 20
inhaled 31
in macrophages 7
in man 21
in marrow 17, 31
metabolism 23
in mice 26
oxide 31
retention 20
retention in mice 23
toxicity 16, 26
pollution 37
post mortem uptake 38
promethium 17
protactinium 17
proteoglycans 1
protraction effects 29

radiation
  dosimetry 24, 25, 27
  exposure 28
  injury 18
Radiochemistry 26
Radiological protection 17, 24
Radionuclide retention 24
Radium 3, 6, 8, 11, 13, 17, 24, 29, 32, 37
  dial workers 8
  distribution in man 13
  in mastoid 13
  metabolism 8
  retention 8
Receptor molecules 1
Relative concentrations 17
Remodelling 3
renal
  dialysis 48
  failure 45, 46, 47, 48
Renkin theory 35
Resorption surface 30, 47
Reticulo-endothelial cells 4